ENNIS AND NANCY HAM LIBRARY
ROCHESTER COLLEGE
800 WEST AVON ROAD
ROCHESTER HILLS, MI 48307

The Dyslexic Brain

The Dyslexic Brain

Edited by Glenn D. Rosen, Ph.D.

*Associate Professor of Neurology
and
Director, Dyslexia Neuroanatomical
Research Laboratory
Beth Israel Deaconess Medical Center
and
Harvard Medical School*

LAWRENCE ERLBAUM ASSOCIATES, PUBLISHERS
2006   Mahwah, New Jersey   London

Acquisitions Editor: Cathleen Petree
Executive Assistant: Erica Kica
Cover Design: Tomai Maridou
Composition: Type Shoppe II Productions, Ltd.

The book was typeset in 10 pt. Stone Serif Roman, Bold, and Italic.
The heads were typeset in Stone Sans Bold and Bold Italic.

Copyright © 2006 by Lawrence Erlbaum Associates, Inc.

All rights reserved. No part of this book may be reproduced in any form, by photostat, microform, retrieval system, or any other means, without prior written permission of the publisher.

Lawrence Erlbaum Assosciates, Inc., Publishers
10 Industrial Avenue
Mahway, New Jersey 07430
www.erlbaum.com

Library of Congress Cataloging-in-Publication Data

CIP information for this volume can be obtained by contacting the Library of Congress.

Books published by Lawrence Erlbaum Associates are printed on acid-free paper, and their bindings are chosen for strength and durability.

Printed in the United States of America
10 9 8 7 6 5 4 3 2 1

Contents

Preface vii
Foreword
    Peggy McCardle ix
Acknowledgments xiii

Section I   The Phenotype of Dyslexia

Introduction 1
From the Sumerians to Images of the Reading Brain:
    Insights for Reading Theory and Intervention
        Maryanne Wolf and Beth O'Brien 5
Neurobiological Studies of Skilled and Impaired
    Reading: A Work in Progress
        Kenneth R. Pugh, Rebecca Sandak, Stephen J. Frost,
        Dina Moore, Jay G. Rueckl, and W. Einar Mencl 21
Process Faster, Talk Earlier, Read Better
        Paula Tallal 49
A Neurological Model of Dyslexia and Other
    Domain-specific Developmental Disorders with
    an Associated Sensorimotor Syndrome
        Franck Ramus 75

Section II   The Genetics of Dyslexia and Cortical Development

Introduction 103
Chromosome 15 and Developmental Dyslexia
        Cecilia Marino and Massimo Molteni 107
Neuronal Migration and Dyslexia Susceptibility
        Joseph J LoTurco, Yu Wang, and
        Murugan Paramasivam 119
Genetic Disorders of Neuronal Migration and Brain
    Wiring
        Joseph Gleeson 129
New Genes Involved in Cortical Development
        Ferran Burgaya, Cristina García-Frigola, Rosa Andrés,
        Nathalia Vitureira, Guillermo López-Domènech,
        Luís de Lecea, and Eduardo Soriano 143
Genomics and Dyslexia: Bridging the Gap
        Robert W. Williams 167

Section III Animal Models of Cortical Development

Introduction 191
Focal Malformations of Cortical Development
    Peter Crino *195*
Excitotoxic Lesions of the Developing Brain
    Frank Plaisant, Romain H. Fontaine, Bettina Mesplès,
    and Pierre Gressens *209*
What a Difference a Day Makes: Linking Timing
to Mechanisms in Epileptogenic Microgyri
    A. Zsombok and K.M. Jacobs *223*
Structural and Functional Deficits in a Rat Model of
Cortical Heterotopia
    Kevin S. Lee, Matthew J. Anzivino, Maro G. Machizawa,
    Fayong Zhang, Cedric Williams, Frank Schottler,
    Sara Tsuchitani, Jessica Drummond, Cindy L. Kinard,
    Edward Bertram, Stacey Trotter, Jaideep Kapur, and
    Zong-Fu Chen *243*
Behavioral Consequences of Focal Anomalies in the
Cerebral Cortex
    R. Holly Fitch and Ann M. Peiffer *259*

Section IV Brain Plasticity

Introduction 289
MRI-based Morphometry in Human Developmental
Disorders: Looking Back in Time
    David N. Kennedy *291*
Cortical Plasticity: The Effects of Sensory Deprivation
    Hugo Théoret and Alvaro Pascual-Leone *307*
Dyslexia: Advances in Cross-level Research
    Albert M. Galaburda *329*

Author Index 355

Subject Index 361

Preface

In 1987, experts from a wide range of fields, including neuroscience, cognitive science, and philosophy, gathered in Florence, Italy, for the first of "The Extraordinary Brain" conferences sponsored by The Dyslexia Foundation (then known as the National Dyslexia Research Foundation). The goal of that conference was to explore issues of neural and cognitive development from a multidisciplinary perspective in the hopes of promoting novel approaches toward research into the neuroscience of dyslexia. The conference itself was an unequivocal success, judging not only from the quality of the scientific discourse and the resulting book (Galaburda, 1989), but also by the wealth of research that emanated from the laboratories of the attending scientists and their students. Prior to that meeting, relatively little was known about the brain and dyslexia, and it has been encouraging to witness the explosive growth of research on this topic in the ensuing years.

The increased interest in understanding the biological substrates of dyslexia is, to some extent, a consequence of the truly remarkable growth of neuroscience research in general that we've seen in the past two decades. The expansion of neuroscience is obvious no matter which metric you choose to use: the number of journals, the membership in scientific societies, the number of publications, not to mention the increased public awareness of issues related to the brain. One of the downsides of the expansion for those of us in the field is that it is difficult to keep up with the speed, volume, and breadth of the data being generated. With regard to study of dyslexia, for example, there are groups that study this problem at a number of different levels—molecular, genetic, physiological, and cognitive—and most of us in the field try to keep abreast of new developments in each of these fields. But we also know that there are key researchers who are studying problems not directly related to dyslexia, but whose results could have a profound impact on the future of our research. Moreover, exposing these researchers to some of the issues related to the study of dyslexia may inspire them or their students to directly address this important problem. With this in mind, we decided to organize an "Extraordinary Brain" conference to bring together neuroscientists in order to foster a more directed dialogue in the hopes of broadening our understanding of developmental dyslexia.

The Development of the Extraordinary Brain took place in June of 2004 in Como, Italy, and this book is a result of this conference.

Our goal in organizing the conference was to bring together leaders in fields of neuroscience that while closely related, weren't necessarily accustomed to talking to one another. We are pleased to note that the conference was eye-opening for a good many of the investigators. To our delight, new collaborations were formed, and a myriad of new research ideas were generated from the high-level interactions that occurred. In this book, we hope to transfer some of this excitement to the reader. The book is grouped into sections, either by scientific discipline or level of analysis, and there is a short introduction at the beginning of each section, which attempts to put the research discussed in the subsequent chapters into a broader context. It is our hope that the changes in research focus and the collaborations that came out of that meeting will have a lasting and meaningful impact on the field, and that these chapters will act as a springboard for the acquisition of more exciting knowledge as to the relationship between the brain and dyslexia.

REFERENCE

Galaburda, A. M. (Ed.) (1989). *From reading to neurons*. Cambridge, MA: MIT Press.

Foreword

This volume documents a momentous symposium sponsored by The Dyslexia Foundation (TDF) entitled "The Development of the Extraordinary Brain." I was accustomed to the fact that TDF had a tradition of sponsoring highly interesting, scientifically valuable symposia, the ultimate goal of which were always to inform participants about developmental dyslexia. I knew that TDF was especially noted for keeping its participants together in a single group for days, bringing together multiple disciplines unused to meeting together, to develop dialogues that were not typical in professional association meetings, and where communication usually was limited to colleagues doing similar types of research on common topics. Yet even with this knowledge, I was unprepared for the level of communication and exchange of ideas that occurred.

On arrival in Como, Italy, I learned that this particular symposium was a revisiting of a meeting—organized by Al Galaburda and held in Florence, Italy, more than 15 years earlier—that had brought together scholars of various disciplines to discuss neural and cognitive development, and the role of these areas in developmental dyslexia. The Como symposium clearly carried on the tradition of TDF symposia, bringing together scholars from a variety of disciplines to take stock of an area, communicate about their own research, brainstorm new approaches and methods to further unlock the intricacies of dyslexia and the brain, and to move the field toward better methods of identification, measurement/assessment, and intervention for developmental dyslexia.

At the Como meeting, under the organizational leadership of Glenn Rosen, TDF brought together neuroscientists, psychologists, neuropsychologists, geneticists, and others who work with both animal and human models in various aspects of behavior, genetics, and neurophysiologic and neurocognitive development. We were there to learn from one another, and to push the frontiers of our respective disciplines and forge a new frontier in bringing those disciplines together. For many of us, it was an intensive course in various aspects of cognitive neuroscience and genetics that we may not deal with on a daily basis. Not all of the researchers were focused on the problem of dyslexia, but that is part

---

The assertions and opinions contained herein represent those of the authors and should not be taken as representing official policies of the NICHD, NIH, or the U.S. Department of Health & Human Services.

of the magic of a TDF symposium: it entices researchers from various disciplines to engage in the intriguing puzzle that is dyslexia. In this way, TDF builds researcher capacity while also encouraging fresh ideas and approaches to an old, well-recognized, but in many respects, still poorly understood problem.

Despite the fact that this symposium included a variety of disciplines and a group of scientists, many of whom had never worked directly together, the presentations were linked thematically to offer a full spectrum of information to help participants fully understand a behaviorally manifested problem such as dyslexia. Presentations included animal models of neurophysiologic and neurocognitive development and neural system plasticity, evidence on typical and dyslexic reading and its remediation, as well as neuroimaging evidence of the brain-behavior link in both typical and struggling readers, the development of behavioral phenotypes, and the genetic techniques that will enable the development of genotypes for aspects of neurocortical and cognitive development, including dyslexia.

The excitement generated by the cutting-edge findings and the discussions that these findings engendered across disciplinary lines would have been sufficient in and of themselves to make the Como meeting worthwhile. But the conversations also entertained potential applications for real children in real classrooms, and the participants often stayed after scheduled sessions to continue discussions and share information beyond what was included in their presentations, to brainstorm new ideas and approaches, and to explore potential research collaborations. And those conversations and the excitement that generated them have not ended.

Glenn Rosen's creative organization of domains and careful selection of scientists who assembled in Como are reflected in this volume. The importance of the symposium is that the excitement, the synergy of the cross-disciplinary interactions, and the sharing that forged new friendships, new approaches, and conceptualizations of problems have resulted in a volume that shares the knowledge generated and the new ideas with a much broader audience. The collaborations that were established across disciplines and laboratories are not restricted to those who were in Como in June of 2004, just as they were not restricted to those who were in Florence in 1987: they can be generated by anyone who reads and shares this volume. Such collaborations will ultimately lead us to a better understanding of how the brain processes information and learns from it, how and why some children develop dyslexia while others learn to read easily, and how we can best tailor reading instruction to the individual needs of every child.

Address correspondence to: Peggy McCardle, Ph.D., MPH, Child Development & Behavior Branch Center for Research for Mothers and Children, National Institute of Child Health and Human Development, 6100 Executive Boulevard, Room 4B05, MSC 7510, Rockville, MD 20852-7510.

Acknowledgments

I would first like to thank The Dyslexia Foundation (TDF) for sponsoring the conference on which this book was based. The "Extraordinary Brain" series of conferences have had a long and impressive history, and it was an honor to serve as the organizer. I would like to thank Phil Pasho and Amanda Harney of TDF for their help in putting the conference together. Special mention must be made to Will Baker, Director of TDF, whose vision and energy drive the foundation and keep the promise of these conferences alive. You won't find Stefany Palmieri's name in the book, but this would never have happened without her. Stefany organized the meeting in Como with exceptional skill and dedication and we would have been lost (literally) without her and her husband Kent Wallace's efforts. The members of my lab, Shira Anconina, Stephanie Chin, Elizabeth Grasso, Karen Heindl, and Chris Pung, also deserve kudos for their role in making sure all the preparations for the conference were completed on time. Finally, I am especially grateful to my friend and mentor Al Galaburda who was an invaluable sounding board throughout the process.

Obviously, the strength of the conference and this book is the direct result of the participants, and I was blessed to have such a diverse and talented group consent to attend and contribute. The speakers were not only at the top of their scientific game, but their congeniality made the interactions both inside and outside of the meeting room informative, stimulating, and, yes, entertaining. Thanks especially to the moderators of the sessions, Al Galaburda, Holly Fitch, Rob Williams, Joe LoTurco, Drake Duane, Maryanne Wolf, and Peggy McCardle for keeping the discussions moving. I also want to thank the generous support of Helen Baker, the Baker Family, Joan McNichols, the John Chany Trust, York Press, Susan Reeves, and Scientific Learning Corporation. I want to make special mention of the support of Keith and Jane Johnson. We in the dyslexia community will always remember Jane's strength and vision, and we will miss her.

I would like to thank Elinor Hartwig for her initial help in getting this book together, Cathleen Petree and Nicole Buchmann at Lawrence Ehrlbaum for their editing work on this book, as well as Lydia Wagner of TypeShoppe 2 for the excellent copyediting. Finally, I would like to thank my family, Anndy, Dan, and Alena, for their support, encouragement, and occasional reference formatting.

Contributors

Rosa Andrés, Ph.D.
Parc Cientific de Barcelona
Developmental Neurobiology and
  Regeneration Group,
Lab A1-S1, Edifici Modular
Josep Samitier, 1-5
Barcelona 08028 SPAIN
Email: @porthos.bio.ub.es

Mathew J. Anzivino
University of Virginia Health Systems
Department of Neuroscience
P.O. Box 801392
Charlottesville, VA 22908-1392 USA
Email: mja7s @virginia.edu

Edward Bertram, M.D.
University of Virginia Health Systems
Department of Neurology
P.O. Box 801392
Charlottesville, VA 22908-1392 USA
Email: ehb2z @virginia.edu

Ferran Burgaya, Ph.D.
Parc Cientific de Barcelona
Developmental Neurobiology and
  Regeneration Group,
Lab A1-S1, Edifici Modular
Josep Samitier, 1-5
Barcelona 08028 SPAIN
Email: burgaya@porthos.bio.ub.es

Zong-Fu Chen, M.D.
University of Virginia Health Systems
Department of Neuroscience
P.O. Box 801392
Charlottesville, VA 22908-1392 USA
Email: zfc6e@yahoo.com

Peter B. Crino, M.D., Ph.D.
University of Pennsylvania
Department of Neurology
3 West Gates Building
3400 Spruce Street
Philadelphia, PA 19104 USA
Email: crinop@mail.med.upenn.edu

Jessica Drummond
University of Virginia Health Systems
Department of Neuroscience
P.O. Box 801392
Charlottesville, VA 22908-1392 USA
Email: drummojm@evms.edu

R. Holly Fitch, Ph.D.
University of Connecticut
Biobehavioral Sciences Graduate
  Degree Program
Box U-154
Storrs, CT 06268 USA
Email: roslyn.h.fitch@uconn.edu

Romain H. Fontaine, M.D., Ph.D.
Hôpital Robert-Debré
Université Paris 7 & Service de
  Neurologie Pédiatrique
INSERM U0676
48 Boulevard Sérurier
F-75019 Paris FRANCE
Email: fontaine@rdebre.inserm.fr

Stephen J. Frost, Ph.D.
Haskins Laboratory
300 George Street
New Haven, CT 06611 USA
Email: frosts@haskins.yale.edu

Albert M. Galaburda, M.D.
Beth Israel Deaconess Medical Center
Division of Behavioral Neurology
330 Brookline Avenue
Boston, MA 02215 USA
Email: agalabur@bidmc.harvard.edu

Cristina Garcia-Frigola, Ph.D.
Salk Institute
SNL-C,
0010 North Torrey Pines Road
La Jolla, CA 92037 USA

Joseph G. Gleeson, M.D.
University of California-San Diego
Department of Neurosciences
Medical Teaching Facility 324
Medical School Campus
9500 Gilman Drive
La Jolla, CA 92093-0624 USA
Email: jogleeson@ucsd.edu

Pierre Gressens, M.D., Ph.D.
Hôpital Robert-Debré
Université Paris 7 & Service de
 Neurologie Pédiatrique
INSERM U0676
48 Boulevard Sérurier
F-75019 Paris FRANCE
Email: gressens@idf.inserm.fr

Kimberle M. Jacobs, Ph.D.
Virgina Commonwealth University
Department of Anatomy and
 Neurobiology
P.O. Box 980709
Richmond, VA 23298-0709 USA
Email: kmjacobs@vcu.edu

Jadeep Kapur, M.D., Ph.D.
University of Virginia Health Systems
Department of Neurology
P.O. Box 801392
Charlottesville, VA 22908-1392 USA
Email: jk8t @virginia.edu

David N. Kennedy, Ph.D.
Massachusetts General Hospital
Department of Neurology
149 13th Street
Room 6014
Charlestown, MA 02129 USA
Email: dave@cma.mgh.harvard.edu

Cindy L. Kinard
University of Virginia Health Systems
Department of Neuroscience
P.O. Box 801392
Charlottesville, VA 22908-1392 USA
Email: clk9s@cms.mail.virginia.edu

Luis de Lecea, Ph.D.
Department of Molecular Biology
The Scripps Institute
10550 North Torrey Pines Road
La Jolla, CA 92037 USA

Kevin S. Lee, Ph.D.
University of Virginia Health Systems
Department of Neuroscience
P.O. Box 801392
Charlottesville, VA 22908-1392 USA
Email: ksl3h@virginia.edu

Guillermo López-Domènech, Ph.D.
Parc Cientific de Barcelona
Developmental Neurobiology and
 Regeneration Group,
Lab A1-S1, Edifici Modular
Josep Samitier, 1-5
Barcelona 08028 SPAIN

Joseph J. LoTurco, Ph.D.
University of Connecticut
Department of Physiology and
 Neurobiology
U-4156
Storrs, CT 06269-4156 USA
Email: loturco@oracle.pnb.uconn.edu

Maro G. Machizawa
University of Virginia Health Systems
Department of Neuroscience
P.O. Box 801392
Charlottesville, VA 22908-1392 USA
Email: maro_g_machizawa @hot
 mail.com

Cecilia Marino, M.D.
Scientific Institute Eugenio Medea
Department of Child
 Psychopathology
Association "La Nostra Famiglia"
20 Don Luigi Monza
Bossiso Parini Lecco 23842 ITALY
Email: cecilia.marino@virgilio.it

Peggy McCardle, Ph.D., MPH
Acting Chief, Child Development &
 Behavior Branch
Center for Research for Mothers &
 Children
National Institute of Child Health
 and Human Development
6100 Executive Boulevard, Suite 4B05
Rockville, MD 20852-7510 USA
Email: pm43q@nih.gov

W. Einar Mencl, Ph.D.
Director of Neuroimaging Research
Haskins Laboratory
300 George Street
New Haven, CT 06511 USA
Email: einar@haskins.yale.edu

Bettina Mesplès, M.D.
Service de Pediatrie
Hôpital Louis Mourier
178, rue des Renouillers
F-92701 COLOMBES Cedex FRANCE
Email: bmesples@noos.fr

Massinmo Molteni, M.D.
Scientific Institute Eugenio Medea
Department of Child Psychopathology
Association "La Nostra Famiglia"
20 Don Luigi Monza
Bossiso Parini Lecco 23842 ITALY
Email: molteni@bp.lnf.it

Dina Moore, Ph.D.
Haskins Laboratory
300 George Street
New Haven, CT 06611 USA
Email: moore@haskins.yale.edu

Beth O'Brien, Ph.D.
Center for Reading and Language
  Research Tufts University
Department of Child Development
Medford, MA 02155 USA
Email: beth.obrien@tufts.edu

Murugan Paramasivam, Ph.D.
University of Connecticut
Department of Physiology and
  Neurobiology
U-4156
Storrs, CT 06269-4156 USA
Email: paramasivam.muru
  gan@uconn.edu

Alvaro Pascual-Leone, M.D., Ph.D.
Beth Israel Deaconess Medical Center
Division of Behavioral Neurology
330 Brookline Avenue
Boston, MA 02215 USA
Email: apleone@bidmc.harvard.edu

Ann M. Peiffer, Ph.D.
Wake Forest University School of
  Medicine
Department of Radiology
Medical Center Boulevard
Winston-Salem, NC 27157 USA
Email: apeiffer@wfubmc.edu

Frank Plaisant, M.D., Ph.D.
Hôpital Robert-Debré
Université Paris 7 & Service de
  Neurologie Pédiatrique
INSERM U0676
48 Boulevard Sérurier
F-75019 Paris FRANCE
Email: plaisant@club-internet.fr

Kenneth R. Pugh, Ph.D.
Haskins Laboratory
300 George Street
New Haven, CT 06511 USA
Email: pugh@haskins.yale.edu

Franck Ramus, Ph.D.
Ecole Normale Supérieure
46 rue d'Ulm
75005 Paris FRANCE
Email: franck.ramus@ens.fr

Jay G. Rueckl, Ph.D.
Department of Psychology
University of Connecticut
406 Babbidge Road, Unit 1020
Storrs, CT 06269-1020 USA
Email: rueckl@psych.psy.uconn.edu

Glenn D. Rosen, Ph.D.
Beth Israel Deaconess Medical Center
Department of Neurology
330 Brookline Avenue
Boston, MA 02215 USA
Email: grosen@bidmc.harvard.edu

Rebecca Sandak, Ph.D.
Haskins Laboratory
300 George Street
New Haven, CT 06511 USA
Email: sandak@haskins.yale.edu

Frank Schottler, Ph.D.
University of Virginia Health Systems
Department of Neuroscience
P.O. Box 801392
Charlottesville, VA 22908-1392 USA
Email: schottlerf@neuro.wustl.edu

Eduardo Soriano, Ph.D.
Parc Cientific de Barcelona
Developmental Neurobiology and
  Regeneration Group,
Lab A1-S1, Edifici Modular
Josep Samitier, 1-5
Barcelona 08028 SPAIN
Email: soriano@porthos.bio.ub.es

Paula Tallal, Ph.D.
Center for Molecular and Behavioral
  Neuroscience
Aidekman Research Center
University of New Jersey Newark
197 University Avenue
Newark, NJ 07102 USA
Email: tallal@axon.rutgers.edu

Hugo Théoret, Ph.D.
Université de Montréal
  Psychology
CP 6128, Succ. Centre Ville
Montreal QC H3C3J7 CANADA
Email: hugo.theoret@umontreal.ca

Stacey Trotter
University of Virginia Health Systems
Department of Neuroscience
P.O. Box 801392
Charlottesville, VA 22908-1392 USA
Email: sat7k@virginia.edu

Sara Tsuchitani
University of Virginia Health Systems
Department of Neuroscience
P.O. Box 801392
Charlottesville, VA 22908-1392 USA
Email: snt3t@cms.mail.virginia.edu

Naathalia Vitureira, Ph.D.
Parc Cientific de Barcelona
Developmental Neurobiology and
  Regeneration Group,
Lab A1-S1, Edifici Modular
Josep Samitier, 1-5
Barcelona 08028 SPAIN

Yu Wang
University of Connecticut
Department of Physiology and
  Neurobiology
U-4156
Storrs, CT 06269-4156 USA
Email: Wang.Yu@uconn.edu

Cedric Williams, Ph.D.
Department of Psychology
University of Virginia
Charlottesville, VA 22908-1392 USA
Email: clw3b@virginia.edu

Robert W. Williams, Ph.D.
University of Tennesee Health
  Science Center
Center for Neuroscience
Department of Anatomy and
  Neurobiology
875 Monroe Avenue
Memphis, TN 38163 USA
Email: rwilliam@nb.utmem.edu

Maryanne Wolf, Ph.D.
Center for Reading and Language
  Research Tufts University
Department of Child Development
Medford, MA 02155 USA
Email: maryanne.wolf@tufts.edu

Fayong Zhang, M.D.
University of Virginia Health Systems
Department of Neuroscience
P.O. Box 801392
Charlottesville, VA 22908-1392 USA
Email: fz3f@cms.mail.virginia.edu

Andrea Zsombok, Ph.D.
Virginia Commonwealth University
Department of Anatomy and
  Neurobiology
P.O. Box 980709
Richmond, VA 23298-0709 USA
Email: azsombok@vcu.edu

Section • I

The Phenotype of Dyslexia

INTRODUCTION

We begin the book with these chapters for somewhat obvious reasons. Because our interest lies in seeing how information from a variety of neuroscience disciplines can impact the study of dyslexia, it makes sense to first understand the state of the art of research on this topic. We are fortunate to have four excellent chapters that cover a wide range of disciplines and perspectives.

I can think of no better way to start off than with the chapter by Maryanne Wolf and Beth O'Brien. These authors lay the foundation for understanding the historical importance of the written word in terms of the cognitive evolution of the human species. They make a compelling case that the brain's ability to read is due to its co-opting of other, preliterary skills, and that appreciating what these skills are can lead to a greater understanding of how the brain learns. This awareness also has a profound impact on what processes might go awry in those students who have difficulty in learning to read. Wolf and O'Brien discuss their research on the well-known "Double-Deficit Hypothesis," which emphasizes the role of phonology and rapid naming (or their combination) in the diagnosis of dyslexia. Of great interest is their discussion of different intervention strategies (the RAVE-O program) that take into account this understanding of how the brain processes language. Preliminary results from these interventions are encouraging, and point out the potential importance of fluency intervention in the treatment of developmental dyslexia.

Functional magnetic resonance imaging (fMRI) has been one of the most dramatic breakthroughs in cognitive neuroscience in the past two decades. Using this technique, researchers can indirectly measure brain activation by assessing blood flow to specific cerebral structures. One of the leaders in using this valuable technique in the study of developmental dyslexia is Ken Pugh from the Haskins Laboratory. Along with his collaborators, Pugh summarizes many years worth of experiments that have led him to postulate a very specific brain network that is necessary for the acquisition of skilled reading. This network is comprised of three distinct regions (dorsal, ventral, and anterior) in the left hemisphere, and each of these areas is hypothesized to contribute uniquely to the process of skilled reading, Of great interest is Pugh et al.'s discussion of their investigations as to how these very complex systems develop in children who acquire skilled reading without difficulty. This is an essential area of investigation, especially when discussing a developmental disorder. While it is important to get a picture, if you will, of the adult state, it is extremely important to study the process whereby this picture gets painted during development. This is a theme that we will return to in other chapters in the book.

Paula Tallal has a long history of involvement in the study of dyslexia and language impairment, and her contribution to this book is a detailed and thoughtful summary of this work. Tallal concentrates her efforts on understanding the processes involved in the acquisition of phonological skill among a population with "Language Learning Impairment" (LLI), which encompasses both dyslexics and individuals with language impairment. It is Tallal's contention that defects in rapid processing of auditory information underlie the phonological impairments of individuals with LLI. Thus, the demonstrable problems that dyslexics have in decoding phonology (using phoneme deletion or rhyming tasks, for example) is hypothesized to be due to the improper encoding of these phonemes by an auditory system that is unable to rapidly process the complex components of speech. As one can imagine, this hypothesis has sparked a good deal of debate in the literature, which is reviewed in this chapter. Tallal believes that much of the controversy surrounding this topic could be resolved by keeping in mind the important developmental aspects of these disorders. When studies are performed on comparable populations, at comparable ages, Tallal argues, the results are more congruent. The chapter concludes with a summary of an intervention program that seeks to retrain the brain's ability to process rapid auditory information.

The last chapter in this section by Franck Ramus is undoubtedly the most controversial in the book. Ramus seeks to bridge the gap between a number of findings concerning the biological substrates of dyslexia. First, Ramus contends that the phonological deficits are the primary problem with dyslexia. Second are the reports (see Fitch & Peiffer, and Galaburda, this volume) that small malformations of the cortex are seen postmortem in individuals with developmental dyslexia. Third are the findings that there are problems with rapid processing of sensory information (see Tallal, this volume). In contrast to Tallal, Ramus believes that cortical malformations are the direct cause of the difficulties in phonological awareness, and that the sensorimotor difficulties that may subsequently occur are related to changes to the thalamus induced by these cortical anomalies. There are obviously a number of points of contention between Tallal and Ramus, and these are carefully considered in both chapters. The beauty of these types of discussions is that they bring the field into sharp focus, which in turn leads to hypotheses that can be directly tested. Although the problems raised by these authors are certainly not resolved, the direction of future experiments that may settle these issues is becoming clearer.

Chapter • **1**

From the Sumerians to Images of the Reading Brain: Insights for Reading Theory and Intervention

Maryanne Wolf and Beth O'Brien

The *genesis* of written language represents one of the major breakthroughs in the cognitive evolution of the human species. It demonstrates the human brain's remarkable capacity to use novel connections within its genetically given physiological structure to create a novel function. Equally remarkable is the development of reading in the child as an example of how the brain learns an evolutionarily recent cognitive skill through the rearrangement of older neurological structures. The study of reading's evolution, development, and pathology contributes to our understanding of how the brain learns, but also, importantly, informs treatment of reading problems for children who struggle to learn to read.

In this chapter, we will describe a research program that uses evidence from reading's evolution, development, and pathology to construct a broadened conceptualization of both reading and reading breakdown in developmental dyslexia. The significance of this view of the reading process is a new, more comprehensive approach to the treatment of reading acquisition difficulty. In the final part of this chapter, we will describe an intervention for struggling beginning readers that is based on the broader conceptualization that there are multiple components involved in reading, and thus multiple, possible sources of breakdown. Preliminary data show that this intervention supports gains in multiple components of reading for various types of dyslexic readers.

EVOLUTION AND READING

Human beings are not born to read. We *are*, however, genetically "hardwired" for other functions like vision, speech, and language, and these functions are reconfigured in reading. Thus, the modern act of reading is based on an ingenious rearrangement of older neuronal circuitries that undergird attentional, perceptual, linguistic, cognitive, and motoric processes that were originally designed for functions other than reading. The human brain's ability to make new connections among these processes is the physiological basis of the reading act.

The history of written language begins with the invention of *symbolic representation*. When human beings first began to represent an object using abstract, visually based signs, as in cave drawings, they were basically rewiring connections among existing neuronal circuits or pathways for visual and conceptual processes (Dehaene, 2003). As symbolic capacities increased (Deacon, 1997), human beings were learning to connect these same areas to areas responsible for linguistic processes. Cave drawings and tokens, tiny markings on pieces of clay dating from 8000 to 4000 BCE, are the first known use of symbols (Schmandt-Besserat, 1992).

It is unknown precisely when or why, but in the fourth millennium BCE, a small subset of symbols began to appear that were used to convey a very limited number of concepts in the oral language. The Sumerian cuneiform system and Egyptian hieroglyphic writing were the first known comprehensive writing systems. From a cognitive viewpoint, both systems employed three major features: first, imagistic logographic symbols to convey a corpus of known concepts and words; second, an unusual, rebus principle that used the first sound of an older symbol to depict the sound of a new word (like a name); and third, a boustrephon (or plowing) directional style, whereby the reader scanned alternating lines of text from left to right, then from right to left. These early systems required a demanding variety of cognitive strategies and scanning styles to decode the symbols (where one symbol might be pictographic and the next rebus-based), as well as a great deal of flexibility by the reader. This is particularly the case as each culture developed both larger sets of symbols and more complex symbols over time. For example, Egyptian hieroglyphs became extremely difficult to decode over the millennia of their use because they possessed ever-increasing layers of encrypted secret meanings.

Perhaps as a direct result of the convoluted demands in early hieroglyph writing, it is believed that a tiny subset of solely sound-based symbols emerged that later would be exploited and developed by Hebrew scribes working in Egypt around 1800 BCE. This earliest known proto-semitic writing is the controversial basis of what some linguists believe to be the first alphabet-like script that was found quite recently in Wadi el Hol, Egypt. Intriguingly, the script has elements of both earlier Egyptian symbols and later semitic symbols found in the Ugarit writing system around 1400 BCE.

Whether or not this script is ever categorized as alphabetic, the invention of the *alphabetic principle* is the most linguistically abstract and complex concept in the history of written language, and is not universal among writing systems. At root, the alphabetic principle represents the profound insight that each word in our oral language consists of a finite group of individual sounds (phonemes) that can be represented by a finite group of individual letters (graphemes). This principle is the basis, therefore, for the ability of every spoken word to be translated into writing.

It took approximately two thousand years of changes in writing between the earliest known cuneiform and hieroglyphic systems, and the more well-established, alphabetic-like, consonantal system among the Ugarits in the latter half of the second millennium BCE. It took an additional millennium before the Greeks created the first, almost perfect alphabet. To do so, the Greeks analyzed the neighboring Phoenician script with an approach that would not embarrass modern speech scientists. First, they analyzed all the phonemes in the neighboring Phoenician language, and the correspondence between that language and their script. Then they systematically isolated all the phonemes in the Greek oral language in order to construct an alphabet of symbols capable of conveying every phoneme in Greek. By the middle of the eighth century BCE, they had created a writing system capable of depicting *all* the phonemes (both consonants and vowels) in the Greek language.

DEVELOPMENT OF READING IN THE CHILD

What is often unrealized by the modern educator is that the prodigious feat by the Greeks requires many of the same basic cognitive insights that every child must achieve before he or she can learn to read. Children must learn three similar concepts: first, symbolic representation; then the idea that a set or system of symbols convey words; and finally (the most difficult and abstract insight), that words are composed of discrete sounds and that letters map these sounds in writing. Children are given six to seven years to discover, understand, and prove their competence in mastering insights that took the species millennia to achieve!

Unappreciated by most people, these insights into reading never just happen in childhood. In fact, the acquisition and development of reading in the child represents the full sum of hundreds of words, thousands of concepts, and tens of thousands of percepts, all of which contribute to the development of a process that demands a great deal of the human brain.

A cognitive model of what it takes for a child to read the word "cat," depicted in Figure 1, includes a range of attentional, memory, visual perceptual, orthographic pattern recognition, auditory perceptual, phonological, semantic, retrieval, and comprehension processes (see also Wolf & Katzir-Cohen, 2001). Each of these sets of processes must function accurately and rapidly in time before they are then integrated within milliseconds to enable the child or adult to read a single word. This view of cognitive and linguistic processes shows the importance not only of decoding-related processes, but also of multiple linguistic and cognitive processes including semantic, syntactic, and comprehension processes. For children to develop into fluent, comprehending analyzers of increasingly sophisticated text, they must develop both decoding skills and their knowledge of words at ever deeper and more linguistically complex levels.

All of these attentional, perceptual, cognitive, and linguistic processes necessary for such fluent, comprehending reading rest on an intricate reorganization of regions in the developing brain. As emphasized, this does not happen because of a preordained genetic program. It happens or fails to happen because of human activity. As linguist Steven Pinker (1997, p. ix-x) states, "Children are wired for sound, but print is an optional accessory that must be painstakingly bolted on." The development of reading involves the *painstaking bolting on* and *bolting together* of the processes in Figure 1. Many learners, replete with a rich preschool history of encounters with "literacy" based materials, are ready to learn, it would seem, almost without effort. Other children, because of environmental reasons or physiological differences in the brain regions subserving reading, have great difficulty acquiring reading. The significant numbers of children in the latter categories require systematic, explicit instruction in the various processes that comprise the components of reading.

A major implication of this particular view of reading is that the multiple components involved in reading can lead to multiple

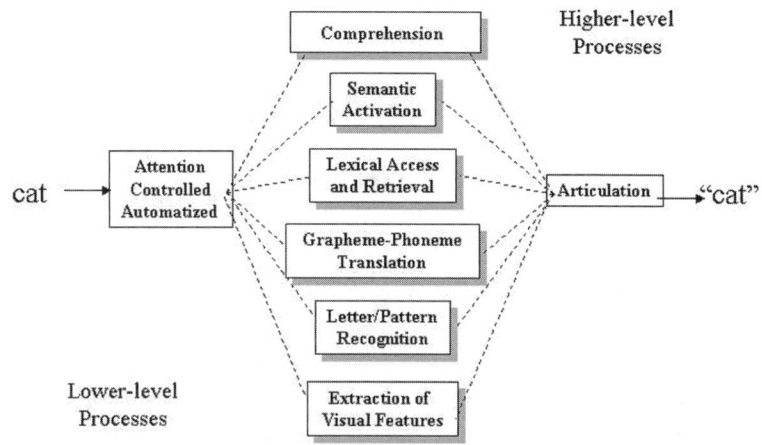

Figure 1. Model of basic reading processes.

possible sources of breakdown that include but go beyond decoding-related impediments. If that is the case, there should be subtypes of children with different causes of reading failure, a conclusion that runs counter to the conventional view of reading failure for the last 30 years. The conventional view assumes that the primary source of reading failure lies in one-half of the processes underlying the child's ability to learn and apply the grapheme-phoneme correspondence rules: that is, the phonological processes. According to this more unidimensional view, a deficit in phonological processes impedes the child's ability to develop phoneme awareness, which impedes the ability to learn grapheme-phoneme correspondence rules, which then impedes learning to decode and comprehend.

It is our position that the phonological core-deficit explanation is necessary but insufficient. An alternative view that emerged from work in the neurosciences on word-retrieval or naming-speed processes in alexia, aphasia, and dyslexia suggests that there are other possible deficits in dyslexia, including those that involve the need for fast, automatic, retrieval processes (Denckla & Rudel, 1976; Geschwind, 1965). These rate-related retrieval processes are independent of phonology and cannot be explained by phonological deficits. There is historical confusion about these rapid retrieval processes because many researchers have conflated the term phonology to include what they call phonological awareness, phonological retrieval, and phonological short-term memory. Based on two decades of research—ranging from multiple regression studies to fMRI differences—our position is that these three sets of processes are largely distinct from one another and should never be subsumed under one term. Indeed our recent imaging studies (Misra, Katzir, Wolf, & Poldrack, in press) show very different brain regions activated for naming speed and phoneme awareness processes, a finding that has been replicated by Eden's group (Turkeltaub, Gareau, Flowers, Zeffiro, & Eden, 2004) and Pugh (see Pugh, Sandak, Frost, Moore, Rueckl, & Mencl, this volume).

SOURCES OF READING BREAKDOWN IN DEVELOPMENTAL DYSLEXIA

The work on naming speed underscored that not only are there different regions in the brain used for rapid name retrieval and phonology processes, but also that there are different types of impaired readers, some with and without phonological impediments to reading. Our effort to capture the heterogeneity found in dyslexic readers originated in what has come to be called the Double-Deficit Hypothesis (DDH) (Bowers & Wolf, 1993; Wolf & Bowers, 1999). Its emphasis is on the description of at least three major subtypes of children, characterized by the presence, absence, or combination of two core deficits in phonology and the processes underlying naming speed. There are now considerable data (Lovett, Steinback, & Frijters, 2000; Manis, Doi, & Bhadha, 2000; Badian, 1996; Ho, Tsang, & Lee, 2002) that there are (a) poor readers who have phonological deficits without problems in naming speed; (b) readers who have adequate phonological and word attack skills, but early naming-speed deficits and later reading fluency and comprehension deficits (Note: these children would be missed by most diagnostic batteries because decoding is accurate); and (c) children with both areas of weaknesses or "double deficits." Children with both core deficits represent the most severely impaired subtype in all aspects of reading—particularly in reading fluency and comprehension—presumably because there are less areas of compensation available.

Wolf and Bowers (1999, 2000) used the term Double-Deficit Hypothesis as an acknowledged transitional vehicle to underscore the need to go beyond an emphasis too exclusively placed on phonological deficits. Unlike phonological deficits, naming-speed deficits can be caused by a variety of possible sources. This is because rapid naming, like the multicomponent view of reading espoused here, is conceptualized as a set of perceptual, cognitive, motoric, and linguistic processes that require seriation, integration, and great rapidity within and across all these processes. Naming speed processes are seen as a subset of the same components and requirements for speed found in reading. Such a view explains the powerful ability of naming speed both to predict reading failure among many children and to differentiate these children from those without reading disabilities.

The Double-Deficit Hypothesis, therefore, can be viewed as an effort to understand several major sources of reading failure. It is not meant to imply that there are only these types of deficit patterns. In every analysis by us and in other colleagues' reanalyses, there are small groups of children who cannot be characterized by either deficit and yet still have severe reading disability (see Lovett, Steinbach, & Frijters, 2000). What the Double-Deficit Hypothesis was meant to underscore is the need to understand how independent these major types of deficits can be in our samples and in our classrooms, with all the implications this has for expanding the foci of existing interventions. The single most important implication is that most children with naming speed deficits have fluency problems at the levels of word and connected text reading. Most existing programs for children with dyslexia focus largely on phonological skills, which are necessary but insufficient emphases for children with processing speed differences. They need additional early and daily emphases on automaticity and fluency at sublexical, lexical, and connected text levels.

The ultimate importance of the Double-Deficit Hypothesis is that it unswervingly emphasizes the need both to understand the role of rate of processing and fluency in reading development, and also to create fluency intervention that addresses these issues. Until recently, children with single, phonological deficits were adequately treated with current programs emphasizing phonological awareness and decoding. However, the other two subtypes with their explicit problems in naming speed and reading fluency were never sufficiently remediated. The next section of this chapter describes a componential reading intervention program that integrates phonological emphases with a new, componential view of "fluency and comprehension."

FLUENCY INTERVENTION: RAVE-O

The consensual view of fluency as "the ability to read connected text rapidly, smoothly, effortlessly, and automatically with little conscious attention to the mechanics of reading such as decoding" (Meyer & Felton, 1999) approaches fluency as an *outcome* of accuracy in decoding processes. In our work, we suggest a figure-ground shift for the conceptualization of fluency specifically, as a developmental process, as well as an outcome. Kame'enui and his colleagues (2001) conceptualized fluency as both the *development* of "proficiency" in underlying lower-level, component skills of reading (e.g., phoneme awareness), and also as the *outcome* of proficiency in higher-level processes and component skills (e.g., accuracy in comprehension). Wolf and Katzir-Cohen (2001) put forth the following developmental definition:

> In its beginnings, reading fluency is the product of the initial development of accuracy and the subsequent development of automaticity in underlying sublexical processes, lexical processes, and their integration in single-word reading and connected text. These include perceptual, phonological, orthographic, and morphological processes at the letter-, letter-pattern, and word-level; as well as semantic and syntactic processes at the word-level and connected-text level. After it is fully developed, reading fluency refers to a level of accuracy and rate, where decoding is relatively effortless; where oral reading is smooth and accurate with correct prosody; and where attention can be allocated to comprehension (p. 219).

Within such a developmental perspective, efforts to address fluency must start at the beginning of the reading acquisition process, not after reading is already acquired.

This definition of fluency further emphasizes its componential nature. Within this new view, fluency demands the development of high-quality orthographic, phonological, semantic, and syntactic representational systems. Second, it requires rapid connections between and among these systems. And third, it demands learning and practice to ensure the rapid retrieval of information from each system. Similarly, in a broader systems-approach to fluency, Berninger and her colleagues (Berninger, Abbott, Billingsley, & Nagy, 2001) give special importance to the role of morphological knowledge about words in facilitating the development of orthographic rate and overall fluency.

Funded by the National Institute of Child Health and Human Development, we designed and tested an experimental, multicomponential approach to fluency instruction. In a twist of historical irony, the instructional method uses a multidimensional approach to words that both incorporates current linguistic insights into the nature of words and also resembles some of the insights into language that the Sumerian pedagogical system contained over four millennia ago. The Sumerians used variously classified lists to show their pupils the multidimensional nature of words; these lists showed students explicitly the shared connections among words that could be classified together in a variety of ways (Cohen, 2003). For example, they taught their pupils evolving lists of words that were categorized by shared semantic or meaning-based features;

others contained shared phonological or sound-based features; still others shared the same logographic root (comparable both to our morphological and orthographic principles).

Described in detail elsewhere (Wolf, Miller, & Donnelly, 2000; Wolf, O'Brien, Adams, et al., 2003), the RAVE-O program (Retrieval, Automaticity, Vocabulary, Engagement with Language, and Orthography) has three large aims for each struggling reader in the second and third grade: first, the development of accuracy and automaticity in letter pattern and word levels; second, increased rate in word attack, word identification, and comprehension; and third, a transformed attitude toward words and language. To these ends, the program simultaneously addresses both the need for automaticity in phonological, orthographic, semantic, syntactic, and morphological systems, and the importance of teaching *explicit connections* among these linguistic systems. This latter feature is based in part on research that stresses the explicit linkages or connections among the orthographic, semantic, and phonological processes (Adams, 1990; Foorman, 1994; Seidenberg & McClelland, 1989). For example, Berninger et al. (2001), Adams (1990), and Moats (2000) stress the connections between morphosyntactic knowledge and these other processes.

The RAVE-O program is taught only in combination with a program that teaches systematic phonological analysis and blending (see Lovett, Steinbach, & Frijters, 2000). Children are taught a group of *core words* each week that exemplify critical phonological, orthographic, and semantic principles. Syntactic and morphological principles are gradually added after initial work has begun in the program. Each core word is chosen on the basis of (a) shared phonemes with the phonological treatment program, (b) sequenced orthographic patterns, and (c) semantic richness (e.g., each core word has at least three different meanings). First, the multiple meanings of core words are introduced through imagistic cards that depict the word in varied semantic contexts. Second, children are taught to connect the phonemes in the core words with the trained orthographic patterns in RAVE-O. For example, children are taught individual phonemes in the phonological program (like "a", "t", and "m") and *orthographic chunks* with the same phonemes in RAVE-O (e.g., "at" and "am" along with their word families; see the work of Goswami, 1999).

There is daily emphasis on practice and rapid recognition of the most frequent orthographic letter patterns in English. Computerized games (see Speed Wizards in Wolf & Goodman, 1996) and a new set of manipulative materials (e.g., letter dice, sound sliders, cards, and the like) were designed to allow for maximal practice and to increase the speed of orthographic pattern recognition (i.e., onset and rime) in an engaging fashion.

There is a simultaneous emphasis on vocabulary and retrieval, based on earlier work in vocabulary development that suggests that one retrieves fastest what one knows best (see Beck, Perfetti, & McKeown, 1982; German, 1992; Kame'enui, Dixon, & Carnine, 1987; Wolf & Segal, 1999). Vocabulary growth is conceptualized as essential to rapid retrieval (in oral *and* written language) and also to improved comprehension, an ultimate goal in the program. Retrieval skills are taught through a variety of ways, including a set of metacognitive strategies.

A series of comprehension stories (e.g., *Minute Mysteries* and *Minute Adventures*) accompany each week of RAVE-O, and directly address fluency and comprehension in several ways. The controlled vocabulary in the timed and untimed stories incorporates the week's particular orthographic and morphological patterns, and also emphasizes the multiple meanings of the week's core words and often their different syntactic uses. The stories provide a superb vehicle for repeated reading practice, which, in turn, helps fluency in connected text. Thus, the Minute Stories are multipurpose vehicles for facilitating fluency in phonological, orthographic, syntactic, and semantic systems at the same time they build comprehension skills. Fluency is our best known bridge to comprehension. The end goal of RAVE-O, therefore, is not about how rapidly children read, but about how well they understand and enjoy what they read.

Connected to this ultimate goal in every daily lesson in RAVE-O is an additional system too little discussed by many researchers; that is, the affective-motivational one. The secret weapon of this program is the game-like *whimsy* in every aspect of the program's activities. We want children to want to read and to play with their oral and written language. We seek to empower what are often linguistically disenfranchised children.

Such a method of instruction demands a special involvement from teachers. Throughout the program, therefore, we strive in as many ways as we can to engage not only the learner, but also the teacher and the teacher's own love of language. Our goal throughout is a group of mutually engaged teachers and engaged learners.

Preliminary results from this randomized treatment-control study strongly support RAVE-O's potential for advancing children's reading performance at the letter-pattern, word, and text levels. In children identified as at risk for developmental reading disability, we compared growth curves for those in a RAVE-O treatment group versus those in a Math-Classroom Survival Skills control condition. During the first year, the latter children received a math curriculum that stressed study skills, which are often negligent in children with learning disabilities. In the second year, they received one of the reading interventions. Each treatment group received 70 one-hour sessions in small groups of four.

Measures of word recognition and decoding accuracy and speed—as well as passage comprehension, spelling, and expressive vocabulary—were taken at pre-, mid-, and posttime points (after 0, 35, and 70 sessions, respectively). The treatment groups differed with respect to change over time on decoding accuracy (*WRMT–R* Word Attack, $p < .001$), word identification accuracy (*WRMT–R* Word Identification, $p < .04$), and reading speed (*TOWRE*—Sight Words, $p < .001$). To evaluate the program's effectiveness with respect to the DDH subtypes with naming speed deficits, initial scores of rapid serial naming speed (RAN letters) were covaried. With the naming speed covariate, growth rates differed between treatment groups on word identification ($p < .03$) and decoding accuracy ($p < .001$), as well as passage comprehension (*WRMT–R* Passage Comprehension, $p < .03$) and vocabulary (Word-R Multiple Definitions Test, $p = .02$). These results indicate the potential of a fluency-based intervention to effect change in fluency comprehension and vocabulary (see Figure 2).

The significance of these results is profound. First, they are some of the few data that demonstrate the potential of a fluency-based intervention to effect change in fluency, comprehension, and vocabulary. For years, there has been an almost universally held assumption that a phonological-based program would ameliorate the word-recognition problems of poor readers and that this, in turn, would pave the way for the amelioration of fluency and comprehension problems. The reality, however, was not so straightforward. As expressed by Lyon and Moats (1997, p. 579):

> Improvements in decoding and word-reading accuracy have been far easier to obtain than improvements in reading and fluency and automaticity. This persistent finding indicates there is much we have to learn about the development of componential reading skills and how such skills mediate reading rate and reading comprehension.

In other words, our best efforts at phonological intervention were insufficient to address the more complex nature of fluency and comprehension. The Double-Deficit Hypothesis provided an alternative perspective on this initial assumption. Seventy percent of children with severe reading impairments exhibit some form of fluency or rate-based difficulty, regardless of the presence of

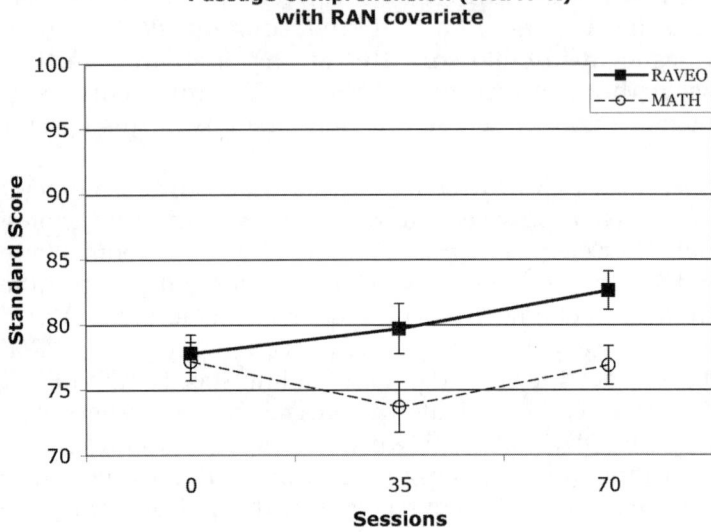

Figure 2. Results for RAVE-O vs. control treatment conditions on passage comprehension.

phonological issues. This view of reading failure insists that intervention that systematically addresses the multiple linguistic and cognitive contributions to fluency is necessary to pursue if we are to move the almost intractable problems underlying fluency and comprehension deficits in children who are struggling readers. The RAVE-O data suggest at a minimum that a multicomponent approach to intervention can simultaneously redress word attack wand word identification and make inroads in fluency, vocabulary, and comprehension. Further, it suggests that the so-called treatment resisters are amenable to change. The data do not ameliorate fluency and comprehension issues, but they point the direction to somewhere new: a conceptualization of reading failure that includes but goes beyond phonological processes in this explanation, and that places particular emphasis on subtype analysis and great understanding of individual reasons for reading failure.

SUMMARY

This chapter described the evolutionarily powerful notion of the brain's ability to *rearrange* itself to learn new cognitive functions. We applied this concept in two ways. First, we presented a conceptualization of the reading brain, in which over the last 5,000 years, the human brain learned to call on an array of regions originally devoted to other things: the perception of tiny, visual features; the hearing and segmenting of the smallest units of sounds in spoken language; the understanding of a symbol; the retrieving of words and their meaning(s); and the integration of all these regions in lightning, almost automatic speeds. Second, we applied the concept of rearrangement to an understanding of heterogeneity in reading disabilities with an emphasis on several major subtypes with different requirements for learning. Third, we applied these concepts to the design of intervention where we illustrated how a developmental view of fluency, in combination with reconfiguration of new and old "best teaching practices," can address fluency and comprehension issues in children with these major types of reading disability. The overarching goal of the RAVE-O intervention program is to help the child integrate the multiple processes activated when we encounter words, in sufficiently rapid time, to allow for accurate decoding and fluent comprehension. In so doing, the RAVE-O program's explicit attempts to depict the multi-dimensional nature of words is, in practice, a new iteration of principles first employed by the Sumerians five thousand years ago!

Address correspondence to: Maryanne Wolf, Ph.D., Center for Reading and Language Research, Miller Hall, Tufts University, Medford, MA 02155; E-mail: maryanne.wolf@tufts.edu

REFERENCES

Adams, M. J. (1990). *Beginning to read: Thinking and learning about print.* Cambridge, MA: MIT Press.

Badian, N. (1996). Dyslexia: Does it exist? Dyslexia, garden-variety poor reading, and the double-deficit hypothesis. Paper presented at the Orton Dyslexia Society, Boston, MA.

Beck, I. L., Perfetti, C. A., & McKeown, M. G. (1982). Effects of long-term vocabulary instructions on lexical access and reading comprehension. *Journal of Educational Psychology, 74,* 506–521.

Berninger, V. W., Abbott, R. D., Billingsley, F., & Nagy, W. (2001). Processes underlying timing and fluency of reading: Efficiency, automaticity, coordination, and morphological awareness. In M. Wolf (Ed.), *Time, fluency, and dyslexia.* Timonium, MD: York Press.

Bowers, P. G., & Wolf, M. (1993). Theoretical links among naming speed, precise timing mechanisms and orthographic skill in dyslexia. *Reading and Writing, 5*(1), 69–85.

Cohen, Y. (2003). Personal correspondence.

Dehaene, S. (2003). Pre-emption of human cortical circuits by numbers and language: The "neuronal" recycling hypothesis. Paper presented at Pontifical Academy of Sciences meeting. Vatican City.

Deacon, T. (1997). *The symbolic species: The co-evolution of language and the human brain.* New York: W.W. Norton & Company.

Denckla, M. B., & Rudel, R. G. (1976). Naming of objects by dyslexic and other learning-disabled children. *Brain and Language, 3,* 1–15.

Eden, G. F., & Moats, L. (2002). The role of neuroscience in the remediation of students with dyslexia. *Nature and Neuroscience, 5*(Suppl.), 1080–1084.

Foorman, B. R. (1994). Phonological and orthographic processing: Separate but equal? In V.W. Berninger (Ed.), *The varieties of orthographic knowledge I: Theoretical and developmental issues* (pp. 319–355). Dordrecht, The Netherlands: Kluwer.

German, D. J. (1992). Word finding intervention for children and adolescents. *Topics in Learning Disorders 13,* 33–50.

Geschwind, N. (1965). Disconnection syndrome in animals and man (Parts I, II). *Brain, 88,* 237–294, 585–644.

Goswami, U. (1999). Causal connections in beginning reading: The importance of rhyme. *Journal of Research in Reading, 22,* 217–240.

Ho Chan, D., Tsang, S.-M., & Lee, S.-H. (2002). The cognitive profile and multiple-deficit hypothesis in Chinese developmental psychology. *Developmental Psychology, 38,* 543–553.

Kame'enui, E. J., Simmons, D. C., Good, R. H., & Harn, B. A. (2001). The use of fluency-based measures in early identification and evaluation of intervention efficacy in schools. In M. Wolf (Ed.), *Time, fluency, and dyslexia.* Timonium, MD: York Press.

Kame'enui, E. J., Dixon, R. C., & Carnine, D. W. (1987). Issues in the design of vocabulary instruction. In M. G. McKeown & M. E. Curtis (Eds.), *The nature of vocabulary acquisition* (pp. 129–145). Hillsdale, NJ: Erlbaum.

Lovett, M. W., Steinbach, K. A., & Frijters, J. C. (2000). Remediating the core deficits of developmental reading disability: A double-deficit perspective. *Journal of Learning Disabilities, 33*(4), 334–358.

Lyon, G. R., & Moats, L. C. (1997). Critical conceptual and methodological considerations in reading intervention research. *Journal of Learning Disabilities, 30,* 578–588.

Manis, F. R., Doi, L. M., & Bhadha, B. (2000). Naming speed, phonological awareness, and orthographic knowledge in second graders. *Journal of Learning Disabilities, 33,* 325–333.

Meyer, M. S., & Felton, R. H. (1999). Repeated reading to enhance fluency: Old approaches and new directions. *Annals of Dyslexia, 49,* 283–306.

Misra, M., Katzir, T., Wolf, M., & Poldrack, R. (in press). Neural systems underlying rapid automatized naming (RAN) in skilled readers: Unraveling the puzzle of RAN-reading relationships. *Scientific Studies of Reading.*

Moats, L. (2000). *Speech to print: Language essentials for teachers.* Baltimore: Paul H. Brookes Publishing Company.

Morris, R., Lovett, M., & Wolf, M. (1996). Treatment of developmental reading disabilities. NICHD grant proposal.

Perfetti, C. A. (1985). *Reading ability.* New York: Oxford Press.

Pinker, S. (1997). Preface to D. McGuinness' *Why our children can't read and what we can do about it: A scientific revolution in reading* (pp. ix–x). University of South Florida, Tampa, FL.

Pugh, K., Sandak, R., Frost, S. J., Moore, D., & Mencl, W. E. (in press). Neurobiological studies of skilled and impaired reading: A work in progress. In G. D. Rosen (Ed.), *The Dyslexic Brain*. Mahwah, NJ: Lawrence Erlbaum Associates.

Schmandt-Besserat, D. (1992). *Before writing: From counting to cuneiform*. College Station, TX: Texas University Press.

Seidenberg, M., & McClelland, J. (1989). A distributed developmental model of word recognition and naming. *Psychological Review, 96*, 35–49.

Teale, W., & Sulzby, E. (Eds.). (1986). *Emergent literacy: Writing and reading*. Norwood, NJ: Ablex, Co.

Wolf, M., O'Brien, B., Adams, K., Joffe, T., Jeffrey, J., Lovett, M., & Morris, R. (2003). Working for time: Reflections on naming speed, reading fluency, and intervention. In B. Foorman (Ed.), *Preventing and remediating reading difficulties: Bringing science to scale*. Timonium, MD: York Press.

Wolf, M., &, Katzir-Cohen, T. (2001). Reading fluency and its intervention. In E. Kame'enui & D. Simmons (Eds.), *Scientific studies of reading (special issue on fluency), 5*, 211–238.

Wolf, M., Miller, L., & Donnelly, K. (2000). The retrieval, automaticity, vocabulary elaboration, orthography (RAVE-O): A comprehensive fluency-based reading intervention program. *Journal of Learning Disabilities, 33*(4), 375–386.

Wolf, M., & Bowers, P. (2000). The question of naming-speed deficits in developmental reading disabilities: An introduction to the double-deficit hypothesis. *Journal of Learning Disabilities, 33*, 322–324.

Wolf, M., & Bowers, P. (1999). The "double-deficit hypothesis" for the developmental dyslexias. *Journal of Educational Psychology, 91*(3), 1–24.

Wolf, M., & Segal, D. (1999). Retrieval-rate, accuracy and vocabulary elaboration (RAVE) in reading-impaired children: A pilot intervention program. *Dyslexia, 5*, 1–27.

Wolf, M., & Goodman, G. (1996). Speed wizards: Computerized games for the teaching of reading fluency. Tufts University and Rochester Institute of Technology.

Chapter • 2

Neurobiological Studies of Skilled and Impaired Reading: A Work in Progress

*Kenneth R. Pugh, Rebecca Sandak,
Stephen J. Frost, Dina Moore, Jay G. Rueckl,
and W. Einar Mencl*

SUMMARY

In recent years, significant progress has been made in studying the neurobiology of reading development and reading disability with the use of functional neuroimaging techniques. There is substantial converging evidence that skilled word recognition is associated with the development of a highly integrated cortical system that includes left hemisphere dorsal, ventral, and anterior subsystems. This paper highlights key findings regarding the functional role of these regions during skilled reading, the developmental trajectory toward this mature reading circuitry in normally developing children, deviations from this trajectory in reading disabled populations, and the ways in which successful reading remediation alters the brain organization for reading. While a number of important brain/behavior relations have been identified to date, much remains to be done in order to progress from largely descriptive toward potentially explanatory accounts.

This research was funded by NICHD grants F32-HD42391 to Rebecca Sandak, R01-HD40411 to Kenneth R. Pugh, and P01-HD01994 to Haskins Laboratories.

Identification of the factors that govern the successful acquisition of literacy skills and identification of the cause(s) of reading failure has long been a high priority for researchers in developmental and educational psychology, and more recently has become a major focus for researchers in the emerging field of cognitive neuroscience. Extensive behavioral research, conducted over many years, has examined these issues, and much progress has been made in identifying important cognitive, linguistic, and perceptual factors associated with reading success or failure (Grigorenko, 2001; Pugh et al., 2000a). Research aimed at identifying neurobiological factors in reading development and reading disability has benefited in recent years from rapid advances in several neuroimaging technologies (e.g., Positron Emission Tomography [PET], functional Magnetic Resonance Imaging [fMRI], and Magnetoencephology [MEG]). These new tools have been used with increasing frequency to examine functional brain organization for language and reading in children and adults with and without reading disability (Papanicolaou et al., 2004).

Both in the history of the human species and in the development of the individual child, spoken language capacity is prior to the secondary, derived language abilities of reading and writing. While brain organization for spoken language perception and production is, to a large degree at least, a biological specialization (Liberman, 1992), reading by contrast is almost certainly not. Indeed, reading skill, unlike speech communication skills, must be explicitly taught. Moreover, while few children will fail to master spoken language communication skills without explicit training, significant numbers of children, for whom spoken language communication skills are adequate, fail to obtain accurate and fluent reading levels, even with intensive training efforts on the part of teachers and parents. When considered from the neurobiological perspective, it seems clear that the challenge for the brain at the onset of literacy instruction is to generate a circuit, comprised of multifunctional visual, language, and associative regions, which can eventually permit rapid translation of visual forms to already well-instantiated language representational systems (Price et al., 2003; Pugh et al., 2000a).

Thus, learning to read fluently places a high premium on brain plasticity, as it involves processing changes across distributed brain systems as reading experience increases. Neuroimaging techniques can help us chart this neurobiological developmental trajectory as well as identify deviation from this trajectory in unsuccessful readers. Moreover, with these trajectories (and deviations) established, we can then determine how different factors in the child's educational environment impact the neurobiological substrate and ultimately, reading performance. Thus, incorporating neuroimaging techniques in this way might facilitate a better understanding of why certain remediation techniques result in improved performance.

While studies identifying neurobiologic markers of reading disability have generated a good deal of enthusiasm lately, it should be remembered that functional neuroimaging measures are not intrinsically explanatory; they simply describe brain organization at a given point in development. To illustrate, we have identified brain regions that develop a reading specialization for normally developing but not for reading-disabled (RD) individuals (see below). We cannot conclude from these data however, that the "cause" of reading failure lies in some sort of neurobiological anomaly at these particular cortical regions. It may be so, but it is just as reasonable to speculate that the locus of the deficit lies elsewhere (outside of the emergent reading circuit) and that the identified regions reflect a kind of "end-state" brain system not obtained when reading fails. Thus, while functional imaging can provide a good description of how the brain solves the problem of building a reading circuit, we will need to use a multiplicity of research tools (at several levels of analysis) and research designs (especially longitudinal studies) to potentially get at the crucial etiological factors in reading disability and how these factors conspire to limit the development of an efficient reading circuit. At minimum, for neurobiological findings to become relevant to our understanding of the causes of reading success or failure, we must establish meaningful links between behavioral/cognitive skills that must be in place to read, and the development of those neural systems that support these skills (Pugh et al., 2000a; Grigorenko, 2001). It is, therefore, of real importance that neuroimaging research be informed by cognitive behavioral theory and research from the outset.

BEHAVIORAL STUDIES OF READING DISABILITY

Reading disability is characterized by the failure to develop age-appropriate reading skill despite normal intelligence and adequate opportunity for reading instruction. Significant progress has been made in understanding the cognitive and linguistic skills that must be in place to ensure adequate reading development in children (Liberman et al., 1974; Brady & Shankweiler, 1991; Rieben & Perfetti, 1991; Bruck, 1992; Shankweiler et al., 1995; Fletcher et al., 1994; Stanovich & Siegel, 1994). With regard to reading disability, it has been shown that for the majority of struggling readers, a core difficulty in reading manifests itself as a deficiency within the language system, and in particular, a deficiency at the level of phonological analysis. Behaviorally, deficits are most evident at the level of single word and pseudoword reading; RD performance is both slow and inaccurate relative to nonimpaired (NI) readers. Many lines of evidence converge on the conclusion that the word and pseudoword reading difficulties in RD individuals are, to a large extent, manifestations of more basic deficits at the level of rapidly assembling the phonological code represented by a token letter string (Bradley & Bryant, 1985). Phonological assembly refers to the decoding operations associated with grapheme-to-phoneme mapping in printed word identification. The failure to develop efficient phonological assembly skill in word and pseudoword reading, in turn, appears to stem from difficulties—at the earliest stages of literacy training—in attaining fine-grained phonemic awareness. Phonological awareness, in general, is defined as the metalinguistic understanding that spoken words can be decomposed into phonological primitives, which in turn can be represented by alphabetic characters (Liberman, Shankweiler, Fischer, & Carter, 1974; Brady & Shankweiler, 1991; Rieben & Perfetti, 1991; Bruck, 1992; Shankweiler et al., 1995; Fletcher et al., 1994; Stanovich & Siegel, 1994). As to why RD readers should have exceptional difficulty developing phonological awareness, there is some support for the notion that the difficulty resides in the phonological component of the larger specialization for language (Liberman, 1992; Liberman, Shankweiler, Fischer, & Carter, 1974). If the phonological system is compromised, its representations will be less than ideally distinct and, therefore, harder to bring to conscious awareness; that in turn will preclude the developmental of efficient decoding routines.

Reading is a complex skill and there can be many reasons why some children fail to learn to read. For example, it has been argued that the reading difficulties experienced by some children may result from difficulties with processing speed (Wolf & Bowers, 1999; Wolf & O'Brien, this volume), rapid auditory processing (Tallal, 1980; Tallal, this volume), general language deficits (Scarborough & Dobrich, 1990), or visual deficits (Cornelissen & Hansen, 1998), among other things. However, as noted above, there is growing consensus that one of the immediate causes of reading failure is the difficulty that many children have in mastering phonemic awareness skills (e.g., Fletcher et al., 1994; Shankweiler et al., 1995; Stanovich & Siegel, 1994). The etiological underpinnings of this difficulty are still actively being investigated, and the question of whether such language-level challenges might, in some children at least, be linked to more basic deficits in one of the above-mentioned domains is much debated. In any event, a large body of evidence directly relates deficits in phonological awareness to difficulties in learning to read: phonological awareness measures predict later reading achievement (Bradley & Bryant, 1985; Torgesen et al., 1994); deficits in phonological awareness consistently separate RD and nonimpaired children (Fletcher et al., 1994; Stanovich & Siegel, 1994); phonological deficits persist into adulthood (Felton, Naylor, & Wood, 1990; Bruck, 1992; Shaywitz et al., 1998) and instruction in phonological awareness promotes the acquisition of reading skills (Bradley & Bryant, 1983; Torgesen, Morgan, & Davis, 1992; Ball & Blachman, 1991; Foorman et al., 1998). For children with adequate phonological skills, the process of phonological assembly in word and pseudoword reading becomes highly automated, efficient, and as a growing body of evidence suggests, this phonological decoding continues to serve as an important component in rapid word identification, even for mature skilled readers (cf., Lukatela & Turvey, 1994; Frost, 1998).

Given this background, our own functional neuroimaging research program, and the studies selected for discussion in this review, involve a comparison of RD and nonimpaired (NI) reading groups on word and pseudoword reading tasks that tap into phonological processing and decoding. For a discussion of functional neuroimaging studies that have examined sensory-level processing deficits in developmental dyslexia (e.g., Eden et al., 1996; Demb, Boynton, Best, & Heeger, 1998), the reader is referred to Eden and Zeffiro (1998) and Habib (2000). For reviews of research examining anatomical/structural brain differences between RD and NI groups, the reader is referred to Filipek (1995), Galaburda (1992), and Habib (2000).

THE CORTICAL READING SYSTEMS AND THEIR ROLES IN SKILLED READING

Recently, functional neuroimaging techniques have been employed in the area of reading development, reading disability, and intervention (see Pugh et al., 2000a; and Sarkari et al., 2002 for reviews). There is substantial converging evidence that skilled word recognition requires the development of a highly organized cortical system that integrates processing of orthographic, phonological, and lexico-semantic features of words. Illustrated in Figure 1, this system broadly includes two posterior subsystems in the left

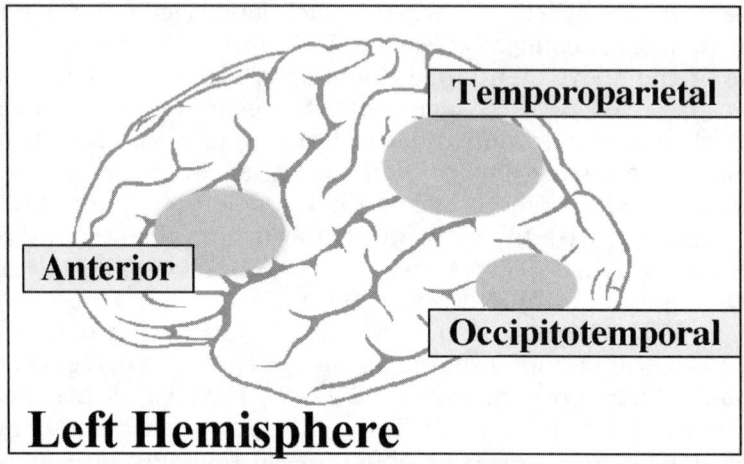

Figure 1. A schematic representation of major cortical regions implicated during reading-related tasks in skilled adult readers.

hemisphere (LH): a ventral (occipitotemporal) and a dorsal (temporoparietal) system, and a third area, anterior to the other two (the IFG).

The ventral system includes a left inferior occipitotemporal/ fusiform area, and extends anteriorly into the middle and inferior temporal gyri. It has been suggested that the occipitotemporal (OT) region functions as a presemantic visual word form area (VWFA) by some researchers (c.f., Cohen et al., 2002, but see Price et al., 2003 for an alternative account). Importantly, the functional specificity of this region appears to be late developing and critically related to the acquisition of reading skill (Booth et al., 2001; Shaywitz et al., 2002). Because of its critical role in skilled reading, we refer to this putative VWFA more neutrally as the ventral "skill zone." More anterior foci within the ventral system, extending into the middle to inferior temporal gyri, appear to be semantically tuned (Fiebach et al., 2002; Tagamets et al., 2000; Simos et al., 2002). The ventral system, particularly more posterior aspects, is also fast-acting in response to linguistic stimuli in skilled readers but not in RD individuals (Salmelin et al., 1996). It should be noted that there is some disagreement in the literature about the precise localization of critical subregions comprising the ventral system (Price et al., 2003; Pammer et al., submitted). Nevertheless, recent studies examining both timing and stimulus-type effects suggest that moving anteriorly through this ventral system, subregions respond to word and word-like stimuli in a progressively abstracted and linguistic manner (Pammer et al., submitted; Tarkiainen, Cornelissen, & Salmelin, 2003; Tagamets et al., 2000).

The more dorsal temporoparietal system broadly includes the angular gyrus and supramarginal gyrus (SMG) in the inferior parietal lobule, and the posterior aspect of the superior temporal gyrus (Wernicke's Area). Among their other functions (e.g., attentionally controlled processing), the areas within this system seem to be involved in mapping visual percepts of print onto the phonological and semantic structures of language (Black & Behrmann, 1994). In skilled readers, certain regions within the LH temporoparietal system (particularly the SMG) respond with greater activity to pseudowords than to familiar words (Price et al., 1996; Simos et al., 2002; Xu et al., 2001). This finding, along with our developmental studies (Shaywitz et al., 2002), suggests that the temporoparietal system plays a role in the types of phonological analyses that are relevant to learning new material.

An anterior system centered in posterior aspects of the inferior frontal gyrus (IFG) appears to be associated with phonological recoding during reading, among other functions (e.g., phonological memory, syntactic processing); the more anterior aspects of IFG seem to play a role in semantic retrieval (Poldrack et al., 1999). The phonologically relevant components of this multifunctional system have been found to function in silent reading and in naming (see Fiez & Petersen, 1998 for a review; Pugh et al., 1997), and like the temporoparietal system, is more strongly engaged by low-frequency words (particularly irregular/exception words) and pseudowords than by high-frequency words (Fiebach et al., 2002; Fiez & Peterson, 1998). We have speculated that this anterior system operates in close conjunction with the temporoparietal system to decode new words during normal reading development (Pugh et al., 2000a).

Of these three systems, the dorsal and anterior systems appear to predominate during initial reading acquisition in normally developing children, with an increased ventral response as proficiency in word-recognition increases. We observed (Shaywitz et al., 2002) that normally developing children younger than 10.5 years of age show strong engagement of dorsal and anterior systems, but limited engagement of the ventral system during reading tasks. In contrast, children older than 10.5 years of age tend to show increased engagement of the ventral system, which in turn is associated with increasingly skilled reading. Indeed, when multiple regression analyses examined both age and reading skill (measured by performance on standard reading tests), the critical predictor was reading skill level: the higher the reading skill, the stronger the response in the LH ventral cortex (with several other areas showing age- and skill-related reductions). Based on these developmental findings, we suggest that a beginning reader on a successful trajectory employs a widely distributed cortical system for print processing including temporoparietal, frontal, and right hemisphere (RH) posterior areas. As reading skill increases, these regions play a somewhat diminished role, while LH ventral sites become more active, and presumably more central to the rapid recognition of printed (word) stimuli (see Booth et al., 2001; Turkeltaub et al., 2003; Tarkanien, Cornelissen, & Salmelin, 2003; McCandliss et al., 2004; for similar arguments).

ALTERED CIRCUITS IN READING DISABILITY

There are clear functional differences between NI and RD readers with regard to activation patterns in dorsal, ventral, and anterior sites during reading tasks. In disabled readers, a number of functional imaging studies have observed LH posterior functional disruption at both dorsal and ventral sites during phonological processing tasks (Brunswick et al., 1999; Paulesu et al., 2001; Pugh et al., 2000; Salmelin et al., 1996; Shaywitz et al., 1998, 2002; Temple et al., 2001). This disruption is instantiated as a relative underengagement of these regions, specifically when processing linguistic stimuli (words and pseudowords) or during tasks that require decoding. This functional anomaly in posterior LH regions has been observed consistently in children (Shaywitz et al., 2002) and adults (Salmelin et al., 1996; Shaywitz et al., 1998). Hypoactivation in three key dorsal and ventral sites, including cortex within the temporoparietal region, the angular gyrus, and the ventral OT skill zone, is detectable as early as the end of kindergarten in children who have not reached important milestones in learning to read (Simos et al., 2002). Indeed, this ventral disruption has been seen as a critical signature of reading disability across several languages (Paulesu et al., 2001; Salmelin et al., 1996).

Most neuroimaging studies have attempted to isolate specific brain regions where activation patterns discriminate RD from NI readers (e.g., Rumsey et al., 1997; Shaywitz et al., 1998; Simos et al., 2002; Temple et al., 2001). However, a deeper understanding of the neurobiology of developmental dyslexia requires that we also consider relations *among* distinct brain regions that function cooperatively as circuits to process information during reading; this issue has been referred to as one of functional connectivity (Friston, 1994). Evidence consistent with the notion of a breakdown in functional connectivity within the posterior reading system in RD readers has been recently reported by Horwitz, Rumsey, and Donohue (1998). Using activation data from the Rumsey et al. (1997) PET study, these authors examined correlations (within task/over subjects) between activation levels in the LH angular gyrus and other brain sites during two reading aloud tasks (exception word and nonword naming). Correlations between the LH angular gyrus and occipital and temporal lobe sites were strong and significant in NI readers and weak in RD readers. Such a result suggests a breakdown in functional connectivity across the major components of the LH posterior reading system.

We also examined functional connectivity between the angular gyrus and other LH posterior regions in a large sample of adult RD and NI readers (Pugh et al., 2000b). We looked at functional connectivity between the angular gyrus and occipital and temporal lobe sites on those tasks that systematically varied demands made on phonological assembly. While for RD readers LH functional connectivity was disrupted on word and nonword reading tasks as also reported by Horwitz et al. (1998), there appeared to be no dysfunction on the tasks that tap metaphonological judgments only (e.g., a single letter rhyme task), or complex visual-orthographic coding only (e.g., an orthographic case judgment task). The results are most consistent with a specific phonological deficit hypothesis. Our data suggest that a breakdown in LH posterior systems functional connectivity manifests only when orthographic to phonological assembly is required. The notion of a developmental lesion, one that would disrupt functional connectivity in this system across all types of cognitive behaviors, is not supported by this result. Moreover, we found that on word and nonword reading tasks, RH homologues appear to function in a compensatory manner for RD readers; correlations were strong and stable in this hemisphere for both reading groups with higher values in RD readers.

Functional connectivity analysis in another sample of 144 good and poor readers, from 7 to 18 years of age, revealed important developmental differences in RD and NI cohorts (Shaywitz et al., 2002; Mencl, Shaywitz, et al., submitted). In this dataset, we initially discovered that only the older (ages 12 to 18) good readers displayed significant connectivity between the ventral skill zone and the reading relevant sites in the IFG; younger good readers (ages 7 to 11) and dyslexics did not. A multivariate analysis was then employed to identify shifts in functional connectivity patterns as a function of age and reading ability. Good readers showed an age-related difference that included (1) increased connectivity between the LH ventral system and IFG, implying integration of orthographic and phonological processing; and (2) decreased connectivity between the OT area and the anterior cingulate gyrus, suggesting more automatic processing. Dyslexic readers showed a distinctly different developmental trend, including (1) increased connectivity between the LH OT area and a set of RH regions, consistent with the notion of compensatory processing strategies (see below); and (2) increased connectivity between the anterior cingulate gyrus and IFG bilaterally, again suggesting a more effortful and attentionally guided reading strategy.

POTENTIALLY COMPENSATORY PROCESSING IN READING DISABILITY

Behaviorally, poor readers compensate for their inadequate phonological awareness and knowledge of letter-sound correspondences by overrelying on contextual cues to read individual words; their word reading errors tend to be visual or semantic rather than phonetic (see Perfetti, 1985 for a review). These behavioral markers of reading impairment may be instantiated cortically by compensatory activation of frontal and RH regions. In our studies (Shaywitz et al., 1998, 2002), we observed processing in RD readers that we interpret as compensatory. We found that on tasks that made explicit demands on phonological processing (pseudoword- and word-reading tasks), RD readers showed a disproportionately greater engagement of IFG and prefrontal dorsolateral sites than did NI readers (see also Brunswick et al., 1999; Salmelin et al., 1996 for similar findings). Evidence of a second, potentially compensatory, shift—in this case to posterior RH regions—comes from several findings. Using MEG, Sarkari et al. (2002) found an increase in the apparent engagement of the RH temporoparietal region in RD children. More detailed examination of this trend, using hemodynamic measures, indicates that hemispheric asymmetries in activity in posterior temporal and temporoparietal regions (the middle temporal and the angular gyri) vary significantly among reading groups (Shaywitz et al., 1998): there was greater right than LH activation in RD readers but greater left than RH activation in NI readers. Rumsey et al. (1999) examined the relationship between RH activation and reading performance in their adult RD and NI participants and found that RH temporoparietal activation was correlated with standard measures of reading performance only for RD readers (see also Shaywitz et al., 2002).

We hypothesize that the reason RD readers tend to strongly engage inferior frontal sites is their increased reliance on covert pronunciation (articulatory recoding) in an attempt to cope with their deficient phonological analysis of the printed word. In addition, their heightened activation of the posterior RH regions with reduced LH posterior activation suggests a process of word recognition that relies on letter-by-letter processing in accessing RH localized visuo-semantic representations (or some other compensatory process) rather than relying on phonologically structured word recognition strategies. These differential patterns, especially the increased activation in frontal regions, might also reflect increased effort during reading; underengagement of LH posterior areas, particularly ventral sites, would not be thought to reflect this increased effort, but rather the failure to engage these areas likely precipitates any change in effort.

NEUROBIOLOGICAL EFFECTS OF SUCCESSFUL READING REMEDIATION

Converging evidence from other studies supports the notion that gains in reading skill resulting from intense reading intervention are associated with a more "normalized" localization of reading processes in the brain. In a recent MEG study, eight young children with severe reading difficulties underwent a brief but intensive phonics-based remediation program (Simos et al., 2002). After intervention, the most salient change observed on a case-by-case basis was a robust increase in the apparent engagement of the LH temporoparietal region accompanied by a moderate reduction in the activation of the RH temporoparietal areas. Similarly, Temple et al. (2003) used fMRI to examine the effects of an intervention (FastForword) on the cortical circuitry of a group of 8- to 12-year-old children with reading difficulties. After intervention, increased LH temporoparietal and inferior frontal increases were observed. Moreover, the LH increases correlated significantly with increased reading scores. In a recent collaborative study with Dr. Benita Blachman of Syracuse University, we examined three groups of young children (average age was 6.5 years at Time 1) with fMRI and behavioral indices (Shaywitz et al., 2004). A treatment RD group received nine months of intensive phonologically analytic intervention (Blachman et al., 2004), and there were two control groups: a typically developing, and an untreated RD group. Relative to RD controls, RD treatment participants showed reliable gains on reading measures (particularly on fluency-related measures such as GORT rate scores). Pre- and post-treatment fMRI employed a simple cross modal (auditory/visual) forced choice letter match task. When RD groups were compared at Time 2 (posttreatment), reliably greater activation increases in LH reading-related sites were seen in the treatment group. When Time 2 and Time 1 activation profiles were directly contrasted for each group, it was evident that both RD treatment and typically developing, but not RD controls, showed reliable increases in LH reading-related sites. Prominent differences were seen in LH IFG, and importantly in LH ventral skill zone. These changes were quite similar to the NI controls as they also learned to read. Importantly, the treatment group also returned one year posttreatment for a follow-up scan, and progressive LH ventral increases along with decreasing RH activation patterns were observed even one year after treatment was concluded. All these initial neuroimaging treatment studies suggest that a critical neurobiological signature of successful intervention, at least in younger children, appears to be increased engagement of major LH reading-related circuits and reduced compensatory reliance on RH homologues.

A PRELIMINARY MODEL OF THE NEUROBIOLOGY OF WORD RECOGNITION

We have proposed a neurobiology of word recognition based on the neurobiological data in which lexical selection is determined largely by the ventral system when the stimulus is familiar and task demands are appropriate, and by the dorsal system, in close conjunction with the IFG, when the stimulus is novel or of low frequency (Pugh et al., 2000). In this early conceptualization, the two systems were thought to correspond (but only loosely) to the two routes of classical dual route theory (Coltheart et al., 1993). While neuroimaging evidence might be taken to support the existence of multiple "routes," there is, as yet, no compelling data to suggest that the faster ventral route involves direct activation of meaning as proposed by standard versions of dual route theory. The phonological representation of the word might still be involved, either in mediating the activation between orthography and lexical meaning or alternatively, as an obligatory consequence after the direct activation of meaning by orthography (Simos et al., 2002).

Our initial neurobiological theory proposed that processing in the dorsal system proceeds relatively slowly, producing phonological representations generated by subword analysis; that is, a result of grapheme-phoneme analysis, onset-body analysis, or other subword phonological analysis. The dorsal system appears to act in concert with the IFG in integrating orthographic and phonological features of words. Direct evidence supporting a critical role of the dorsal system in subword phonological analysis comes from electrocortical stimulation studies. For example, Simos et al. (2000) found that electrical interference within a small portion of the posterior superior temporal gyrus consistently impaired patients' ability to decode pseudowords. Whereas this ability relies primarily on the slower (dorsal) system, the ability to read real words with exceptional spellings, which could be accomplished by the faster (ventral) system, remained unaffected. There is additional, albeit indirect, evidence that the IFG and at least one other component of the dorsal system (the SMG) support subword phonological analysis. Activity in both regions is stronger for (1) reading pseudowords compared to real words, (2) low-frequency words relative to high-frequency words, (3) tasks that require phonological analysis such as rhyme judgment, and (4) tasks that involve phonological priming (Mencl, Frost, et al., submitted). Moreover, during reading tasks, beginning and early readers show dorsal and anterior activity, but do not show substantial ventral activity, unlike more skilled readers (Booth et al., 2001; Shaywitz et al., 2002; Turkeltaub et al., 2003). When present, activity in ventral OT regions, which shows strong left-hemisphere lateralization in adults, appears to be bilaterally symmetric in children, a finding consistent with the notion of a progressive specialization of the ventral system in the LH with reading experience (Simos et al., 2001). In response to a printed word, the ventral system responds more rapidly than the dorsal, suggesting that it is a faster-acting system (Breier et al., 1999; Salmelin et al., 1996; Simos et al., 2001). As noted earlier, several studies have also reported greater activation to real words than to pseudowords within the ventral system, particularly at middle and inferior temporal sites (Fiebach et al., 2002; Tagamets et al., 2000). And, as noted above, reading-related activation in ventral regions increases with age and reading skill (Shaywitz et al., 2002).

Further Partitioning of the Three Major Systems

This initial, speculative taxonomy of three broad LH systems (dorsal, ventral, and anterior) and their computational processing roles is obviously very coarse-grained and underspecified. Indeed, each of these component systems consists of distinct subregions that most likely engage in different types of processing. In order to refine our basic theoretical framework, we have recently conducted a series of experiments aimed at obtaining a more detailed understanding of the information-processing characteristics of the major LH reading-related regions. One line of studies involves a series of manipulations of theoretically relevant psycholinguistic variables aimed at refining our understanding of the functional properties of the subregions and how they operate in relation to one another. A second line of experiments is aimed at obtaining a better understanding of the neurobiological foundations of adaptive learning in the context of reading. We feel that this set of studies provides important constraints on our understanding of the functional neuroanatomy of reading. However, we must note that these studies are currently under review; therefore, appropriate conservatism should be employed when interpreting them.

Phonological Priming. We have recently completed an fMRI study of phonological and orthographic priming effects in printed word recognition (Mencl, Frost, et al., submitted). Participants performed a primed lexical decision task. Primes were either (1) both orthographically and phonologically similar to the targets (bribe-TRIBE), (2) orthographically similar but phonologically dissimilar (couch-TOUCH), or (3) unrelated (lunch-SCREEN). Results indicate that condition (2) evoked more activation than (1) in several LH cortical areas hypothesized to underlie phonological processing: this modulation was seen in IFG, Wernicke's area, and the SMG. Notably, this phonological priming effect was also obtained within the early-activating LH OT skill zone, consistent with the claim that phonological coding influences lexical access at its earliest stages (but see Development of Multimodal Imaging Techniques below).

Tradeoffs between Phonology and Semantics. Many previous studies have attempted to identify the neural substrates of orthographic, phonological, and semantic processes in NI (Fiebach et al., 2002) and RD (Rumsey et al., 1997) cohorts. RD readers have acute problems in mapping from orthography to phonology and appear to rely on semantic information to supplement deficient decoding skills (Plaut & Booth, 2000). NI readers, too, appear to show a trade-off between these component processes. Strain, Patterson, and Seidenberg (1996) provided behavioral confirmation of this, demonstrating that the standard consistency effect on low-frequency words (longer naming latencies for words with inconsistent spelling-to-sound mappings such as PINT relative to words with consistent mappings such as MILL) is attenuated for words that are highly imageable/concrete. Importantly, this interaction reveals that semantics can facilitate the processes associated with orthographic-to-phonological mapping in word recognition. Using fMRI, we sought to identify the neurobiological correlates of this phenomenon (Frost et al., submitted). A go/no-go naming paradigm was employed in an event-related fMRI protocol. Word stimuli represented the crossing of frequency, imageability, and spelling-to-sound consistency. Higher activation for high-imageable words was found in middle temporal and posterior parietal sites. In contrast, higher activation for inconsistent relative to consistent words was found in the IFG (a critical area for articulatory recoding), replicating findings by Fiez et al. (1999) and Herbster et al. (1997). Critically, analyses revealed that imageability was associated with reduced consistency-related activation in IFG but increased posterior parietal activation; this appears to be the principal neural signature of the behavioral trade-off between semantics and phonology revealed by Strain and colleagues (1996). This finding serves as an important step in the linking of neurobiological and computational models of reading.

Adaptive Learning. Previous studies have demonstrated that both increased familiarity with specific words and increased reading skill are associated with a shift in the relative activation of the cortical systems involved in reading from predominantly dorsal to predominantly ventral. In another line of research, we are carrying out functional neuroimaging experiments in order to provide a more precise characterization of the means by which practice with unfamiliar words results in this shift, and to gain insights into how these systems learn to read new words. In one study from our lab group (Katz et al., submitted), we found evidence for this shift as skilled readers acquired familiarity for words via repetition. In that study, we examined repetition effects (comparing activation for thrice repeated tokens relative to unrepeated words) in both lexical decision and overt naming. Across tasks, repetition was associated with facilitated processing as measured by reduced response latencies and errors. Many sites, including IFG, SMG, supplementary motor area, and cerebellum, showed reduced activation for highly practiced tokens. Critically, a dissociation was seen within the ventral system: the OT skill zone showed practice-related reduction (like the SMG and IFG sites) whereas more anterior ventral sites, particularly MTG, were stable or even showed increased activation with repetition. Thus, we concluded that a neural signature of increased efficiency in word recognition is more efficient processing in dorsal, anterior, and posterior ventral sites, with stable or increased activation in more anterior middle and inferior temporal sites.

A second experiment (Sandak et al., 2004) tested the hypothesis that the type of processing engaged in when learning a new word mediates how well that word is learned, and the cortical regions engaged when that word is subsequently read. We suspected that repetition alone is not sufficient to optimize learning; rather, we hypothesized that the quality of the lexical representations established when new words are learned is affected by the type of processing engaged in during learning. Specifically, we predicted that, relative to attending to the orthographic features of novel words, learning conditions that stress phonological or semantic analysis would speed naming, and in turn, cortical activation patterns similar to those characteristic of increased familiarity with words (as seen in Katz et al., submitted). Prior to MRI scanning, participants completed a behavioral session in which they acquired familiarity for three sets of pronounceable pseudowords while making orthographic (consonant/vowel pattern), phonological (rhyme), or semantic (category) judgments. Note that in the semantic condition, participants learned a novel semantic association for each pseudoword. Following training, participants completed an event-related fMRI session in which they overtly named trained pseudowords, untrained pseudowords, and real words.

As predicted, we found that the type of processing (orthographic, phonological, or semantic) engaged in when learning a new word influences how well that word is learned and the cortical regions engaged when that word is subsequently read. Behaviorally, phonological and semantic training resulted in speeded naming times relative to orthographic training. Of the three training conditions, we found that only phonological training was associated with both facilitated naming and the pattern of cortical activations previously implicated as characteristic of increased efficiency for word recognition (Katz et al., submitted). We suggest that for phonologically trained items, learning was facilitated by engaging in phonological processing during training; this in turn resulted in efficient phonological processing (instantiated cortically as relatively reduced activation in IFG and SMG) and efficient retrieval of presemantic lexical representations during subsequent naming (instantiated cortically as relatively reduced activation in the OT skill zone). Semantic training also facilitated naming but was associated with increased activation in areas previously implicated in semantic processing, suggesting that the establishment and retrieval of semantic representations compensated for less efficient phonological processing for these items.

Implications of our Recent Findings

Initially, we had speculated that the temporoparietal and anterior systems are critical in learning to integrate orthographic, phonological, and semantic features of words, whereas the ventral system develops, as a consequence of adequate learning during reading acquisition, to support fluent word identification in normally developing, but not RD, individuals (Pugh et al., 2000). Our recent experiments examining phonological priming, phonological/ semantic trade-offs, and critical factors associated with adaptive learning in reading have yielded findings that require us to refine our initial taxonomy. These data allow for the development of a more fine-grained picture of the functional neuroanatomy and subspecializations within these systems, illustrated in Figure 2. Across these studies, identical sets of voxels in the SMG (within the temporoparietal system), IFG (within the anterior system), and the OT skill zone (within the ventral system) showed (1) increased activation for pseudowords relative to words, (2) strong phonological priming effects, and (3) repetition-related reductions that were most salient in the phonologically analytic training condition. This pattern strongly suggests a phonological "tuning" in these subregions. It is particularly noteworthy that the developmentally critical OT skill zone—the putative VWFA—by these data, appears to be phonologically tuned. It makes good sense that this region should be so structured given the failure to develop this system in reading disability when phonological deficits are one of the core features of this population. By contrast, the angular gyrus (within

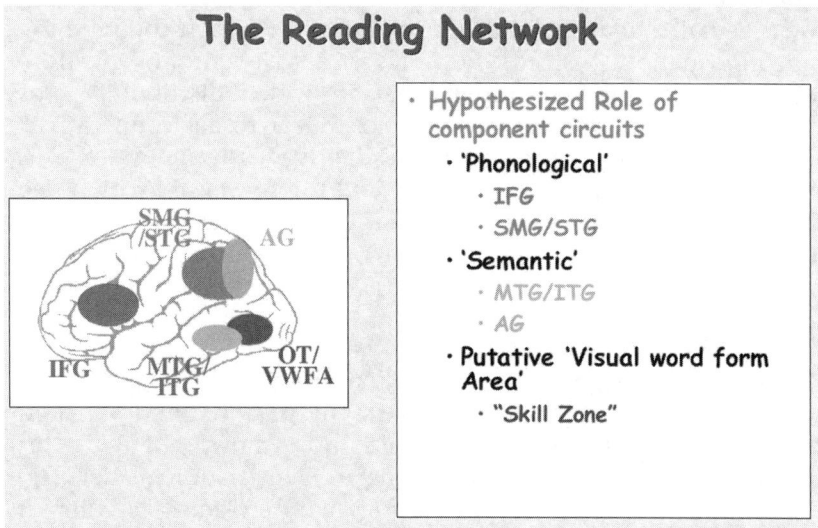

Figure 2: A schematic representation of subregions thought to be associated with different component processes in reading.

the temporoparietal system) and the middle/inferior temporal gyri (within the ventral system) appear to have more abstract lexico-semantic functions across our studies (see Price et al., 1997 for similar claims).

From these findings, we speculate that subregions within SMG and IFG operate in a yoked fashion to bind orthographic and phonological features of words during learning; these systems also operate in conjunction with the angular gyrus where these features are further yoked to semantic knowledge systems distributed across several cortical regions. Adequate binding, specifically adequate orthographic/phonological integration, enables the development of the presemantic OT skill zone into a functional pattern identification system. As words become better learned, this area becomes capable of efficiently activating lexico-semantic subsystems in MTG/ITG, enabling the development of a rapid ventral word identification system. RD individuals, with demonstrable anomalies in temporoparietal function (and associated difficulties with phonologically analytic processing on behavioral tests), fail to adequately "train" ventral subsystems (particularly the OT skill zone) and thus develop compensatory responses in frontal and RH systems. In our view, this revised account better lends itself to the architectural assumptions put forward in interactive models (e.g., Harm & Seidenberg, 1999) than with classic dual route models. The findings on stimulus-type effects, and especially the data on adaptive learning, do not readily support the notion of independent dorsal and ventral reading pathways, with each coding different information. Instead, they suggest a set of phonologically or semantically tuned subsystems that are widely distributed across both dorsal and ventral cortex, and appear to act cooperatively during fluent word reading and in adaptive learning. In our view, a crucial next step is to begin to attend to the ways in which neurobiological findings and computational models may constrain one another.

NEW DIRECTIONS

In recent years, significant progress has been made in the study of reading and reading disability with the use of functional neuroimaging techniques. A good deal is now known about the distributed neural circuitry for reading in skilled adult readers, the developmental trajectory toward this mature reading circuitry in normally developing children, deviations from this trajectory in reading disability, and the ways in which intensive training for struggling younger readers alters brain organization for reading.

Further advancement in developing an adequate theory of the neurobiology of reading demands considerable progress in a number of domains:

Development of Multimodal Imaging Technologies

The development of a neurobiologically grounded, computational model of reading requires that we obtain information regarding not only the localization of reading-related neural systems, but also the relative timing for and connectivity among these systems. This can be accomplished by taking the best aspects of several imaging modalities and systematically combining them. Hemodynamic information from fMRI and PET yields excellent localization; however, the millisecond-level temporal resolution for neural activity obtained with EEG or MEG provides crucial information as well. Much work on optimizing communication between these approaches is underway (c.f., Dale et al., 2000). Given that hemodynamic and electrophysiological methods yield distinct but necessarily related types of information, finding a way to use both approaches in a mutually constraining fashion would be ideal. To illustrate the pressing need for this fusion of technologies, consider the question of the role of phonological processing in skilled reading. Some cognitive studies suggest that phonological coding plays a role at the earliest stages of lexical access, though the issue continues to be debated (c.f., Coltheart et al., 1993; Frost, 1998). As noted earlier, we have identified phonologically driven activation in the ventral skill zone in our priming experiment (Mencl, Frost, et al., submitted). Given that this region operates very early in word processing, such a finding is logically consistent with the early phonology hypothesis. However, given the time scale on which fMRI measures operate, we cannot know whether the observed phonologically modulated hemodynamic response occurred early or late in processing (i.e., as a result of feedback from other language regions to the ventral skill zone). By combining hemodynamic and electrophysiological measures during task performance, we may be able to shed light on the theoretically important issue of whether phonology mediates fast time-scale processing in LH ventral cortex.

Work in reading disability (Horwitz, Rumsey, & Donohue, 1998; Pugh et al., 2000) employing functional connectivity analyses has been promising. However, this approach is still in its early stages of development. Moreover, studies using both hemodynamic and electrophysiological data to isolate correlated activation can be combined with emerging findings from diffusion-weighted tensor imaging (DTI), which reveals axonal tracts connecting distributed neural subsystems across cortex. Indeed, a recent study using diffusion-weighted imaging analysis has documented structural anomalies in white matter tracts within the LH temporoparietal region, suggesting a possible neural basis for the often seen functional anomalies in disabled readers (Klingberg et al., 2000). In addition, new developments in spectroscopic imaging techniques can support more careful analyses of the basic operations of regions targeted by functional studies to investigate the etiology of abnormal development. More deeply, reading disability is a genetically linked syndrome (Grigorenko et al., 1997; Pennington et al., 1991). Links between genetic polymorphisms, brain structure and function, and cognitive deficits promise to constitute the core scientific foundation for our understanding of neurodevelopmental disorders in the coming years, to progressive from descriptive neurobiological findings to potentially explanatory models.

Extending Research on Intervention, Populations, and Skilled Reading

To date, there appears to be substantial convergence that successful reading interventions in at-risk children result in increased response in critical LH posterior regions (Shaywitz et al., 2003b; Simos et al., 2002; Temple et al., 2003). Each of these studies has utilized training programs that emphasize phonological awareness training to differing degrees. However, several pressing questions remain. First, will similar remediation effects be obtained for older populations with persistent reading difficulties? Moreover, are there specific etiological factors that distinguish children who demonstrate only minimal gains with treatment from responders? If so, might alternative instructional approaches be more effective for these children? These are complex issues and demand large-scale studies that compare and contrast various interventions and examine interactions with individual difference or subtype dimensions. Such contrastive research will greatly extend the utility of brain-based developmental research.

In addition, there is a real need to find better markers of abnormal trajectories in very young (preschool-age) children, as well as to develop appropriate early interventions. Whereas it is known that the development of phonemic awareness is strongly and causally related to the development of reading skill (e.g., Bradley & Bryant, 1985; Wagner & Torgesen, 1987), little is known about the cognitive primitives underlying the development of phonemic awareness. Some researchers have suggested that deficits in phonemic awareness in reading impaired children may arise from a more basic deficit in speech perception (e.g., Mody, Studdert-Kennedy, & Brady, 1997) or auditory temporal processing (e.g., Tallal, 1980). Future behavioral and neuroimaging work needs to continue to examine the development of phonological awareness and reading in order to understand the etiology of reading disabilities at multiple levels of analysis.

Finally, whereas much behavioral research has compared reading processes across languages and orthographies, most neuroimaging research to date has been carried out on participants reading or listening to English words or pseudowords (but see Nakamura et al., 2002; Paulesu et al., 2001; Tan et al., 2000). Given the significant variability in orthographic form, orthographic regularity, methods of reading instruction, and manifestations of reading disability across languages and cultures, more work needs to be done in the area of cross-linguistic studies of reading, both in order to identify the neurobiological universals of reading and to understand how the functional organization of reading varies with language-specific features.

Address correspondence to: Ken Pugh, Ph.D., 270 Crown Street, New Haven, CT 06611; E-mail: pugh@haskins.yale.edu

REFERENCES

Ball, E. W., & Blachman, B. A. (1991). Does phoneme awareness training in kindergarten make a difference in early word recognition and developmental spelling? *Reading Research Quarterly, 26*, 49–66.

Blachman, B., Schatschneider, C., Fletcher, J. M., Francis, D. J., Clonan, S., Shaywitz, B. A., & Shaywitz, S. E. (2004). Effects of intensive reading remediation for second and third graders and a one year follow up. *Journal of Educational Psychology, 96*, 444–461.

Black, S. E., & Behrmann, M. (1994). Localization in alexia. In A. Kertesz (Ed.), *Localization and neuroimaging in neuropsychology*. New York: Academic Press.

Booth, J. R., Burman, D. D., Van Santen, F. W., Harasaki, Y., Gitelman, D. R., Parrish, T. B., & Mesulam, M. M. (2001). The development of specialized brain systems in reading and oral-language. *Neuropsychology Development in Cognition, Sect. C Child Neuropsychology, 7*(3), 119–141.

Bradley, L., & Bryant, P. (1985). *Rhyme and reason in reading and spelling*. Ann Arbor, MI: University of Michigan Press.

Brady, S. A., & Shankweiler, D. (1991). *Phonological processes in literacy: A tribute to Isabelle Y. Liberman*. Hillsdale, NJ: Erlbaum Associates.

Breier, J. I., Simos, P. G., Zouridakis, G., & Papanicolaou, A. C. (1999). Temporal course of regional brain activation associated with phonological decoding. *Journal of Clinical and Experimental Neuropsychology, 21*, 465–476.

Bruck, M. (1992). Persistence of dyslexics' phonological deficits. *Developmental Psychology, 28,* 874–886.
Brunswick, N., McCrory, E., Price C., Frith, C. D., & Frith, U. (1999). Explicit and implicit processing of words and pseudowords by adult developmental dyslexics: A search for Wernicke's Wortschatz. *Brain, 122,* 1901–1917.
Cohen, L., Lehericy, S., Chochon, F., Lemer, C., Rivaud, S., & Dehaene, S. (2002). Language-specific tuning of visual cortex? Functional properties of the visual word form area. *Brain, 125,* 1054–1069.
Coltheart, M., Curtis, B., Atkins, P., & Haller, M. (1993). Models of reading aloud: Dual-route and parallel-distributed-processing approaches. *Psychological Review, 100,* 589–608.
Cornelissen, P. L., & Hansen, P. C. (1998). Motion detection, letter position encoding, and single word reading. *Annals of Dyslexia, 48,* 155–188.
Dale, A. M., Liu, A. K., Fiscal, B. R., Buckner, R. L., Belliveau, J. W., Lewine, J. D., & Halgren, E. (2000). Dynamic statistical parametric mapping: Combining fMRI and MEG for high-resolution imaging of cortical activity. *Neuron, 26,* 55–67.
Demb, J. B., Boynton, G. M., Best, M., & Heeger, D. J. (1998). Psychophysical evidence for a magnocellular pathway deficit in dyslexia. *Vision Research, 38*(11), 1555–1559.
Eden, G. F., Vanmeter, J. W., Rumsey, J. M., Maisog, J. M., Woods, R. P., & Zeffiro, T. A. (1996). Abnormal processing of visual motion in dyslexia revealed by functional brain imaging. *Nature, 382*(6586), 66–69.
Eden, G. F., & Zeffiro, T. A. (1998). Neural systems affected in developmental dyslexia revealed by functional neuroimaging. *Neuron, 21,* 279–282.
Felton, R. H., Naylor, C. E., & Wood, F. B. (1990). Neuropsychological profile of adult dyslexics. *Brain and Language, 39*(4), 485–497.
Fiebach, C. J., Friederici, A. D., Mueller, K., & von Cramon, D. Y. (2002). fMRI evidence for dual routes to the mental lexicon in visual word recognition. *Journal of Cognitive Neuroscience, 14,* 11–23.
Fiez, J. A., Balota, D. A., Raichle, M. E., & Petersen, S. E. (1999). Effects of lexicality, frequency, and spelling-to-sound consistency on the functional anatomy of reading. *Neuron, 24,* 205–218.
Fiez, J. A., & Petersen, S. E. (1998). Neuroimaging studies of word reading. *Proceedings of the National Academy of Sciences, 95,* 914–921.
Filipek, P. A. (1995). Neurobiologic correlates of developmental dyslexia: How do dyslexics brains' differ from those of normal readers? *Journal of Child Neurology, 10*(Suppl. 1), S62–S69.
Fletcher, J., Shaywitz, S. E., Shankweiler, D. P., Katz, L., Liberman, I. Y., Stuebing, K. K., Francis, D. J., Fowler, A. E., & Shaywitz, B. A. (1994). Cognitive profiles of reading disability: Comparisons of discrepancy and low achievement definitions. *Journal of Educational Psychology, 86,* 6–23.
Foorman, B. R., Francis, D., Fletcher, J. K., Schatschneider, C., & Mehta, P. (1998). The role of instruction in learning to reading: Preventing reading failure in at-risk children. *Journal of Educational Psychology, 90,* 37–55.
Friston, K. (1994). Functional and effective connectivity: A synthesis. *Human Brain Mapping, 2,* 56–78.

Frost, R. (1998). Toward a strong phonological theory of visual word recognition: True issues and false trails. *Psychological Bulletin, 123,* 71–99.
Frost, S. J., Mencl, W. E., Sandak, R., Moore, D. L., Mason, S. A., Rueckl, J. G., Katz, L., & Pugh, K. R. (Manuscript submitted for publication). Capturing interactions between semantics and phonology in brain.
Galaburda, A. M. (1992). Neurology of developmental dyslexia. *Current Opinion in Neurology and Neurosurgery, 5*(1), 71–76.
Grigorenko, E. L., Wood, F. B., Meyer, M. S., Hart, L. A., Speed, W. C., Shuster, A., & Pauls, D. L. (1997). Susceptibility loci for distinct components of developmental dyslexia on chromosomes 6 and 15. *American Journal of Human Genetics, 60,* 27–39.
Grigorenko, E. L. (2001). Developmental dyslexia: An update on genes, brain, and environments. *Journal of Child Psychology and Psychiatry, 42,* 91–125.
Habib, M. (2000). The neurological basis of developmental dyslexia: An overview and working hypothesis. *Brain, 123,* 2372–2399.
Harm, M. W., & Seidenberg, M. S. (1999). Computing the meanings of words in reading: Cooperative division of labor between visual and phonological processes. *Psychological Review, 106,* 491–528.
Herbster, A., Mintun, M., Nebes, R., & Becker, J. (1997). Regional cerebral blood flow during word and nonword reading. *Human Brain Mapping, 5,* 84–92.
Horwitz, B., Rumsey, J. M., & Donohue, B. C. (1998). Functional connectivity of the angular gyrus in normal reading and dyslexia. *Proceedings of the National Academy of Sciences, 95,* 8939–8944.
Katz, L., Lee, C., Frost, S. J., Mencl, W. E., Rueckl, J., Sandak, R., Tabor, W., Mason, S., & Pugh, K. R. (Manuscript submitted for publication). Effects of printed word repetition in lexical decision and naming on behavior and brain activation.
Klingberg, T., Hedehus, M., Temple, E., Salz, T., Gabrieli, J. D., Moseley, M. E., & Poldrack, R. A. (2000). Microstructure of temporo-parietal white matter as a basis for reading ability: Evidence from diffusion tensor magnetic resonance imaging. *Neuron, 25,* 493–500.
Liberman, A. M. (1992). The relation of speech to reading and writing. In R. Frost & L. Katz (Eds.), *Orthography, phonology, morphology, and meaning.* Amsterdam: Elsevier.
Liberman, I. Y., Shankweiler, D., Fischer, W., & Carter, B. (1974). Explicit syllable & phoneme segmentation in the young child. *Journal of Child Psychology, 18,* 201–212.
Lukatela, G., & Turvey, M. T. (1994). Visual lexical access is initially phonological: 1. Evidence from associative priming by words, homophones, and pseudohomophones. *Journal of Experimental Psychology: General, 123,* 107–128.
Mencl, W. E., Frost, S. J., Sandak, R., Lee, J. R., Jenner, A. R., Mason, S., Rueckl, J. G., Katz, L., & Pugh, K. R. (Manuscript submitted for publication). Effects of orthographic and phonological priming in printed word identification: An fMRI study.
Mencl, W. E., Shaywitz, B. A., Shaywitz, S. E., Pugh, K. R., Fulbright, R. K., Skudlarski, P., Constable, R. T., Marchione, K. E., Fletcher, J. M., & Gore, J. C. (Manuscript submitted for publication). Developmental changes in functional connectivity in nonimpaired and dyslexic readers.

Mody, M., Studdert-Kennedy, M., & Brady, S. (1997). Speech perception deficits in poor readers: Auditory processing or phonological coding? *Journal of Experimental Child Psychology, 64*, 199–231.

Nakamura, K., Honda, M., Hirano, S., Oga, T., Sawamoto, N., Hanakawa, T., Inoue, H., Ito, J., Matsuda, T., Fukuyama, H., & Shibasaki, H. (2002). Modulation of the visual word retrieval system in writing: A functional MRI study on the Japanese orthographies. *Journal of Cognitive Neuroscience, 14*, 104–115.

Pammer, K., Hansen, P. C., Kringelbach, M. L., Holliday, I., Barnes, G., Krish, S. D., & Cornelissen, P. (Manuscript submitted for publication). Visual word recognition: The first half second.

Papanicolaou, A. C., Pugh, K. R., Simos, P. G., & Mencl, W. E. (2004). Functional brain imaging: An introduction to concepts and applications. In P. McCardle and V. Chhabra (Eds.), *The voice of evidence in reading research*. Baltimore: Paul H. Brookes Publishing Company.

Paulesu, E., Demonet, J.-F., Fazio, F., McCrory, E., Chanoine, V., Brunswick, N., Cappa, S. F., Cossu, G., Habib, M., Frith, C. D., & Frith, U. (2001). Dyslexia: Cultural diversity and biological unity. *Science, 291*, 2165–2167.

Pennington, B. F., Gilger, J. W., Pauls, D., Smith, S. A., Smith, S. D., & DeFries, J. C. (1991). Evidence for major gene transmission of developmental dyslexia. *Journal of the American Medical Association, 266*, 1527–1534.

Perfetti, C. A. (1985). *Reading ability*. New York: Oxford University Press.

Plaut, D. C., & Booth, J. R. (2000). Individual and developmental differences in semantic priming: Empirical and computational support for a single-mechanism account of lexical processing. *Psychological Review, 107*, 786–823.

Poldrack, R. A., Wagner, A. D., Prull, M. W., Desmond, J. E., Glover, G. H., & Gabrieli, J. D. (1999). Functional specialization for semantic and phonological processing in the left inferior prefrontal cortex. *Neuroimage, 10*, 15–35.

Price, C. J., More, C. J., Humphreys, G. W., & Wise, R. J. S. (1997). Segregating semantic from phonological processes during reading. *Journal of Cognitive Neuroscience, 9*, 727–733.

Price, C. J., Winterburn, D., Giraud, A. L., Moore, C. J., & Noppeney, U. (2003). Cortical localization of the visual and auditory word form areas: A reconsideration of the evidence. *Brain and Language, 86*, 272–286.

Price, C. J., Wise, R. J. S., & Frackowiak, R. S. J. (1996). Demonstrating the implicit processing of visually presented words and pseudowords. *Cerebral Cortex, 6*, 62–70.

Pugh, K. R., Mencl, W. E., Jenner, A. R., Katz, L., Frost, S. J., Lee, J. R., Shaywitz, S. E., & Shaywitz, B. A. (2000a). Functional neuroimaging studies of reading and reading disability (developmental dyslexia). *Mental Retardation & Developmental Disabilities Research Reviews, 6*, 207–213.

Pugh, K., Mencl, E. W., Shaywitz, B. A., Shaywitz, S. E., Fulbright, R. K., Skudlarski, P., Constable, R. T., Marchione, K., Jenner, A. R., Shankweiler, D. P., Katz, L., Fletcher, J., Lacadie, C., & Gore, J. C. (2000b). The angular gyrus in developmental dyslexia: Task-specific differences in functional connectivity in posterior cortex. *Psychological Science, 11*, 51–56.

Pugh, K. R., Shaywitz, B. A., Shaywitz, S. A., Shankweiler, D. P., Katz, L., Fletcher, J. M., Skudlarski, P., Fulbright, R. K., Constable, R. T., Bronen, R. A., Lacadie, C., & Gore, J. C. (1997). Predicting reading performance from neuroimaging profiles: The cerebral basis of phonological effects in printed word identification. *Journal of Experimental Psychology: Human Perception and Performance, 2*, 1–20.

Rieben, L., & Perfetti, C. A. (1991). *Learning to read: Basic research and its implications.* Hillsdale, NJ: Erlbaum Associates.

Rumsey J. M., Horwitz, B., Donohue, B. C., Nace, K. L., Maisog, J. M., & Andreason, P. A. (1999). Functional lesion in developmental dyslexia: Left angular gyral blood flow predicts severity. *Brain and Language, 70*, 187–204.

Rumsey, J. M., Nace, K., Donohue, B., Wise, D., Maisog, J. M., & Andreason, P. (1997). A positron emission tomographic study of impaired word recognition and phonological processing in dyslexic men. *Archives of Neurology, 54*, 562–573.

Salmelin, R., Service, E., Kiesila, P., Uutela, K., & Salonen, O. (1996). Impaired visual word processing in dyslexia revealed with magnetoencephalography. *Annals of Neurology, 40*, 157–162.

Sandak, R., Mencl, W. E., Frost, S. J., Mason, S. A., Rueckl, J. G., Katz, L., Moore, D. L., Mason, S. A., Fulbright, R., Constable, R. T., & Pugh, K. R. (2004). The neurobiology of adaptive learning in reading: A contrast of different training conditions. *Cognitive Affective and Behavioral Neuroscience, 4*, 67–88.

Sarkari, S., Simos, P. G., Fletcher, J. M., Castillo, E. M., Breier, J. I., & Papanicolaou, A. C. (2002). The emergence and treatment of developmental reading disability: Contributions of functional brain imaging. *Seminars in Pediatric Neurology, 9*, 227–236.

Scarborough, H., & Dobrich, W. (1990). Development of children with early language delay. *Journal of Speech and Hearing Research, 33*, 70–83.

Shankweiler, D., Crain, S., Katz, L., Fowler, A. E., Liberman, A. M., Brady, S. A., Thornton, R., Lundquist, E., Dreyer, L., Fletcher, J. M., Stuebing, K. K., Shaywitz, S. E., & Shaywitz, B. A. (1995). Cognitive profiles of reading-disabled children: Comparison of language skills in phonology, morphology, and syntax. *Psychological Science, 6*, 149–156.

Shaywitz, B. A., Shaywitz, S. E., Blachman, B. A., Pugh, K. R., Fulbright, R. K., Skudlarski, P., et al. (2004). Development of left occipitotemporal systems for skilled reading in children after a phonologically-based intervention. *Biological Psychiatry, 55*(9), 926–933.

Shaywitz, B., Shaywitz, S., Blachman, B., Pugh, K. R., Fulbright, R., Skudlarski, P., Mencl., W. E., Constable, T., Holahan, J., Marchione, K., Fletcher, J., Lyon, R., & Gore, J. (2003b). Development of left occipitotemporal systems for skilled reading following a phonologically-based intervention in children. Poster presented at the 9th International Conference on Functional Mapping of the Human Brain, New York.

Shaywitz, S. E., Shaywitz, B. A., Fulbright, R. K., Skudlarski, P., Mencl, W. E., Constable, R. T., Pugh, K. R., Holahan, J. M., Marchione, K. E., Fletcher, J. M., Lyon, G. R., & Gore, J. C. (2002). Disruption of posterior brain systems for reading in children with developmental dyslexia. *Biological Psychiatry, 52*, 101–110.

Shaywitz, S. E., Shaywitz, B. A., Fulbright, R. K., Skudlarski, P., Mencl, W. E., Constable, R. T., Pugh, K. R., Holahan, J. M., Marchione, K. E.,

Fletcher, J.M., Lyon, G. R., & Gore, J. C. (2003a). Neural systems for compensation and persistence: Young adult outcome of childhood reading disability. *Biological Psychiatry, 54*, 25–33.

Shaywitz, S. E., Shaywitz, B. A., Pugh, K. R., Fulbright, R. K., Constable, R. T., Mencl, W. E., Shankweiler, D. P., Liberman, A. M., Skudlarski, P., Fletcher, J. M., Katz, L., Marchione, K. E., Lacadie, C., Gatenby, C., & Gore, J. C. (1998). Functional disruption in the organization of the brain for reading in dyslexia. *Proceedings of the National Academy of Sciences, 95*, 2636–2641.

Simos, P. G., Breier, J. I., Fletcher, J. M., Foorman, B. R., Castillo, E. M., & Papanicolaou, A. C. (2002). Brain mechanisms for reading words and pseudowords: An integrated approach. *Cerebral Cortex, 12*, 297–305.

Simos, P. G., Breier, J. I., Fletcher, J. M., Foorman, B. R., Mouzaki, A., & Papanicolaou, A. C. (2001). Age-related changes in regional brain activation during phonological decoding and printed word recognition. *Developmental Neuropsychology, 19*, 191–210.

Simos, P. G., Breier, J. I., Wheless, J. W., Maggio, W. W., Fletcher, J. M., Castillo, E., & Papanicolaou, A. C. (2000). Brain mechanisms for reading: The role of the superior temporal gyrus in word and pseudoword naming. *Neuroreport, 11*, 2443–2447.

Simos, P. G., Fletcher, J. M., Bergman, E., Breier, J. I., Foorman, B. R., Castillo, E. M., Davis, R. N., Fitzgerald, M., & Papanicolaou, A. C. (2002). Dyslexia-specific brain activation profile becomes normal following successful remedial training. *Neurology, 58*, 1203–1213.

Stanovich, K. E., & Siegel, L. S. (1994). Phenotypic performance profile of children with reading disabilities: A regression-based test of the phonological-core variable-difference model. *Journal of Educational Psychology, 86*, 24–53.

Strain, E., Patterson, K., & Seidenberg, M. S. (1996). Semantic effects in single-word naming. *Journal of Experimental Psychology: Learning, Memory, and Cognition, 21*, 1140–1154.

Tagamets, M. A., Novick, J. M., Chalmers, M. L., & Friedman, R. B. (2000). A parametric approach of orthographic processing in the brain: An fMRI study. *Journal of Cognitive Neuroscience, 1*, 281–297.

Tallal, P. (1980). Auditory temporal perception, phonics, and reading disabilities in children. *Brain and Language, 9*, 182–198.

Tan, L. H., Spinks, J. A., Gao, J. H., Liu, H. L., Perfetti, C. A., Xiong, J., Stofer, K. A., Pu, Y., Liu, Y., & Fox, P. T. (2000). Brain activation in the processing of Chinese characters and words: A functional MRI study. *Human Brain Mapping, 10*, 16–27.

Tarkiainen, A., Cornelissen, P. L., & Salmelin, R. (2003). Dynamics of visual feature analysis and object-level processing in face versus letter-string perception. *Brain, 125*, 1125–1136.

Temple, E., Deutsch, G. K., Poldrack, R. A., Miller, S. L., Tallal, P., Merzenich, M. M., & Gabrieli, J. D. E. (2003). Neural deficits in children with dyslexia ameliorated by behavioral remediation: Evidence from functional MRI. *Proceedings of the National Academy of Sciences, 100*, 2860–2865.

Temple, E., Poldrack, R. A., Salidis, J., Deutsch, G. K., Tallal, P., Merzenich, M. M., & Gabrieli, J. D. (2001) Disrupted neural responses to phonological and orthographic processing in dyslexic children: An fMRI study. *NeuroReport, 12*, 299–307.

Torgesen, J. K., Morgan, S. T., & Davis, C. (1992). Effects of two types of phonological awareness training on word learning in kindergarten children. *Journal of Educational Psychology, 84*, 364–370.

Turkeltaub, P. E., Gareau, L., Flowers, D. L., Zeffiro, T. A., & Eden, G. F. (2003). Development of neural mechanisms for reading. *Nature Neuroscience, 6*, 767–773.

Wagner, R. K., & Torgesen, J. K. (1987). The nature of phonological processing and its causal role in the acquisition of reading skills. *Psychological Bulletin, 101*, 192–212.

Wolf, M., & Bowers, Greig, P. (1999). The double-deficit hypothesis for the developmental dyslexias. *Journal of Educational Psychology, 91*, 415–438.

Xu, B., Grafman, J., Gaillard, W. D., Ishii, K., Vega-Bermudez, F., Pietrini, P., Reeves-Tyer, P., DiCamillo, P., & Theodore, W. (2001). Conjoint and extended neural networks for the computation of speech codes: The neural basis of selective impairment in reading words and pseudowords. *Cerebral Cortex, 11*, 267–277.

Chapter • 3

Process Faster, Talk Earlier, Read Better

Paula Tallal

INTRODUCTION

It is a discouraging fact that despite substantially increased funding over the past 20 years, literacy scores in the United States have remained flat with less than one-third of fourth grade students achieving a proficient reading level (Campbell, Hombo, & Mazzeo, 1999).

To acknowledge the importance of this literacy problem, the United States government has sponsored the No Child Left Behind legislation that mandates that all children in public schools must pass a state-wide reading proficiency test by third grade or be retained. Yet past experience has shown that increased funding, educational focus, and even political clout has failed to solve the reading problem. What is needed is a better understanding of how the brain learns (specifically how the brain learns language), how oral and written language are linked through common neural systems, and how this information can be used to develop neuroscience informed intervention strategies aimed at improving the reading outcomes of children.

Research derived from languages around the world has demonstrated that proficiency in decoding words into their

---

I thank April Benasich, Holly Fitch, Albert Galaburda, Glenn Rosen, Elise Temple, Russell Poldrack, John Gabrieli, Dorothy Bishop, and Michael Merzenich for insightful discussions and collaborations. I thank the National Institute of Deafness and Communication Disorders, National Institute of Neurological Disorders and Stroke, National Institute of Child Health & Human Development, March of Dimes, and Santa Fe Institute Consortium for funding.

phonemic segments is one of the keys to developing reading skills, and is considered by many to be the core deficit in dyslexia (Carrol & Snowling, 2004; Castles & Coltheart, 2004; Lyon, 1995). Becoming aware that words can be subdivided into individual sounds (phonological awareness) not only predicts future literacy skills, but also significantly differentiates dyslexic readers from typical readers (Lundberg, Olofsson, & Wall, 1980; Elbro, Borstrøm, & Petersen, 1998). While it is widely accepted that dyslexia is characterized by both orthographic and phonological deficits, with phonological deficits predominating, the precise etiology of these deficits remains the focus of intense research. Central research questions have focused on: (1) whether phonological deficits related to reading failure are speech specific or derived from more basic auditory processing deficits; (2) whether dyslexia is a deficit specific to written language or may be the outcome of oral language weakness in the language in which a child is trying to learn to read; (3) whether dyslexia constitutes a distinct disability or the disadvantageous end of individual differences within a normal distribution; (4) whether dyslexia results from genetic, neurological, social and/or educational causes, or more likely, a combination of many of the above; and (5) whether dyslexia is a unitary condition, or more likely, is comprised of a variety of different subgroups of children showing many different clinical profiles that change with maturation and experience.

While there are many similarities between children with specific language impairments (SLI) and dyslexia, there are also differences (Bishop & Snowling, 2004). For the purpose of this discussion, I will use the more inclusive term Language Learning Impairment (LLI) to focus on areas of similarity. However, further research is needed to better understand both the similarities and differences between SLI and dyslexia, and specifically how clinical profiles can change in the same individual as a function of maturation.

Although it is widely accepted that LLI is characterized by phonological deficits, the precise etiology of these deficits remains the focus of intense research and often heated theoretical debate. A central research question is whether phonological deficits are "speech specific" or rather derive from more basic attention/perception/memory and/or motor constraints. Research aimed at addressing this question has led to the development of several different models of LLI including the rate-processing constraint hypothesis (Fitch & Tallal, 2003; Habib, 2000; Kraus et al., 1996; Talcott et al., 2000; Witton et al., 1998), the magnocellular deficit hypothesis (Stein & Talcott, 1999; Wright, Bowen, & Zecker, 2000), the cerebellar deficit hypothesis (Nicolson, Fawcett, &

Dean, 2001), the double-deficit hypothesis (Wolf & Obregon, 1992; Wolf & O'Brien, this volume), the attentional dwell time hypothesis (Hari, Vlata, & Uutela, 1999), and the maturational lag hypothesis (Bishop & McArthur, 2004). Interestingly, all of these hypotheses have in common a constraint in the speed of information processing and/or production that is postulated to disrupt essential components of language learning, beginning with the acquisition of phonological representations.

Others have argued that these nonlinguistic deficits occur in only a minority of individuals with LLI, may not be specific to spectrotemporal processing constraints or to the auditory modality and, as such, are neither necessary nor sufficient to be causative (Bishop, Carlyon, Deeks, & Bishop, 1999; Mody, Studdert- Kennedy, & Brady, 1997; Ramus, 2003; Ramus, this volume; Rosen, 2003; Rosen & Manganari, 2001). It is interesting to note, however, that most of the subjects participating in these studies were much older; usually college students or adults. Thomas and Karmiloff-Smith (2002) recently suggested that much of the confusion in this literature may derive from a failure to take a developmental neuroscience perspective. While most early studies of developmental dyslexia focused almost exclusively on young children who were failing to learn to read, more recent research has been dominated by studies of much older individuals (primarily college students) with a lifelong history of developmental language and/or reading problems. Not only do college students fail to be representative of the typical population of individuals who experience severe language and reading disabilities, it is not possible to address the initial causes of a developmental disability such as dyslexia in older individuals who have spent a lifetime developing alternate brain strategies to cope with their earlier disabilities. Similarly, Thomas and Karmiloff-Smith (2002) argue that many current theories and models of developmental language and reading disorders adopt a modular view derived from studies of adults with acquired focal brain lesions that disrupt language and/or reading. However, in their extensive review of this issue, they present considerable data both from experimental studies with human subjects as well as computational models that mitigate against taking a modular view of developmental learning disabilities such as SLI and dyslexia. Specifically, they emphasize that focal lesions sustained in infancy do not result in similar patterns of deficits, particularly language deficits, to those seen in adults with comparable focal lesions. Rather, the developing brain adapts to insult quite differently than does the adult brain.

Neuroplasticity research has demonstrated that altered sensory input during critical periods of development not only disrupts cellular organization within sensory neural maps but also significantly alters brain structure as well. These changes endure into adulthood and can only be altered by explicit neuroplasticity-based intervention (Chang & Merzenich, 2003; Recanzone, Schreiner, & Merzenich 1993; Zhang, Bao, & Merzenich, 2002). However, key theories pertaining to dyslexia have rarely taken into account the likely changes in brain structure and function that would result from altered learning during critical periods of development.

As mentioned previously, it is possible to predict with considerable accuracy which children are going to struggle to learn to read based on their ability to manipulate phonemes within words. To discover this, you can play simple word games that do not involve any letters, but rather require the ability to manipulate speech sounds within words. For example, in a typical phoneme deletion task, you can ask a child, "How would you say the word 'plate' without the /p/ sound?" The answer is "late". "Okay, now how would you say the word 'plate' if you take away the /t/ sound?" The answer is "play". In order to perform this task correctly, at a minimum, a child must first correctly perceive the whole word. Next, the word must be segmented into the individual sounds (phonemes) that comprise it. Then, the identified sound must be deleted from the word, the remaining sounds must be put back together, and the motor/articulatory sequence must be executed in order to achieve the correct pronunciation. Of course, you can begin with much easier words for younger children such as, "How do you say the word 'cat' without the /c/ sound?" The answer would be the word "at", but the same complex sensory, perceptual, motor, and cognitive mechanisms must be engaged in order to arrive at the correct response. While considerable attention has been placed on metacognitive aspects of phonological awareness deficits in dyslexics, it is important to emphasize that lower level speech perception has also been shown to play a substantial role (Chiappe, Chiappe, & Siegel, 2001). These authors demonstrated that variance in phoneme identification accounts for significant variance in phoneme deletion, and conclude that deficits in speech perception play a causal role in the deficient phonological processing of poor readers and that insufficient differentiated phonological representations are a mediating link between speech perception and deficient phonological awareness. Considerable research has demonstrated that difficulty with these phonological aspects of spoken language are not only predictive of children who are likely to struggle to learn to read (dyslexia), but also characterize individuals with SLI (Gathercole & Baddeley, 1990; Leitão, Hogben, & Fletcher, 1997).

SPECIFIC LANGUAGE IMPAIRMENT (SLI)

A recent epidemiological study assessed the oral language development of a random sample of five-year-old children just prior to entering school. Children with other identifiable deficits or syndromes known to impede language development (e.g., hearing impairment, mental retardation, seizure disorder, neurologic anomalies, motor disabilities, autism) were excluded from the sample. This epidemiological study demonstrated that even after children with other identifiable known causes of developmental language impairment were excluded, approximately 7.4% of the five-year-olds tested were shown to demonstrate significant delays (1.25 standard deviation or more below the mean of normal) in language development (Tomblin et al., 1997). These specific language impairments manifested as disabilities in expressive language, receptive language, or both. Perhaps even more surprising was the finding that only 29% of these children had been identified previously either by their parents or physician as having language problems.

This epidemiological study demonstrated two very important findings. First, the number of children identified with SLI at school entry (7.4%) is more than twice as high as previous estimates (2%–3%) generally discussed in the research and clinical literature. Second, the vast majority (71%) of children who meet the clinical diagnosis of SLI are not diagnosed or treated before they enter school. Furthermore, when they do begin to struggle in school, rarely is the focus on their oral language abilities. Rather, they are identified as having difficulty with reading. Thus, a minimum of 7.4% of five-year-olds enter school without sufficient oral language skills upon which literacy depends. This number is substantially increased if the deficient linguistic skills of many second language learners are included.

Specific language deficits are characterized by difficulties in two main domains of language: phonology and grammatical morphology (see Bishop, 1997; Leonard, 1998 for reviews). Similarly, deficits in these same components of language also characterize dyslexics. As discussed previously, phonological processing is critical for beginning readers' ability to learn word attack and decoding skills. Morphology, on the other hand, has been shown to be the most important variable related to improving written vocabulary, comprehension, and fluency beyond the early stages of reading development, particularly in middle and high school (Mann & Singson, 2000; Singson, Mahony, & Mann, 2000; Mahony, Singson, & Mann, 2000). Unfortunately, only a few studies on dyslexia have actually reported formal assessment data on either the current oral language proficiency of their subjects or, more importantly, acquired accurate historical data pertaining to oral language development prior to the development of the reading problem (Bishop & Snowling, in press; McArthur et al., 2000). On the other hand, many prospective longitudinal studies have demonstrated a strong link between early oral language deficits and subsequent literacy and other academic achievement problems (Aram, Ekelman, & Nation, 1984; Bishop & Adams, 1990; Catts, Fey, Tomblin, & Zhang, 2002; Flax et al., 2003; Scarborough, 1990; Stark et al., 1984; Tallal, Allard, Miller, & Curtiss, 1997). Given the link between oral and written language deficits, the epidemiological findings that relatively few oral language deficits are ever diagnosed, and the growing awareness of the pivotal importance that phonological analysis and awareness abilities play in both oral language development as well as in breaking the alphabetic code for reading, it seems imperative that we understand better the neural basis of phonological development and disorders.

HOW DO SPEECH SOUNDS COME TO BE REPRESENTED IN THE BRAIN?

To break the code for reading alphabetic language such as English, the beginning reader needs to learn that words can be broken down into smaller sounds (phonemes), and it is these sounds that are represented by letters. But how do phonemes come to be represented in the brain to begin with? It is obvious from observing deaf children that disruption in the sensory registration of sound in the peripheral auditory system impairs speech perception, giving rise to a global oral language disorder. What may be less obvious is that hearing impairment is also likely to significantly limit the acquisition of reading, even in individuals who are fluent in a visual sign language (Rapin, 1978). This may be because in order to learn to perceive and produce oral language, the acoustic waveform of speech must travel from the peripheral to the central auditory nervous system. The ongoing speech stream must be chunked into individual phonemes (the smallest unit of sound that can change the meaning of the word), and these individual phonemes must acquire distinct neural representation so that they can subsequently be extracted from words and associated with letters. Clearly, this is problematic for deaf children. But is there similar evidence of reading deficits in children with normal peripheral hearing but with central auditory processing disorders (CAPD)?

One of the most prominent debates in language research concerns whether phonological processes are specific to linguistic systems (modules) in the brain (often referred to as the "speech is special" hypothesis) or rather rely on general purpose spectral (frequency) and temporal analysis in the central auditory system. Taking a developmental perspective is critical to addressing this often hotly contested debate empirically. While some aspects of language may be innate, an infant does not know which language he or she will need to learn. It is clear that infants must learn from experiencing the acoustic waveform produced by the articulators or speakers around them which speech sounds (phonemes) will form the basis of their native language (Jusczyk, 2002; Kuhl, 2000). Furthermore, each language has its own set of phonemes that must be learned from experiencing the ongoing speech stream of the native language and represented as distinct neural firing patterns in the brain. Donald Hebb (1949) proposed that when neurons are excited *nearly simultaneously in time*, they wire together as a unit. The more often the same pattern of neurons are excited nearly simultaneously, the more likely it will be that they will bind together (be represented) as a unit. Repeated exposure to consistent sensory inputs such as speech will increase the probability that a particular neural firing pattern will come to be distinctly represented (Recanzone, Schreiner, & Merzenich, 1993). This type of statistical learning is referred to as Hebbian learning or neuroplasticity (Hebb, 1949; Sejnowski, 1999).

The acoustic waveform of speech is complex and is represented by several frequency bands known as formants. As we move our speech articulators when producing ongoing speech, the acoustic waveform that is produced is characterized by continuous and very rapid acoustic changes in frequency and intensity. Physiological single cell recordings in animals have demonstrated that spectral, temporal, and "inseperable" temporospectral acoustic features are exquisitely organized in the central auditory cortex, based on experience-dependent learning (Blake et al., 2002; Linden et al., 2003; Orduna Mercado, Guck, & Merzenich, 2001; Schreiner, 1991). Thus, it would be easy to understand how phonemes could come to be represented in the brain of infants based on their distinct acoustic features and the infants' experience with speech input of their native language. However, within the ongoing acoustic waveform of speech, the temporospectral pattern of each phoneme differs acoustically within different contexts. Furthermore, there are no clear boundaries between phonemes that occur within syllables or words. Thus, we have hypothesized that in order to learn to represent the acoustic waveform of speech, the brain must first segment the acoustic signal into chunks of time and then form neural representations based on the consistency and frequency of occurrence (the statistical probability) of neural firing patterns (Tallal, Merzenich, Miller, & Jenkins, 1998). Importantly, consistencies within the speech waveform can occur in chunks of various durations. Chunking within the 10s of msec. time window (short duration) will allow for the fine grain analysis needed to represent the acoustic differences between individual phonemes such as /b/ and /d/, while chunking over longer periods of time (100s of msec) will result in firing patterns consistent with syllable or word length representations.

Over 30 years of behavioral as well as electrophysiological research has demonstrated that children with language based learning deficits are more likely than typical children to require more time to process and/or produce rapidly successive or dynamic sensory (auditory, visual, tactile) and motor stimuli (Bishop & McArthur, 2004; Farmer & Klein, 1995; Johnston, Stark, Mellits, & Tallal, 1981; Kraus et al., 1996; Stark & Tallal, 1988; Stein & Talcott, 1999; Talcott et al., 2000; Tallal, Galaburda, vonEuler, & Llinas, 1993; Witton et al., 1998; Wright et al., 1997). Furthermore, at least when young, these children demonstrate particular difficulty discriminating and producing precisely those speech sounds that are characterized by rapidly changing spectrotemporal cues such as stop consonants differing in place of articulation and/or VOT (Breier et al., 2001; Stark & Tallal, 1979; Tallal & Stark, 1981). However, these children are unimpaired, or less impaired, both perceiving and producing speech contrasts based on longer duration acoustic cues or multiple cues (Tallal & Piercy, 1974; Stark & Tallal, 1988; Mody, Studdert-Kennedy, & Brady, 1997).

In a recent study, Breier et al. (2001) investigated the relationship between auditory temporal processing, phoneme perception, and reading disability. Tasks assessing perception of a phonemic contrast based on voice onset time (VOT) and a nonspeech analog of a VOT contrast using tone onset time (TOT) were administered to school age dyslexic and control children (ages 7.5 to 15.9 years). Results showed that the dyslexic children were impaired on both tasks. These authors concluded that, "The presence of a deficit in perception of onset asynchrony in speech and nonspeech stimuli containing analogous acoustic cues is consistent with the hypothesis that a low level deficit in the auditory system is present in children with reading disability and that this deficit could account for observed difficulty in perception of speech stimuli" (Breier et al., 2001, pp. 264). Interestingly, these authors also demonstrated that differential patterns of deficits, as well as correlations between variable, occurred for dyslexic subjects with or without co-morbid attention deficits hyperactivity disorder (ADHD). These results underscore the importance of both stimulus characteristics as well as differential subject profiles in addressing the relationship between auditory temporal processing, phonological perception, phonological awareness, and reading.

This study highlights several important issues that may help resolve discrepancies across studies. To investigate these issues in a meaningful way, it is essential that comparable acoustic cues to those engaged in speech perception be used in selecting nonspeech analog stimuli for study. To highlight this issue, we can contrast the results obtained in Breier et al. (2001) with those obtained by Ramus and colleagues (Ramus et al., 2003; for review, see Ramus, this volume) who failed to detect significant deficits on auditory processing tasks in the majority of their dyslexic subjects, and also failed to find a significant correlation between auditory processing and phonological skills. In their study with dyslexic college students, Ramus et al., (2003) investigated temporal order judgment (TOJ) perception by asking subjects to listen to either long or short duration environmental sounds (a dog bark versus a horn honk), presented rapidly in succession, and report which sound came first. However, merely determining which of two sounds comes first is not a test of TOJ as this task can be done by perceiving the first sound only. Furthermore, there is little relationship between the neural mechanisms engaged in processing environmental sounds such as the difference between a dog bark and a horn honk, and the rapid spectrotemporal formant transitions or brief acoustic cues such as VOT that characterize speech processing. Environmental sounds differ across a multitude of acoustic cues throughout their entire acoustic spectrum (regardless of their duration). Furthermore, both neuropsychological and neural imaging studies have demonstrated that environmental sounds such as these, as well as features associated with pitch, are processed in the right cerebral hemisphere of the brain, and speech *as well as nonspeech* stimuli, characterized by spectrotemporal changes occurring in the tens of millisecond range, are processed in the left cerebral hemisphere (Belin et al., 1998; Fiez et al., 1995; Zatorre, 2003; Zatorre, Evans, Meyer, & Gjedde, 1992). Thus, when investigating the role of nonlinguistic acoustic processing in speech perception, it is essential to develop nonspeech analog stimuli that mimic the acoustic properties of speech, and thus are likely to engage similar acoustic processing mechanisms in the brain. Directly comparing VOT and TOT is a direct test of the hypothesis under investigation. Asking subjects to determine whether a dog bark or a horn honk came first, regardless of the rate of presentation, or engaging subjects in other acoustic tasks that bear little relationship to the neural mechanisms involved in speech perception, is not.

A DEVELOPMENTAL VIEW OF DEVELOPMENTAL READING DISABILITIES

Research with individuals with developmental disabilities has rarely taken a true developmental perspective in exploring theories pertaining to etiology. According to Hebbian learning (Hebb, 1949; Sejnowski, 1999) as well as neurophysiological studies of sensory mapping, neurons that fire nearly simultaneously in time wired together, result in exquisitely organized sensory neural maps (Recanzone, Schreiner, & Merzenich, 1993). For example, the individual representation of the fingers on the hand in the somatosensory cortex will closely approximate the actual physical representation of the hand because stimulation occurring at one particular location of the finger will likely occur more nearly simultaneously in time than stimulation occurring on a different finger as an animal explores its environment. Jenkins et al. (1990) demonstrated the importance of temporal input to the neural representation of fingers in the somatosensory cortex by demonstrating that the normal neural representation can be dramatically altered by temporally controlled tactile stimulation delivered intensely and repeatedly on the fingers. This experiment represents the dynamic neuroplasticity of the cortex as well as the essential role played by temporal input of sensory stimulation.

But what time period is encompassed by "nearly simultaneous?" Furthermore, are there individual differences across brains in what this time window of integration is? To investigate this question, April Benasich and I developed a method for establishing individual rapid auditory processing (RAP) thresholds for six-month-old infants (Benasich & Tallal, 1996). Infants were operantly trained (using their natural propensity to move their eyes to explore the world) to look to a toy located on their right side when they heard one acoustic sequence (a low tone followed by a high tone), and to their left when they heard a different sequence (a low tone followed by another low tone). Once infants had learned this task to criterion using a training stimulus incorporating 70 msec duration tones and a 500 msec interstimulus interval (ISI), the duration of the silence gap (ISI) between the end of the first tone and the beginning of the second tone was systematically reduced for correct responses or increased for incorrect responses until an individual threshold was established for each infant.

Two groups of infants have been studied using this procedure. One group had a family history of a parent and/or a sibling with a diagnosed LLI (family history positive, FH+) while a second group had no family members who had ever experienced a language or learning problem (family history negative, FH-). Family aggregation studies have demonstrated that approximately 50% of infants born into families with a positive history of language learning impairments will also have similar impairments (see Flax et al., 2003 for review). Thus, it is of considerable interest that these psychophysical studies demonstrated that approximately 50% of the infants in the family history positive group had elevated thresholds (needed longer ISIs between tones) to respond correctly to brief, rapidly successive acoustic stimuli (Benasich & Tallal, 1996). There was a highly significant group difference in rapid auditory processing (RAP) thresholds between infants born into the family history positive as compared to the family history negative group. However, further inspection of the data indicated that there were considerable individual differences, not only within the family history positive group of infants, but also within the control group of infants without a family history of language learning problems. Based on these results, we hypothesized that individual differences in RAP thresholds, which can be observed in infancy, would affect what each brain binds together as nearly simultaneous. This, in turn, would have a significant impact on the grain of analysis of the acoustic waveform of speech, leading to differential rates and patterns of phonological and language development.

In order to investigate this developmental hypothesis both prospectively and longitudinally, these same babies were followed from six months of age to three years of age, assessing in great detail their perceptual, cognitive, and linguistic development (Benasich & Tallal, 2002). Results of these studies demonstrated that within the broad battery of sensory, perceptual, memory, and cognitive abilities assessed, individual differences in RAP thresholds were the single best predictor of both receptive and expressive language development in children. While there was a disproportionate number of FH+ infants who showed higher RAP thresholds as well as delayed language development at the age of two and three years, there were children without a family history who showed similar patterns both for nonlinguistic acoustic processing in infancy and subsequent language delay. Importantly, across the entire sample, there was a highly significant, predictive correlation between early RAP thresholds and subsequent language development. Indeed, the correlation between infant RAP threshold and language development was significantly greater than the correlation between infant speech discrimination and subsequent language development.

Further analyses demonstrated that not only was RAP threshold and family history at 7.5 months of age significantly correlated with outcomes on standardized language tests, but also these variables were highly predictive of which individual children would fall within the normal range as compared to the impaired range (one or more standard deviations below the mean) on the Stanford-Binet verbal reasoning scales. Discriminative function analysis demonstrated that RAP threshold, together with being male, quite accurately identified at infancy those children who would be "impaired" at age three on the language-specific subscales of the Stanford-Binet as well as overall verbal intelligence as indexed by the verbal reasoning standard age score. Overall, classification accuracy of impaired versus nonimpaired children at 36 months was over 90% on the verbal reasoning scales (Benasich & Tallal, 2002).

It could be argued that the most alert infants on any variable assessed in infancy may have been equally predictive to any cognitive outcomes subsequently in life, rather than demonstrating a specific link between RAP thresholds and subsequent language and verbal reasoning abilities. In order to assess this possibility, similar analyses were run to determine whether any other variables assessed in infancy (such as recognition memory or visual habituation) were able to significantly predict outcomes at age three. No significant prediction was found for any other infant variable to scores on any of the Stanford-Binet scales at age 36 months, demonstrating the specificity of the relationship between RAP threshold, male gender, and verbal outcomes (Benasich & Tallal, 2002). These results are consistent with results by Trehub and Henderson (1996) showing temporal resolution in infancy predicts subsequent language development in normal infants.

FOR SPEECH PROCESSING, TIME IS OF THE ESSENCE

We can conclude from behavioral studies that infants who need more time between rapidly successive acoustic events are highly likely to develop poorer verbal reasoning and linguistic skills. We also know from similar studies with preschool and school-age children with diagnosed specific language impairment that most of these children require more time between acoustic events differing in frequency to process them accurately. Similarly, we know both from infant studies as well as studies with very young children that there is a high correlation between RAP thresholds and the ability to process speech syllables that are characterized by rapid spectrotemporal acoustic changes. High correlations also have been found between RAP abilities and phonological awareness abilities in children with LLI (Farmer & Klein, 1995; Tallal, 1980; Wright, Bowen, & Zecker, 2000). It should be emphasized that while similar correlations have been found in some, but not all older children and adults with dyslexia, and deficits also have been found in other nontemporal specific aspects of auditory and visual processing, the relationship may be weaker and more difficult to uncover with behavioral techniques alone (Ahissar, Protopapas, Reid, & Merzenich, 2001; Hari & Kiesla, 1996; McArthur & Bishop, 2004; Stark et al., 1984; Wright, Bowen, & Zecker, 2000).

However, as noted previously, some studies have failed to demonstrate deficits in rapid auditory processing in children (Mody, Studdent-Kennedy, & Brady, 1997; but for critique see Denenberg 1999) and adults with SLI and/or dyslexia (Baily & Snowling, 2003; McArthur & Bishop, 2004; Ramus, 2003; Rosen, 2003; Rosen & Manganari, 2001). In these studies, only a minority of subjects showed deficient rapid auditory processing, and there was no significant correlation found between RAP thresholds, speech perception, and/or phonological decoding and reading skills.

In an attempt to better understand discrepancies across studies, converging methodologies (behavioral/psychoacoustic/ electrophysiological) have been used to study rapid auditory processing. Benasich, Thomas, Choudhury, and Leppänen (2002) studied infants with or without a family history of language disorder using both behavioral and event related potential (ERP) paradigms. They demonstrated that in infants, behavioral and electrophysiological data yielded similar results. Both methods showed that rapid auditory processing differed as a function of family history and was predictive of later language outcome. Taking a similar approach, Bishop and McArthur (2004) directly compared the responses of 10- to 19-year-old individuals with SLI to two closely separated auditory stimuli differing in frequency. Surprisingly, they obtained quite different results from electrophysiological scalp recordings than they had obtained previously from a behavioral measure of backward recognition masking using the same stimuli (McArthur & Bishop, 2004). Specifically, no significant difference was found between the behavioral responses of the SLI and control groups on tone pairs at any inter-stimulus-interval (ISI). However, a significant group difference *was* found for the *same* tone pairs based on ERP recording data, with virtually *all* of the subjects with SLI showing aberrant ERP responses to these stimuli. Significant effects of ISI duration as well as age were found. For example, at 50 msec ISI, a differential brain response to two tones versus one tone was greater for younger than for older participants. Furthermore, age and ISI interacted significantly with SLI status. ERPs of older participants with SLI differed from age-matched controls and resembled ERPs of controls four years younger. These data are consistent with longitudinal data first reported by Stark et al. in 1984 that had shown rapid auditory spectrotemporal processing deficits in four- to eight-year-old subjects with SLI but failed to be able to demonstrate deficits on the same task with the same subjects four years later. They also are consistent with several recent studies suggesting that subjects' age and maturation might affect results of studies of auditory processing deficits in subjects with LLI (Wright & Reid, 2002; Hautus, Setchell, Waldie, & Kirk, 2003; Bishop & McArthur, 2004).

In conclusion, results from converging methodologies suggest that much of the controversy that has surrounded this area of research may be resolved by taking a more developmental perspective. These studies highlight the fact that intervening maturational effects, coupled with the profound experiential differences across children, make it difficult—if not impossible—to address questions of etiology in older subjects. This is not to suggest that individual differences in the manner in which sensory information is segmented and thus represented early in development does not leave a lasting legacy on the manner in which higher-level complex information such as speech is processed in the brain later in life. Rather, the ability to demonstrate these direct relationships using simple correlational analyses may become increasingly obscured with increasing development and maturation. The use of electrophysiological recordings and other functional neural imaging technologies, as well as a variety of converging methodologies in subjects of various ages, may provide a more sensitive means for addressing the relationship between individual differences in lower-level sensory information processing and higher-level cognitive operations involved in language and reading.

The data derived from prospective longitudinal studies of at-risk infants give us perhaps the most compelling evidence of the developmental impact of RAP thresholds on language development and disorders. Other compelling data are coming from studies of animals with induced or genetic anomalies of neocortical migration designed to mimic those found in LLI (for reviews, see

Fitch & Tallal, 2003; Galaburda, this volume; Fitch & Peiffer, this volume). These animal models show a strikingly similar pattern of thalamocortical magnocellular disruption, as well as behavioral RAP deficits, to those seen in individuals with LLI. These animal data not only contribute additional converging evidence to the human studies, but they also open the door for a more rigorous exploration of the neurobiological substrates underlying LLI, than can be investigated in humans.

PLASTICITY AND REMEDIATION

It has long been thought that Hebbian learning primarily occurs during early critical periods of development when sensory neural maps are established for a lifetime. However, single cell physiological studies demonstrating that these maps can be substantially altered at the cortical level, by intensive behavioral training in adult animals, has significantly challenged that perspective. Of particular relevance to our focus on language learning are animal studies demonstrating that the grain of analysis for segmenting rapidly changing auditory events can be significantly sharpened by behavioral training, based on Hebbian learning principles (Kilgard & Merzenich, 1998; Recanzone, Schreiner, & Merzenich, 1993).

In the early 1990s, my colleagues Michael Merzenich, Steve Miller, Bill Jenkins, and I began discussing whether the results of the neuroplasticity-based behavioral training studies in animals that he had been conducting in his laboratory, particularly those pertaining to enhancing the capacity to segment rapidly successive auditory events, might be applied to children with language learning impairments and rapid auditory processing problems. These discussions led to a series of laboratory studies, and subsequently to the development of a novel, computerized training approach called Fast ForWord®. Fast ForWord® incorporates two simultaneous approaches to intervention. In one approach, subjects indicate the temporal order of sweep tones that are either rising or falling in pitch. These stimuli were specifically designed to cover the range of frequencies and speeds that typify the acoustic frequency changes that occur in formant transitions in consonants. The exercise begins at an easy level with longer duration stimuli presented relatively slowly (with long ISIs). The computer program adaptively changes (increases or decreases) the duration of stimulus presentation based on each subject's trial-by-trial performance. The goal of the exercise is to increase the ability to process more rapidly changing acoustic stimuli to obtain levels typically found in the acoustic changes that characterize phonemes within syllables and words. In the second approach, we use a computer algorithm to acoustically modify (temporally extend and emphasize) the rapidly successive acoustic changes that occur with ongoing speech. This acoustically modified speech algorithm is used in a series of exercises designed to train individual components of language and reading at all levels, from the phoneme to the whole sentence. Within all of these exercises, as linguistic performance improves, the amount of acoustic modification adaptively decreases so that the stimuli becoming increasingly more natural. The goal of the entire series of Fast ForWord® exercises is to improve multiple aspects of oral and written language comprehension and fluency.

In our original laboratory studies, two matched groups of children with significant language learning impairments participated in daily training for approximately three hours per day for four weeks. Only the Fast ForWord® language exercises were evaluated in this study. The experimental group was trained with the two approaches described above. The treatment control group received the same language intervention, but with speech that was not modified, and instead of the auditory tone sequencing exercise, the control group played nontemporally adapted visual computer games. After training, the experimental group showed significantly greater improvement than the control group on rate of acoustic processing, speech discrimination, and performance on standardized language tests. The language gains made by the experimental group were dramatic, bringing many, but not all, of these children into the normal range (Merzenich et al., 1996; Tallal et al., 1996).

These results have significant theoretical as well as practical implications. They provided strong empirical support for the hypothesis that basic acoustic spectrotemporal processing constraints play a significant role in language learning impairment by demonstrating that when the precision of spectrotemporal processing is significantly enhanced, phonological processing, as well as higher-level aspects of linguistic processing, significantly improves. Furthermore, results showed a strikingly high correlation between the degree of improvement in rapid spectrotemporal acoustic analysis and the degree of improvement in language comprehension.

These results were first replicated and extended to the treatment of dyslexia in an independent study with French children using a similar acoustic modification algorithm to train phonological awareness abilities (Habib et al., 2002). More recently, additional Fast ForWord® intervention programs have been designed to move children from language to reading, and then through multiple levels of reading skills, further extending this intervention approach to struggling readers. Thus, in addition to the theoretical implications, these laboratory studies have had considerable practical implications. They led to the development of a series of commercially available neuroplasticity-based computer intervention programs for treating a wide variety of language and reading problems that have been extensively field tested in schools and clinics. To date, these intervention procedures have been applied to over 375,000 children in over 2,000 schools and clinics in English speaking countries (for school and clinic results, see www.scientificlearning.com/results).

As is the case with any intervention, not all children improved to the same extent, and some not at all. Furthermore, many children in the control group who received the same intensive language intervention, but without the benefit of the acoustically modified speech or RAP training, also improved, leading to questions about the specificity of the results to the temporal manipulations per se. Aspects of this intervention share some features in common with many other successful treatment approaches, specifically the intensity and consistency of treatment as well as explicit training of one or more components of language or reading (Ehri et al., 2001; Gillam & Van Kleek, 1996; Torgesen, 2000; Wise, Ring, & Oslon, 1999). However, these factors were explicitly addressed in our randomized, treatment control laboratory studies. While both groups showed significant gains over baseline performance on language measures, the experimental group receiving language training with acoustically modified speech, coupled with RAP training, showed a statistically significant advantage over the treatment control group (Tallal et al., 1996). Thus, these results cannot simply be attributed to more general factors such as novelty of computer intervention, intensity of intervention, or amount of reinforcement as these variables were controlled across groups.

Despite good overall success with these first-generation neuroplasticity-based computerized training approaches, there remains a percentage of children who improve only slightly, or not at all. And, as is the case with all intervention strategies, specifically those applied in multiple types of classroom settings, compliance to protocol and the percent of program completion will significantly alter outcomes and efficacy. Long-term follow up studies of trained children are needed, together with a better understanding of individual difference in outcomes that may be influenced by the clinical profile and learning environment of each child. Studies focusing on more effective ways to translate laboratory research into clinical and education practice are also sorely needed. Finally, additional research is needed to better understand which specific components of this and other intervention programs drive which specific outcomes, and for which specific children.

THE LANGUAGE TO LITERACY LINK

The laboratory and field trials described above demonstrated that a novel form of neural plasticity-based training can be highly successful in increasing the oral language skills of children with a variety of language-based learning disorders. Other investigators have hypothesized that phoneme awareness deficits, that are widely accepted to be the core deficit of dyslexia, derived from "fuzzy" neural representations for distinct phonemes. We have hypothesized that the Fast ForWord® training programs, that explicitly focuses on sharpening neural representations for distinct phonemes, would sharpen neural representation in the auditory system, leading to enhanced ability to segment words into component sounds, thus improving decoding and other reading skills. However, until recently, this hypothesis had not been put to an empirical test in a controlled laboratory study.

Recently, a group at Stanford University (Temple et al., 2000, 2003) used behavioral as well as functional magnetic resonance imaging (fMRI) to evaluate the effectiveness of Fast ForWord® language training in remediating reading abilities in a group of adult dyslexic subjects as well as children with dyslexia. Previous studies by a number of researchers using fMRI have demonstrated consistently that both adults and children with dyslexia have aberrant metabolic activity during phonological processing tasks in language areas in the temporal-parietal region of the left hemisphere (for review, see Temple, 2002). The goal of the Stanford studies was to determine whether the aberrant metabolic activity in temporoparietal cortex, observed in individuals with dyslexia while performing phonological awareness tasks, would be ameliorated after neuroplasticity-based training (Temple et al., 2000, 2003). In the latter study, 20 children who met clinical criteria for developmental dyslexia and 12 typical readers matched for age, socioeconomic status, and intelligence, received two fMRI scans at approximately eight weeks apart while performing a letter rhyming task. Between scans, the dyslexic children completed the Fast ForWord® language training program. Recall that this version of Fast ForWord® focuses on increasing the rate of auditory processing as well as improving attention, memory, and oral language skills. After training, performance on all measures of oral language (receptive and expressive) as well as *all* measures of *reading* (word identification, word attack, passive comprehension) showed significant improvement in the group of subjects with dyslexia. Of particular importance, word attack skills (representing the core deficit of phonological awareness) moved from one standard deviation below the mean (below average) before Fast ForWord® language training to well within the normal range after approximately eight weeks of Fast ForWord® training. The control group who received the same battery of language and reading standardized tests approximately eight weeks apart showed no significant change, demonstrating that these post-training results cannot be attributed to regression to the mean, normal maturation, or test-retest practice affects.

In addition to significant changes in reading observed with standardized behavioral measures, fMRI results demonstrated that after training, the dyslexia readers also showed increased metabolic activity during the letter rhyming task in left hemisphere temporoprietal language regions, bringing the brain activation in these regions closer to that seen in children with normal reading skills. This result is consistent with other recent studies similarly demonstrating "normalization" of brain function after extensive acousic/phonological training (Shaywitz et al., 2004; Tremblay & Kraus, 2002). Interestingly, the magnitude of increased activation in the left temporoparietal cortex was significantly correlated with the magnitude of improvement in language skills. Other areas of the brain also showed significant changes in metabolic activity after training, specifically homologous areas in the right hemisphere (Temple et al., 2003). These findings are being further investigated in a current study incorporating a randomized control group of dyslexic subjects receiving a different form of intervention.

The significant improvements in reading following Fast ForWord® language training provide strong support for the theoretical premise initially driving the hypothesis linking rapid auditory processing, language, and reading. Recall that this series of training exercises does not incorporate any letters at all, but rather was designed to improve the rate of auditory sequential processing, attention, memory, phonological processing, and grammatical skills. The finding of improved *reading* immediately following this training demonstrates the importance of these essential building blocks, not only for language development but also for reading success.

CONCLUSION

The role of rapid auditory processing in developmental language and reading impairments has become a central focus of research.

Several significant methodological issues that have clouded this area of research are increasingly being resolved, leading to increased understanding of the etiology of these developmental language-based learning disabilities. Specifically, it is becoming increasingly clear that we need to better understand the long-term effects of early individual differences in experience and brain maturation. Patterns that may be seen in infants or very young children may fail to replicate in school-age children, college students, or adults. Even well after early patterns of deficit/difference/maturation of sensory information processing may have resolved, or become recalcitrant to behavioral assessment, they are likely to leave a lasting legacy on the way the brain has organized itself for phonological processing, language, and reading throughout life. With the advent of more sophisticated neuroimaging procedures, specifically those that can track real-time neural processing in the time range of speech, future research may be better able to address issues pertaining to similarities and differences in the way speech and nonspeech acoustic signals are processed in the human brain. Such studies should lead to a better understanding of the types of stimuli, ages of subjects, and clinical subgroups that may be most effective in addressing the most relevant questions pertaining to the neurobiological origins of language-based learning disabilities. Finally, the development of animal models that mimic anatomical, physiological, and behavioral features associated with language-based learning disabilities offer new avenues for exploring the complex interaction of neurobiological, genetic, and environmental factors that contribute to these impairments.

Address correspondence to: Paula Tallal, Ph.D., Center for Molecular and Behavioral Neuroscience, Rutgers University, 197 University Avenue, Newark, NJ 07102; E-mail: tallal@axon.Rutgers.edu

DISCLOSURE STATEMENT

Paula Tallal is a founder and director, and has a financial interest in, Scientific Learning Corporation (http://www.scientificlearning.com), the company that developed and markets the Fast ForWord® family of training programs. She is also a consultant to Neuroscience Solutions Corporation (http://www.neurso.com).

REFERENCES

Aram, D. M., Ekelman, B. L., & Nation, J. E. (1984). Preschoolers with language disorders: 10 years later. *Journal of Speech and Hearing Research, 27*, 232–244.

Ahissar, M., Protopapas, A., Reid, M., & Merzenich, M. M. (2001). Auditory processing parallels reading abilities in adults. *Proceedings of the National Academy of Sciences of the United States of America, 97,* 6832–6837.
Baily, P., & Snowling, M. (2003). Auditory processing and the development of language and literacy. *British Medical Bulletin, 63,* 135–146.
Belin, P., Zilbovicius, M., Crozier, S., Thivard, I., Fontaine, A., Masure, M. C., et al. (1998). Lateralization of speech and auditory temporal processing. *Journal of Cognitive Neuroscience, 10,* 536–540.
Benasich, A. A., & Tallal, P. (1996). Auditory temporal processing thresholds, habituation and recognition memory over the first year. *Infant Behavior and Development, 19,* 339–357.
Benasich, A. A., & Tallal, P. (2002). Infant discrimination of rapid auditory cues predicts later language impairment. *Behavioral Brain Research, 136,* 31–49.
Benasich, A., Thomas, J. J., Choudhury, N., & Leppänen, P. H. (2002). The importance of rapid auditory processing abilities to early language development: Evidence from converging methodologies. *Developmental Psychobiology, 40,* 278–292.
Bishop, D. V. M. (1997). *Uncommon understanding.* Hove, England: Psychology Press.
Bishop, D. V. M., & Snowling, M. J. (2004). Developmental dyslexia and specific language impairment: Same or different? *Psychological Bulletin, 130,* 858–886.
Bishop, D. V. M., & Adams, C. (1990). A prospective study of the relationship between specific language impairment, phonological disorders and reading retardation. *Journal of Child Psychology and Psychiatry, 31,* 1027–1050.
Bishop, D. V. M., Carlyon, R. P., Deeks, J. M., & Bishop, S. J. (1999). Auditory temporal processing impairment: Neither necessary nor sufficient for causing language impairment in children. *Journal of Speech and Hearing Research, 42,* 1295–1310.
Bishop, D. V. M., & McArthur, M. (2004). Immature cortical responses to auditory stimuli in specific language impairment: Evidence from ERPs to rapid tone sequences. *Developmental Science, 7*(3), F11–F18.
Blake, D. T., Strata, F., Churchland, A., & Merzenich, M. M. (2002). Neural correlates of instrumental learning in primary auditory cortex. *Proceedings of the National Academy of Sciences of the United States of America, 99*(15), 10114–10119.
Breier, J. I., Gray, L., Fletcher, J. M., Diehl, R. L., Klaas, P., Foorman, B. R., & Molis, M. R. (2001). Perceptions of voice and tone onset time continua in children with dyslexia with and without attention deficit/hyperactivity disorder. *Journal of Experimental Child Psychology, 80,* 245–270.
Campbell, J. R., Hombo, C. M., & Mazzeo, J. (1999). Trends in academic progress: Three decades of student performance. U.S. Department of Education, Office of Educational Research and Improvement. National Center for Education Statistics. Washington DC.
Carrol, J. M., & Snowling, M. J. (2004). Language and phonological skills in children at high-risk of reading difficulties. *Journal of Child Psychology and Psychiatry, 45,* 631–640.

Castles, A., & Coltheart, M. (2004). Is there a causal link from phonological awareness to success in learning to read? *Cognition, 91*, 77–111.

Catts, H. W., Fey, M. E., Tomblin, J. B., & Zhang, X. (2002). A longitudinal investigation of reading outcomes in children with language impairments. *Journal of Speech, Language, and Hearing Research, 45*, 1142–1157.

Chang, E. F., & Merzenich, M. M. (2003). Environmental noise retards auditory cortical development. *Science, 300*(5618), 498–502.

Chiappe, P., Chiappe, D. L., & Siegel, L. (2001) Speech perception, lexicality and reading skill. *Journal of Experimental Child Psychology, 80*, 58–74.

Denenberg, V. H. (1999). A critique of Mody, Studdert-Kennedy and Brady's "Speech perception deficits in poor readers: Auditory processing or phonological coding?" *Journal of Learning Disabilities, 32*, 379–383.

Ehri, L. C., Nunes, S. R., Willows, D. M., Schuster, B., Yaghoub-Zadeh, Z., & Shanahan, T. (2001). Phonemic awareness instruction helps children learn to read: Evidence from the national reading panel's meta-analysis. *Reading Research Quarterly, 36*, 250–287.

Elbro, C., Borstrøm, I., & Petersen, D. K. (1998). Predicting dyslexia from kindergarten: The importance of distinctness of phonological representations of lexical items. *Reading Research Quarterly, 33*, 36–60.

Farmer, M. E., & Klein, R. M. (1995). The evidence for a temporal processing deficit linked to dyslexia: A review. *Psychonomic Bulletin & Review, 2*(4), 460–493.

Fiez, J. A., Raichle, M. F., Miezin, F. M., Petersen, S. E., Tallal, P., & Katz, W. F. (1995). PET studies of auditory and phonological processing: Effects of stimulus characteristics and task demands. *Journal of Cognitive Neuroscience, 7*(3), 357–375.

Fitch, R. H., & Tallal, P. (2003). Neural mechanisms of language-based learning impairments: Insights from human populations and animal models. *Behavioral and Cognitive Neuroscience Reviews, 2*(3), 155–178.

Flax, J. F., Realpe-Bonilla, T., Hirsch, L. S., Brzustowicz, L., Bartlett, C., & Tallal, P. (2003). Specific language impairment in families: Evidence for co-occurrence with reading impairments. *Journal of Speech, Language, and Hearing Research, 46*, 530–543.

Gathercole, S. E., & Baddeley, A. D. (1990). Phonological memory deficits in language disordered children: Is there a causal connection? *Journal of Memory and Language, 29*, 336–360.

Gillam, R. B., & Van Kleek, A. (1996). Phonological awareness training and short-term working memory: Clinical implications. *Topics in Language Disorders, 17*, 72–81.

Habib, M. (2000). The neurological basis of developmental dyslexia: An overview and working hypothesis. *Brain, 123*(12), 2373–2399.

Habib, M., Rey, V., Daffaure, V., Camps, R., Espeser, R., Joly-Pottus, B., & Demonet, J. (2002). Phonological training in children with dyslexia using temporally modified speech: A three-step pilot investigation. *International Journal of Language and Communication Disorder, 37*, 289–308.

Hari, R., & Kiesla, P. (1996). Deficit of temporal auditory processing in dyslexic adults. *Neuroscience Letters, 205*, 138–140.

Hari, R., Vlata, M., & Uutela, K. (1999). Prolonged attentional dwell time in dyslexic adults. *Neuroscience Letters 271*, 202–204.

Hautus, M., Setchell, G., Waldie, K., & Kirk, I. (2003). Age-related improvements in auditory temporal resolution in reading-impaired children. *Dyslexia, 9,* 37–45.
Hebb, D. O. (1949). *The organization of behavior: A neuropsychological theory.* New York: Wiley.
Johnston, R. B., Stark, R., Mellits, D., & Tallal, P. (1981). Neurological status of language-impaired and normal children. *Annals of Neurology, 10,* 159–163.
Jenkins, W. M., Merzenich, M. M., Ochs, M. T., Allard, T., & Guic, R. E. (1990). Functional reorganization of primary somatosensory cortex in adult owl monkeys after behaviorally controlled tactile stimulation. *Journal of Neurophysiology, 63,* 82–104.
Jusczyk, P. W. (2002). How infants adapt speech processing capacities to native-language structure. *Current Directions in Psychological Science, 11,* 15–18.
Kilgard, M. P., & Merzenich, M. M. (1998). Plasticity of temporal information processing in the primary auditory cortex. *Nature Neuroscience, 1*(8), 727–731.
Kraus, N., McGee, T. J., Carrell, T. D., Zecker, S. G., Nicol, T. G., & Koch, D. B. (1996). Auditory neurophysiologic responses and discrimination deficits in children with learning problems. *Science, 273,* 971–973.
Kuhl, P. (2000). A new view of language acquisition. *Proceedings of the National Academy of Sciences of the United States of America, 97,* 11850–11857.
Leitão, S., Hogben, J., & Fletcher, J. (1997). Phonological processing skills in speech and language impaired children. *European Journal of Disorders of Communication, 32,* 73–93.
Leonard, L. B. (1998). *Children with specific language impairment.* Cambridge, MA: MIT Press.
Linden, J. F., Liu, R. F., Sahani, M., Schreiner, C. E., & Merzenich, M. M. (2003). Spectrotemporal structure of receptive fields in areas A1 and AAF of the mouse auditory cortex. Journal of *Neurophysiology, 90,* 2660–2675.
Lundberg, I., Olofsson, A., & Wall, S. (1980). Reading and spelling skills in the first school years predicted from phonemic awareness skills in kindergarten. *Scandinavian Journal of Psychology, 121,* 159–173.
Lyon, G. R. (1995). Towards a definition of dyslexia. *Annals of Dyslexia 45,* 3–27.
Mahony, D., Singson, M., & Mann, V. (2000). Reading ability and sensitivity to morphological relations. *Reading and Writing, 12,* 191–198.
McArthur, G. M., Hogben, J. H., Edwards, V. T., Heath, S. M., & Mengler, E. D. (2000). On the "specifics" of specific reading disability and specific language impairment. *Journal of Child Psychology and Psychiatry, 41,* 869–874.
McArthur, G., & Bishop, D. (2004). Which people with specific language impairment have auditory processing deficits? *Cognitive Neuro psychology, 21,* 79–94.
Merzenich, M., Jenkins, W. M., Johnston, P., Schreiner, C., Miller, S. L., & Tallal, P. (1996). Temporal processing deficits of language learning impaired children ameliorated by training. *Science, 271,* 77–81.

Mody, M., Studdert-Kennedy, M., & Brady, S. (1997). Speech perception deficits in poor readers: Auditory processing or phonological coding? *Journal of Experimental Child Psychology, 64*(2), 199–231.

Nicolson, R. I., Fawcett, A. J., & Dean, P. (2001). Developmental dyslexia: The cerebellar deficit hypothesis. *Trends Neuroscience, 24*(9), 508–511.

Orduna, I., Mercado, E., Guck, M. A., & Merzenich, M. M. (2001). Spectrotemporal sensitivities in rat auditory cortical neurons. *Hearing Research, 160*, 47–57.

Ramus, F. (2003). Developmental dyslexia: Specific phonological deficit or general sensorimotor dysfunction? *Current Opinion in Neurobiology, 13*, 212–218.

Ramus, F., Rosen, S., Dakin, S. C., Day, B. L., Castellote, J. M., White, S., & Frith, U. (2003). Theories of developmental dyslexia: Insights from a multiple case study of dyslexic adults. Brain, 126(Pt. 4), 841–865.

Rapin, I. (1978). Consequences of congenital hearing loss—A long term view. *Journal of Otolaryngology 7*(6), 473–483.

Recanzone, G. H., Schreiner, C. E., & Merzenich, M. M. (1993). Plasticity in the frequency representation of primary auditory cortex following discrimination training in adult owl monkeys. *The Journal of Neuroscience, 13*, 87–104.

Rosen, S. (2003). Auditory processing in dyslexia and specific language impairment. *Journal of Phonetics, 31*, 509–527.

Rosen, S., & Manganari, E. (2001). Is there a relationship between speech and nonspeech auditory prcessing in children with dyslexia? *Journal of Speech Language Hearing Research, 44*, 720–736.

Scarborough, H. S. (1990). Very early language deficits in dyslexic children. *Child Development, 61*, 1728–1743.

Schreiner, C. E. (1991). Functional topographies in the primary auditory cortex of the cat. *Acta Otolaryngolgy Supplement, 491*(7–15): discussion 16.

Sejnowski, T. (1999). The book of Hebb. *Neuron 24*, 773–776.

Shaywitz, B. A., Shaywitz, S. E., Blachman, B. A., Pugh, K. R., Fulbright, R. K., Skudlarski, P., Mencl, W. E., Constable, R. T., Holahan, J. M., Marchione, K. E., Fletcher, J. M., Lyon, G. R., & Gore, J. C. (2004). Development of left occipitotemporal systems for skilled reading in children after a phonologically-based intervention. *Biological Psychiatry, 55*(9), 926–933.

Singson, M., Mahony, D., & Mann, V. (2000). The relation between reading ability and morphological skills: Evidence from derivational suffixes. *Reading and Writing, 12*, 219–252.

Stark, R., & Tallal, P. (1979). Analysis of stop consonant production errors in developmentally dysphasic children. *Journal of the Acoustical Society of America, 66*, 1703–1712.

Stark, R. E., & Tallal, P. (1988). *Language, speech, and reading disorders in children: Neuropsychological studies.* Boston: Little, Brown and Co., Inc.

Stark, R. E., Bernstein, L. E., Condino, R., Bender, M., Tallal, P., & Catts, H. (1984). Four-year follow-up study of language impaired children. *Annals of Dyslexia, 34*, 49–68.

Stein, J., & Talcott, J. (1999). Impaired neuronal timing in developmental dyslexia—The magnocellular hypothesis. *Dyslexia, 5*, 59–77.

Talcott, J. B., Witton, C., McLean, M. F., Hansen, P. C., Rees, A., Green, G. G. R., et al. (2000). Dynamic sensory sensitivity and children's word decoding skills. *Proceedings of the National Academy of Sciences of the United States of America, 97*, 2952–2957.

Tallal, P. (1980). Auditory temporal perception, phonics, and reading disabilities in children. *Brain and Language, 9*, 182–198.

Tallal, P., Allard, L., Miller, S., & Curtiss, S. (1997). Academic outcomes of language impaired children. In C. Hulme & M. Snowling (Eds.), *Dyslexia: Biology, cognition and intervention*. London: Whurr.

Tallal, P., Galaburda, A., vonEuler, C., & Llinas, R. (1993). *Temporal information processing in the nervous system*. New York: New York Academy of Sciences Press.

Tallal, P., & Piercy, M. (1974). Developmental aphasia: Rate of auditory processing and selective impairment of consonant perception. *Neuropsychologia, 12*, 83–93.

Tallal, P., & Stark, R. (1981). Speech acoustic cue discrimination abilities of normally developing and language impaired children. *Journal of the Acoustical Society of America, 69*, 568–574.

Tallal, P., Merzenich, M. M., Miller, S., & Jenkins, W. (1998). Language learning impairment: Integrating basic science technology and remediation. *Experimental Brain Research, 123*, 210–219.

Tallal, P., Miller, S. L., Bedi, G., Byma, G., Wang, X., Nagaragan, S. S., Schreiner, C., Jenkins, W. M., & Merzenich, M. M. (1996). Language comprehension in language-learning impaired children improved with acoustically modified speech. *Science, 271*, 81–84.

Temple, E. (2002). Brain mechanisms in normal and dyslexic readers. *Current Opinion in Neurobiology, 12*, 178–183.

Temple, E., Deutsch, G. K., Poldrack, R. A., Miller, S. L., Tallal, P., Merzenich, M. M., & Gabrieli, J. D. E. (2003). Neural deficits in children with dyslexia ameliorated by behavioral remediation: Evidence from functional MRI. *Proceedings of the National Academy of Sciences of the United States of America, 100*, 2860–2865.

Temple, E., Poldrack, R. A., Protopapas, A., Nagarajan, S., Salz, T., Tallal, P., Merzenich, M. M., & Gabrieli, J. D. E. (2000). Disruption of the neural response to rapid acoustic stimuli in dyslexia: Evidence from fMRI. *Proceedings of the National Academy of Sciences of the United States of America, 97*(25), 13907–13912.

Thomas, M., & Karmiloff-Smith, A. (2002). Are developmental disorders like cases of adult brain damage? Implications from connectionist modelling. *Behavioural Brain Science, 25*(6), 727–750.

Tomblin, J. B., Records, N. I., Buckwalter, P., Zhang, X., Smith, E., & O'Brien, M. (1997). Prevalence of specific language impairment in kindergarten children. *Journal of Speech, Language and Hearing Research, 40*, 1245–1260.

Trehub, S. E., & Henderson, J. L. (1996). Temporal resolution in infancy and subsequent language development. *Journal of Speech and Hearing Research, 39*, 1315–1320.

Torgesen, J. K. (2000). Individual differences in response to early interventions in reading: The lingering problem of treatment registers. *Learning Disabilities Research and Practice, 15*, 55–64.

Tremblay, K. L., & Kraus, N. (2002). Auditory training induces asymmetrical changes in cortical neural activity. *Journal of Speech, Language, and Hearing Research, 45*, 564–572.

Wise, B. W., Ring, J., & Olson, R. K. (1999). Training phonological awareness with and without explicit attention to articulation. *Journal of Experimental Child Psychology, 72*, 271–304.

Witton, C., Talcott, J. B., Hansen, P. C., Richardson, A. J., Griffiths, T. D., Rees, A., et al. (1998). Sensitivity to dynamic auditory and visual stimuli predicts nonword reading ability in both dyslexic and normal readers. *Current Biology, 8*, 791–797.

Wolf, M., & Obregon, M. (1992). Early naming deficits, developmental dyslexia, and a specific deficit hypothesis. *Brain and Language, 42*(3), 219–247.

Wright, B. A., Bowen, R. W., & Zecker, S. G. (2000). Nonlinguistic perceptual deficits associated with reading and language disorders. *Current Opinion in Neurobiology, 10*, 482–486.

Wright, B. A., Lombardino, L. J., King, W. M., Puranik, C. S., Leonard, C. M., & Merzenich, M. M. (1997). Deficits in auditory temporal and spectral resolution in language-impaired children. *Nature, 387*, 176–178.

Wright, B., & Reid, M. (2002). Excessive auditory masking in children with language or listening impairments interpreted as a developmental delay (abstract). Association for research in otolaryngology 74. http://www.aro.org/archives/(2002)/(2002)74.html

Zatorre, R. J. (2003). Sound analysis in auditory cortex. *Trends in Neuroscience, 26*, 229–230.

Zatorre, R. J., Evans, A. C., Meyer, E., & Gjedde, A. (1992). Lateralization of phonetic and pitch discrimination in speech processing. *Science, 256*, 846–849.

Zhang, L. I., Bao, S., & Merzenich, M. M. (2002). Disruption of primary auditory cortex by synchronous auditory inputs during a critical period. *Proceedings of the National Academy of Sciences of the United States of America, 99*(4), 2309–2314.

Chapter •4

A Neurological Model of Dyslexia and Other Domain-specific Developmental Disorders with an Associated Sensorimotor Syndrome

Franck Ramus

SUMMARY

Given mounting evidence that auditory, visual and/or motor dysfunction may not cause developmental dyslexia, but are often associated with it, the present paper proposes a new neurological model of dyslexia that explains how a specific phonological deficit might arise, and sometimes occur together with a more general sensorimotor syndrome. Based on a review of the neurology of dyslexia, the model specifies that: (1) genetically determined focal cortical anomalies in specific left perisylvian language areas are the underlying cause of the phonological deficit; (2)

This work was supported by a Marie Curie fellowship of the European Community programme Quality of Life (QLGI-CT 1999-51305) and a research grant from the Fyssen Foundation. I thank Al Galaburda, Uta Frith, John Morton, Alfonso Caramazza, and all participants of the Extraordinary Brain workshop for much discussion, feedback, and encouragement, and Sarah White for comments on a previous version of this paper. The present chapter elaborates on Ramus, F. (2004). Neurobiology of dyslexia: A reinterpretation of the data. *Trends in Neurosciences* 27(12), 720–726.

this phonological deficit is the primary cause of reading impairment; (3) under certain hormonal conditions during gestation, these cortical anomalies induce secondary disruption in sensory pathways, notably in the thalamus. The disruption may even extend to further areas, like the posterior parietal cortex and even the cerebellum; and (4) when this happens, the individual affected displays one or several components of a sensorimotor syndrome, which may in some cases aggravate the reading impairment. The model generalizes to specific language impairment and possibly to other domain-specific developmental disorders, each particular disorder characterized by the specific location of the brain anomalies.

INTRODUCTION

Certain developmental disorders, including dyslexia, specific language impairment (SLI), and autism are the subject of considerable controversy regarding their neurological and cognitive origins. Certain theoreticians consider them to be domain-specific disorders, arising from congenital dysfunctions circumscribed to certain cognitive components such as phonology, syntax, or mentalizing, respectively (Snowling, 2000; Gopnik, 1997; Frith, 2003; van der Lely, Rosen, & McClelland, 1998). Others think that these disorders are much more general, and that the seemingly specific components affected are, in fact, part of a more extended syndrome, usually encompassing the sensory and motor domains (Stein & Walsh, 1997; Karmiloff-Smith, 1998; Tomblin & Pandich, 1999; Gepner & Mestre, 2002). Some of these researchers even hold that domain-specific developmental disorders are, in principle, unlikely to exist at all (Thomas & Karmiloff-Smith, 2002).

In the case of developmental dyslexia, the predominant theory is that it is due to a specific phonological deficit (Snowling, 2000). Nevertheless, this view has been challenged by increasing evidence of sensory and motor disorders in dyslexics, leading to competing theories implicating auditory/temporal processing deficits (Tallal, 1980; Farmer & Klein, 1995; Tallal, this volume), visual/magnocellular dysfunction (Lovegrove, Bowling, Badcock, & Blackwood, 1980; Livingstone, Rosen, Drislane, & Galaburda, 1991; Stein & Walsh, 1997), or motor/cerebellar dysfunction (Nicolson & Fawcett 1990; Nicolson, Fawcett, & Dean, 2001). In the face of this highly diverse and inconsistent data set, only one theory so far has attempted to account for all the empirical evidence: the general magnocellular theory, in which a generalized dysfunction of magno-cells affects all sensory pathways and further spreads to the posterior parietal cortex and the cerebellum, thereby encompassing all the known cognitive, sensory, and motor manifestations of dyslexia (Stein & Walsh 1997; Stein, 2001).

However, as I have argued elsewhere (Ramus et al., 2003; Ramus, 2003), the magnocellular theory only partly succeeds in explaining the whole data set. In particular, it fails to explain why the prevalence of sensorimotor dysfunction is so much lower than that of the phonological deficit in the dyslexic population. Even within the subset of dyslexics affected by sensory and/or motor disorders, the causal relationship with the reading impairment is far from clear (Ramus, 2003; Rosen, 2003). On the basis of a comprehensive review of the literature, I have previously advocated that dyslexia is, in most individuals, explained by a specific phonological deficit; furthermore, a more general sensorimotor syndrome occurs more often in the dyslexic than in the general population, but does not by itself play a causal role in the etiology of the reading impairment (Ramus, 2003). According to this view, a complete theory of dyslexia must explain both how a specific phonological deficit might arise, and why a sensorimotor syndrome should be significantly associated with it.

In this paper, I propose a neurological model that serves this purpose. Specifically, it potentially explains how a phonological deficit may arise from genetically determined brain anomalies, in isolation in certain individuals or in conjunction with sensorimotor impairments in others. This model is compatible with all the known genetic, neurological, and cognitive data available on dyslexia. It easily generalizes to SLI and possibly to other domain-specific developmental disorders. It further suggests explanations for a few puzzling issues like comorbidity between and heterogeneity within disorders, and makes a number of specific predictions yet to be tested.

INSIGHTS FROM ANATOMICAL STUDIES AND ANIMAL MODELS

Postmortem examination and brain imaging studies have documented many differences between dyslexic and control brains in the left perisylvian cortex (Galaburda, Sherman, Rosen, Aboitiz, & Geschwind, 1985; Rae et al., 1998; Eliez et al., 2000; Brown et al., 2001; Leonard et al., 2001), the underlying white matter (Klingberg et al., 2000), the thalamus (Livingstone et al., 1991; Galaburda, Menard, & Rosen, 1994), the corpus callosum (Rumsey et al., 1996; Robichon & Habib, 1998), the cerebellum (Rae et al., 2002; Finch, Nicolson, & Fawcett, 2002), and so on (see Habib, 2000 for a comprehensive review). In most cases, the functional significance of these brain differences has not been elucidated. It is not even clear which of those differences are specifically relevant to dyslexia, considering the well-known comorbidity between dyslexia and many other disorders (Kadesjö & Gillberg, 2001; Kaplan, Wilson, Dewey, & Crawford, 1998; McArthur, Hogben, Edwards, Heath, & Mengler, 2000). Nevertheless, the functional significance of two types of brain anomalies has been studied in greater detail.

Anomalies of cell migration called molecular layer ectopias and focal microgyri have been observed by Galaburda and colleagues in the perisylvian cortex of dyslexic brains (Galaburda & Kemper, 1979; Galaburda et al., 1985; Humphreys, Kaufmann, & Galaburda, 1990; Galaburda, this volume), predominantly in the left hemisphere and with a much greater prevalence than in control brains (Kaufmann & Galaburda, 1989). Ectopias consist of up to hundreds of neurons and glia that have escaped into the molecular layer of the cortex through a breach in the external glial limiting membrane, accompanied by mild disorganization of the subjacent cortical layers. Microgyria are more severe disturbances where the organization of all layers of the cortex is severely affected. Cytoarchitectonic anomalies have also been observed in dyslexics' thalamus: in the lateral geniculate nucleus, the magnocellular layers were more disorganized, with overall smaller cell bodies (Livingstone et al., 1991). Similarly, there was a disproportionate number of small neurons in dyslexics' left medial geniculate nucleus (MGN) (Galaburda, Menard, & Rosen, 1994).

It is quite natural to hypothesize that anomalies in the magnocellular layers of the lateral geniculate are the cause of visual deficits, and that anomalies in the medial geniculate are the cause of auditory deficits. There is at least evidence for the latter causal link in rats (Herman, Galaburda, Fitch, Carter, & Rosen, 1997). Similarly, it is easy to see cortical anomalies in left perisylvian areas as the underlying cause of phonological, and perhaps other cognitive difficulties.

In this anatomical evidence, one can, therefore, see direct neurological support for auditory and magnocellular theories of dyslexia. The implicit causal (bottom-up) scenario is that anomalies in the thalamus engender ectopias and microgyria in certain cortical areas to which the thalamus is connected. At the cognitive level, this would translate into the auditory deficit causing a phonological deficit, and into the basic visual deficit causing visual attention/planning problems as prescribed by the magnocellular theory. However, this scenario may well be incorrect (Galaburda, 1999). Indeed, Galaburda and colleagues have found that, at least in animal models, the causal direction seems to be the opposite (top-down); that is, that the cortical anomalies engender the thalamic anomalies.

The evidence comes from a whole series of studies on rats and mice. Indeed, it is possible to surgically induce ectopias and microgyria by poking a hole in the external glial limiting membrane of the developing cortex of rats during late neocortical neuronal migration. There are also strains of mutant mice that spontaneously develop similar malformations. Investigation of these animal models have led to a number of important findings.

First of all, newborn rats with surgically induced microgyria in the frontal, parietal, or occipital cortex subsequently develop anomalies in the MGN: they have more small and fewer large neurons in the MGN than rats receiving sham lesions, an anomaly similar to that found in dyslexics' MGN (Herman et al., 1997; Peiffer, Rosen, & Fitch, 2002a; Fitch & Peiffer, this volume). This suggests that the direction of causation is indeed top-down, from the cortex to sensory relays in the thalamus. Furthermore, rats with such an abnormal MGN were found to perform less well in an auditory discrimination task (Herman et al., 1997; Fitch, Tallal, Brown, Galaburda, & Rosen, 1994; Fitch, Brown, Tallal, & Rosen, 1997; Peiffer, Rosen, & Fitch, 2002a; Fitch & Peiffer, this volume), which confirms that the observed disruption in the MGN has an impact on auditory capacities. Similar auditory disorders are found in ectopic mice, regardless of the localization of ectopias (Peiffer et al., 2001), which suggests that this top-down scenario may also occur when cortical malformations have a genetic origin.

Another interesting aspect uncovered in these studies is that only male rats were initially found to have impaired auditory function following early inducement of microgyria (Fitch et al., 1997; Fitch & Peiffer, this volume). Indeed, female rats showed normal auditory performance and did not show a similar anatomical disruption of the MGN in response to the microgyria, even though their cortical lesions were as extended (Herman et al., 1997). Similarly, only male ectopic mice show auditory deficits (Peiffer, Rosen, & Fitch, 2002b). It was then found that this sex difference had a hormonal basis; indeed, female rats that were androgenized by injection of testosterone during gestation showed disrupted MGN like males (Rosen, Herman, & Galaburda, 1999).

Finally, the cortical anomalies themselves seem to have an impact on cognitive function: ectopic mice and rats with spontaneous or induced ectopias and microgyria exhibit a variety of learning deficits (Denenberg, Sherman, Schrott, Rosen, & Galaburda, 1991; Schrott et al., 1992; Balogh, Sherman, Hyde, &

Denenberg, 1998; Rosen, Waters, Galaburda, & Denenberg, 1995), including problems with working memory (Boehm, Sherman, Rosen, Galaburda, & Denenberg, 1996; Waters, Sherman, Galaburda, & Denenberg, 1997; Hyde, Sherman, Hoplight, & Denenberg, 2000). Furthermore, the location of the cortical disruption influences the specific type of learning deficit exhibited by the animal (Hyde et al., 2001; Hyde, Stavnezer, Bimonte, Sherman, & Denenberg, 2002), but not the likelihood of further thalamic disruption and sensory impairment.

To summarize, these results suggest that, in animal models at least, (1) cortical anomalies (microgyria, ectopias) induce secondary anomalies in sensory relays in the thalamus, but (2) only under certain fetal hormonal conditions. Leaping to the human case, and assuming that early cortical anomalies are directly related to dyslexics' future phonological deficit, these findings suggest that (1) the neural basis for a phonological deficit may exist *prior* to the neural basis for any auditory impairment, and that (2) it may exist *in the absence of* any auditory impairment (when the disruption does not propagate to the thalamus, like in female rats: Herman et al., 1997). Obviously, there are many more conceivable neurodevelopmental models of dyslexia than the one most directly suggested by these particular neurological observations and animal models. But limited as these data are, they seem more compatible with the idea of a specific phonological deficit optionally associated with additional sensorimotor disorders than with any theory requiring causation of the phonological deficit through other sensory/cognitive disturbances.

I will now spell out and discuss in further detail what a plausible neurological model of dyslexia and other developmental disorders might be, based on this reinterpretation of the anatomical and animal data. It should be emphasized that this model is largely speculative; it attempts to be compatible with all the available data, but given that the available data are not excessively constraining, alternative models are perfectly viable. The goal here is mainly to provide a plausible, testable model that makes specific predictions.

A NEUROLOGICAL MODEL OF DYSLEXIA

Focal Anomalies and the Phonological Deficit

The main claim of the model is that congenital anomalies in specific left perisylvian areas are the direct cause of a phonological deficit, which itself is the direct cause of reading impairment.

A simple version of this model attributes the main responsibility to cortical ectopias and microgyria. Galaburda et al. (1985) found most ectopias in the left perisylvian cortex. This is indeed where the main brain areas involved in phonology seem to be located: mainly the supramarginal and angular gyri, the posterior superior temporal gyrus, the insula, and the inferior frontal gyrus, although there is debate as to which areas are involved specifically in phonological representations, and which are more concerned with reading or speaking (Paulesu et al., 1996; Paulesu et al., 2001; Poldrack et al., 1999; Binder et al. 2000[DR1]; Simos et al., 2000; Shaywitz et al., 2002; Temple, 2002; Habib, 2000; Jacquemot, Pallier, LeBihan, Dehaene, & Dupoux, 2003). Note that this does not exclude areas that become more specifically dedicated to reading (like the left fusiform gyrus; e.g., Cohen et al., 2002) might also be the targets of ectopias, although there is currently no such evidence. More generally, the multiplicity of areas involved in phonology and reading, together with the multiple differences found between dyslexic and control brains, makes it plausible that several different patterns of cortical disruption will lead to a reading impairment; this diversity may actually underlie the various manifestations of the phonological deficit in dyslexia.

Unfortunately, work on ectopias and focal microgyria in dyslexia has been scarce (only eight brains have been dissected so far), so the reality of their involvement needs to be confirmed. However this criticism equally applies to all other neurological differences found in dyslexics. The interest of ectopias is that they have been replicated in animal models, and this work provides us with some cues about their genetic origin, and their further neurological and functional consequences. Furthermore, their implication in the etiology of dyslexia is further supported by recent findings by LoTurco and colleagues (this volume; Wang et al., submitted) that a dyslexia susceptibility gene is involved in neural migration, and that the deletion found in a dyslexic family disrupts its function. Nevertheless, given the current state of the research on the neurology of dyslexia, it remains entirely possible that other brain anomalies might be as, or even more strongly, implicated. In fact, many other brain anomalies might themselves be related to ectopias and microgyria, which may indeed be just one manifestation of a wider disruption. For instance, the planum temporale has been argued to be excessively symmetric in dyslexics (Galaburda et al., 1985; Larsen, Høien, Lundberg, & Ødegaard, 1990), and this is thought to be closely linked with the presence of ectopias and microgyria (Rosen, Sherman, Mehler, Emsbo, & Galaburda, 1989; Galaburda, 2001). Furthermore, increased callosal connections (Rumsey et al., 1996; Robichon & Habib, 1998) are also interpretable as a consequence of the excessive symmetry of the planum temporale and/or other cortical areas, as this symmetry is typically manifested by an enlargement of the usually smaller side (Galaburda et al., 1987). Finally, ectopias and microgyria may also be related to the disruption of underlying white matter tracts (Klingberg et al., 2000). Many of the brain anomalies observed in dyslexia may, therefore, be associated with ectopias and microgyria, and be part of the same disruption. Exactly which part of this disruption plays a significant functional role remains to be established. Quite plausibly, cortical ectopias and microgyria in specific left perisylvian areas might affect phonological representations; so might a disrupted planum temporale, as this area is thought to underlie speech representations (Liégeois-Chauvel, de Graaf, Laguitton, & Chauvel, 1999; Jäncke, Wüstenberg, Scheich, & Heinze, 2002; Scott & Johnsrude, 2003); and disrupted white matter might affect interfaces between phonological and orthographic representations, or between different levels of phonological representation (Paulesu et al., 1996; Klingberg et al., 2000).

Given the current uncertainty on structure/function relationships, the more general version of the present model is not committed to one particular type of brain anomaly, nor to a particular functional interpretation of each anomaly. However, it specifically hypothesizes (1) that the disruption is related to ectopias and microgyria, and, therefore, that it appears very early in development (before the fifth month of gestation in humans); (2) that the functionally significant part of the disruption is *focal*, specific to certain cortical areas or cortico-cortical connections; (3) that these focal anomalies specifically affect the development of phonological and/or orthographic representations/processing; and (4) that they are a sufficient cause of reading impairment, without the help of broader sensorimotor dysfunction (see Figure 1). In essence, this pattern of neurological dysfunction, analogous to that observed in the female rat, gives rise to "pure phonological dyslexia."

Sex Hormones and the Sensorimotor Syndrome

The second claim of the model is that when the focal anomalies already discussed are present, *and* under certain hormonal conditions at an early stage of brain development, additional disruptions arise in sensory pathways, notably the thalamus, and perhaps subsequently in other areas like the posterior parietal cortex and the cerebellum (Stein & Walsh, 1997). These disruptions

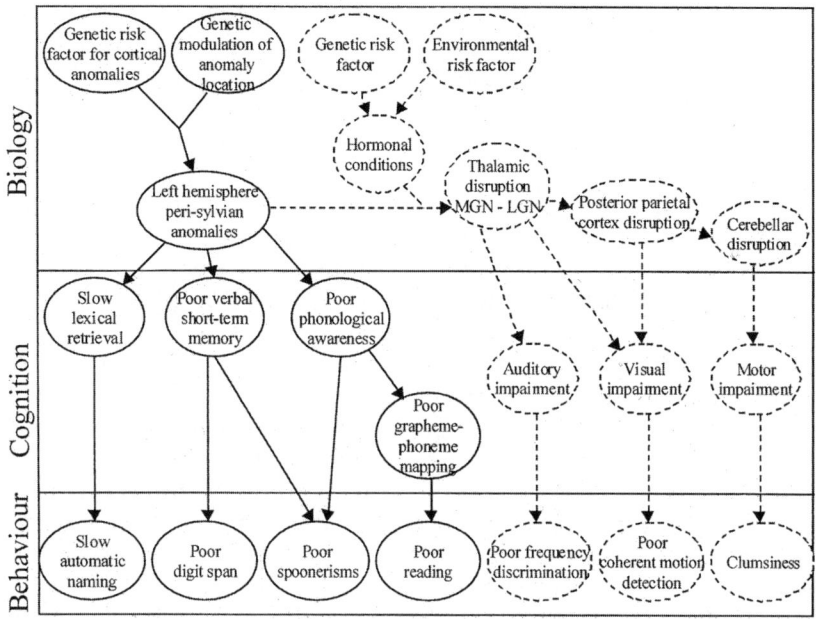

Figure 1. A causal model of the etiology of developmental dyslexia. Bubbles represent traits at the biological, cognitive, and behavioral levels of description. Arrows represent causal relationships between traits. Solid lines are used for core traits of developmental dyslexia, dashed lines for optional, associated traits. Only a subset of all possible behavioral manifestations are represented. Cases of comorbidity with other developmental disorders (e.g., SLI) are not represented. LGN: lateral geniculate nucleus. MGN: medial geniculate nucleus.

are responsible for a syndrome consisting of a constellation of sensory, motor, and perhaps attentional difficulties.

The research just reviewed suggests that the "hormonal conditions" may reduce to an elevated concentration of testosterone in the fetal environment (Rosen, Herman, & Galaburda, 1999). More generally, it has been proposed that testosterone plays an important role in brain development, notably by slowing the growth of the left hemisphere, and that it is involved in a number of brain and cognitive anomalies (Geschwind & Behan, 1982). There is also indirect evidence that a high concentration of fetal testosterone is associated with autism (Manning, Baron-Cohen, Wheelwright, & Sanders, 2001), another disorder with a high incidence of the sensorimotor syndrome (Spencer et al., 2000; Milne et al., 2002; Milne et al., in press). Fetal testosterone is, therefore, a likely candidate as a mediator for the sensorimotor syndrome. Nevertheless, the situation may be more complex. Indeed, other gonadal steroids like progesterone and estrogen have been shown to influence brain development, usually in positive ways (Hall, Pazara, & Linseman, 1991; Roof, Duvdevani, Braswell, & Stein, 1994). It may be that testosterone acts by attenuating the protective effects of these other hormones (Fitch et al., 1997), which suggests that sex differences in the neurophysiological response to cortical damage may result from a complex interaction of several hormones. Finally, it could also be that these "hormonal conditions" are a matter of hormone receptors in the brain rather than hormone concentration per se (Geschwind & Galaburda, 1985). This will all be matter for future research.

The hypothesis is, therefore, that under certain hormonal conditions to be precisely defined, focal cortical anomalies may induce further disruption in the thalamus, and more particularly in the medial geniculate nucleus (as demonstrated in male rats: Rosen, Herman, & Galaburda, 1999), as well as in the lateral geniculate nucleus (as suggested by dyslexics' brains: Livingstone et al., 1991). This would be the direct cause of subtle auditory and visual deficits. Although it has been suggested that sensory dysfunction might be specifically or predominantly magnocellular (Galaburda, Menard, & Rosen, 1994; Livingstone et al., 1991; Stein & Walsh, 1997), as pointed out earlier, the empirical evidence seems inconclusive. The model is, therefore, neutral to this issue. The sensory disorders in question might well be magnocellular, parvocellular, a combination of the two, or perhaps this dichotomy serves no meaningful purpose in the characterization of the deficit: this is a matter for future research. The main claim is that these sensory disorders arise optionally, under certain conditions in certain individuals only, and on top of the phonological deficit.

Similarly, Stein, and Walsh (1997) proposed that the magnocellular disruption further extends to the posterior parietal cortex and to the cerebellum. Again, this might well be true, but the model is neutral to this issue. If this is true (and even if the abnormalities are not specifically magnocellular), this might explain further visuo-attentional (Hari, Renvall, & Tanskanen, 2001) and motor (Fawcett, Nicolson, & Dean, 1996) problems also evidenced in some dyslexics (see Figure 1).

Obviously, when present, the sensorimotor syndrome may in principle aggravate the situation of the dyslexic child. In particular, a severe auditory deficit might aggravate the phonological deficit (Ramus et al., 2003). Visual or visuo-attentional deficits might also aggravate the reading impairments (Stein & Walsh,

1997). However, it should be noted that in both cases, the proposed causal links are still speculative and await further evidence.

Extension of the Model to Other Developmental Disorders

Dyslexia and SLI have two features in common: first, relatively specific cognitive deficits; and second, the additional presence of a sensorimotor syndrome in part of the population. The model presented here seems perfectly suited to explain all disorders that share these two features.

Indeed, nothing in this model restricts the possible loci of focal anomalies to areas subserving language. I hypothesize that in humans, like in mice (Hyde et al., 2001), what makes each developmental disorder unique is the location of the focal anomalies. In this view, what makes, say, a dyslexic child qualitatively different from an SLI child, has little to do with differences in low-level perception or the like, but depends on whether the cortical areas affected implement, say, processing of speech sounds, or of syntactic structure or lexical items. The model proposed for dyslexia, therefore, generalizes quite naturally to SLI, and possibly to other specific disorders like developmental dyscalculia (Shalev & Gross-Tsur, 2001) or prosopagnosia (Galaburda & Duchaine, 2003). Certain cases of autism, dyspraxia, and ADHD might also be explained within the same framework, insofar as the focal anomalies under discussion may arise in the brain areas involved in mentalizing, motor control, or attention, respectively. On the other hand, disorders like Williams, Down, or fragile-X syndromes clearly do not fit into this class of specific developmental disorders (Donnai & Karmiloff-Smith, 2000; Korenberg et al., 2000).

In the rat model, thalamic disruption arises under high fetal testosterone conditions, whether microgyria are located in the parietal, frontal, or occipital lobe (Herman et al., 1997). Similarly, in male ectopic mice, auditory deficits are found, regardless of ectopia location (Peiffer et al., 2001). According to the present model, this further explains why a similar sensorimotor syndrome seems to appear across a whole range of developmental disorders, and typically only in a subset of individuals within each disorder, whether dyslexia, SLI, or other (Hill, 2001; Kadesjö & Gillberg, 2001; McArthur & Bishop, 2001; Milne et al., 2002; Ramus, 2003; O'Brien, Spencer, Atkinson, Braddick, & Wattam-Bell, 2002; Milne et al., in press). I specifically hypothesize that the sensorimotor syndrome arises in any individual who presents with both the focal brain anomalies and the hormonal conditions discussed in the preceding section, regardless of the specific type of cognitive deficit.

Heterogeneity and Comorbidity

In the brains examined by Galaburda and colleagues (Galaburda et al., 1985), several dozens of ectopias spread over large cortical areas were found in each subject. This may seem at odds with the presumed specificity of the cognitive deficit. But this depends on the precise functional consequences of such cortical anomalies: it may well be that only a critical concentration of ectopias in one area produces any significant cognitive disruption, or that disruption occurs only when an area is affected bilaterally. Nevertheless, it is perfectly likely that several distinct cognitive systems are disrupted within a dyslexic individual: indeed, as already mentioned, there is more than one component to the phonological and reading systems, and nothing prevents a dyslexic from presenting other cognitive deficits unrelated to reading. Together with clinicians' strategy of sorting cases into a few basic diagnostic categories, this seems consistent both with the well-known heterogeneity within disorder and comorbidity between disorders.

Within Disorder. It seems to be the case that none of the usual diagnostic categories reflect homogeneous cognitive profiles. For instance, dyslexics' phonological deficit typically has three main manifestations: poor phonological awareness, poor verbal short-term memory, and slow automatic naming, which are significantly associated but may be partly independent (Wolf et al., 2002; Wolf & O'Brien, this volume). This is consistent with the view that this triad of impairments reflects distinct disruptions of, say, the left posterior superior temporal gyrus, the left inferior frontal gyrus, and the angular/supra-marginal gyri, respectively. Similarly, SLI is typically characterized by any combination of poor grammar, vocabulary, and/or speech articulation, which can be seen as reflecting distinct impairments of the syntactic, lexical, or articulatory systems. Finally, assuming that the number of focal anomalies may vary between individuals, the model is consistent with the existence of both individuals with a multifaceted disorder, and others with a purer subtype like pure phonological dyslexia (Wolf et al., 2002) or Grammatical-SLI (van der Lely & Stollwerk, 1997).

Between Disorders. Of course, multiple focal anomalies may span several cognitive domains as well as subsystems of the same domain. For instance, both phonological and syntactic systems may be affected, in which case the resulting disorder can be interpreted as a comorbid case of dyslexia and SLI. This helps explain why between one-third and one-half of children with a developmental disorder also qualify for the diagnosis of another one (Kadesjö & Gillberg, 2001; Kaplan, Wilson, Dewey, & Crawford, 1998; Hill, 2001; McArthur et al., 2000).

PREDICTIONS OF THE MODEL

Brain Anomalies in Other Developmental Disorders

Further research should reveal much more on the brain anomalies underlying dyslexia and other developmental disorders. While the present model is specified sufficiently loosely to accommodate a variety of outcomes, it also makes specific predictions: that a whole class of domain-specific disorders are characterized by focal brain anomalies, the differences between disorders reducing to differences in the localization of the anomalies. As far as SLI is concerned, the sample studied by Galaburda et al. (1985) actually included individuals whose profile was more that of comorbid dyslexia and SLI than of pure dyslexia, which is consistent with the observed distribution of cortical anomalies across language areas. More generally, MRI anatomical studies are globally consistent with the idea that brain anomalies of a similar nature, but not identical, are present in SLI and dyslexia (Plante, Swisher, Vance, & Rapcsak, 1991; Jernigan, Hesselink, Sowell, & Tallal, 1991; Gauger, Lombardino, & Leonard 1997; Leonard et al., 2002). The little that is known about developmental dyscalculia suggests that it might also fit into the same class of neurodevelopmental disorders, possibly with abnormalities in inferior parietal cortex (Levy, Reis, & Grafman, 1999; Dehaene, Piazza, Pinel, & Cohen, 2003); so might developmental prosopagnosia and associated visual recognition difficulties, with abnormalities in posterior inferior temporal cortex (Galaburda & Duchaine, 2003). However, much more research is needed to confirm the hypothesis that all these disorders are the product of similar neurological disruptions but in different anatomical localizations or configurations. On the other hand, research on such disorders as autism and ADHD has led to rather different neurological hypotheses (Bailey et al., 1998; Kemper & Bauman, 2002; Krause, Dresel, Krause, la Fougere, & Ackenheil, 2003; Castellanos et al., 2002), but this does not exclude the possibility that certain cases of these disorders might be explained by focal anomalies of the same nature as dyslexia in relevant brain areas. Furthermore, the model predicts that thalamic abnormalities will be found in a subpopulation only of each disorder, in parallel with the sensorimotor syndrome, but unrelated to the specific nature of the cognitive deficits.

Postmortem dissection, high-resolution MRI, diffusion-tensor imaging, and proton-MR spectroscopy studies will all be important tools to test these predictions. But they will be useful only insofar as the anatomical measures are matched with comprehensive and reliable cognitive testing in order to test precisely the postulated structure-function correspondences within each individual.

Sex-ratio

It is commonly accepted that males are more affected by dyslexia than females (e.g., Flannery Liederman, Daly, & Schultz, 2000), although this has been challenged (Shaywitz, Shaywitz, Fletcher, & Escobar, 1990). Within the magnocellular theory, the finding that thalamic disruption was mediated by fetal testosterone in the mouse model has been interpreted as a possible explanation for the uneven sex-ratio in dyslexia (e.g., Herman et al., 1997).

In the present model, the cause of reading impairment has been shifted away from the thalamus to the cortical anomalies. In this view, the sex-ratio of dyslexia has little to do with fetal hormones but is tightly related to possible sex differences in cortical anomalies. It turns out that the female dyslexic brains that were dissected showed fewer ectopias than male ones, and were characterized instead by a large number of small myelinated glial scars (Humphreys, Kaufmann, & Galaburda, 1990). This may imply that females are less likely to have a phonological deficit and that the deficit will be less severe on average in females, or alternatively that females require more severe neuropathology in order to exhibit behavioral problems, thereby explaining the uneven sex-ratio. But the exact functional significance of these differences in cortical anomalies is unknown, so it is at present impossible to predict the theoretical sex-ratio of the phonological deficit.

However, because of the hormonal mediation leading to the thalamic disruption, the model does predict an increased prevalence of the sensorimotor syndrome in males. More precisely, irrespective of the actual male/female ratio in dyslexia, it predicts that this ratio will be increased in the subpopulation with a sensorimotor syndrome compared to the subpopulation without it. And it predicts just the same for the sensorimotor syndrome in other developmental disorders. Such predictions could be easily tested by carrying out post-hoc analyses on already existing data sets including reliable individual data on sensory and/or motor measures.

Markers of Fetal Hormonal Conditions

Another prediction of the model is that if one could measure the relevant hormonal conditions in human fetuses and relate these measures to later outcome measures of sensorimotor functions, there would be significant correlations to be found (more than with measures of each specific cognitive deficit). Unfortunately, only major longitudinal studies including all the relevant measures will be able to test this prediction.

In the meantime, one may want to look for markers of fetal hormonal conditions that would still be measurable in the child or even in the adult. One such marker has been proposed: the ratio between the length of the second digit and that of the fourth digit (2D:4D ratio) would be inversely correlated to fetal testosterone levels (Manning, Scutt, Wlson, & Lewis-Jones, 1998), and has been shown to be significantly lower in autism than in the general population (Manning et al., 2001). Furthermore, a recent study replicated this result and found that within a group of autistic-spectrum disorder children, the 2D:4D ratio was correlated with their performance in coherent motion detection and in manual dexterity (Milne et al., in press). Obviously, such results are to be taken with caution considering the very indirect relationship between the two measures. Their interpretation may be further complicated by the fact that, as was evoked earlier, the determining hormonal conditions might not be simply a matter of testosterone concentration.

Genetics

Because developmental disorders like dyslexia and SLI have a strong genetic basis, the model predicts that ectopias and other relevant focal anomalies must arise under genetic control. This is indeed confirmed by studies of autoimmune mice that spontaneously develop ectopias (Sherman, Morrison, Rosen, Behan, & Galaburda, 1990; Sherman, Stone, Denenberg, & Beier, 1994), and by recent findings on the role of the Dyx1c1 dyslexia susceptibility gene (Wang et al., submitted; LoTurco et al., this volume). Furthermore, unless total cross-heritability across different disorders is shown, the model also predicts that the precise location of cortical anomalies is under genetic control. This is consistent with the fact that different strains of mutant mice have ectopias in different locations (Denenberg, Sherman, Schrott, Rosen, & Galaburda, 1991), but the exact mechanisms influencing their location are not known yet.

On the other hand, fetal hormonal conditions may be partly genetically determined, but are also more likely to be influenced by external factors. The model, therefore, predicts a lower heritability of the sensorimotor syndrome than of specific cognitive deficits. The possibility that some cases of sensorimotor dysfunction are due to genetically determined cortical anomalies in visual, auditory, or motor cortex, or in the cerebellum, may attenuate this prediction. Nevertheless, it is currently consistent with the finding that the phonological deficit is highly heritable (both in dyslexia and SLI), while auditory and visual deficits are not, or to a much lower extent (Bishop et al., 1999; Davis et al., 2001; Olson & Datta, 2002).

It is also notable that all the specific cognitive disorders under consideration here have a complex genetic etiology involving several regions on different chromosomes (e.g., Fisher & DeFries, 2002), unlike Williams, Fragile-X, Down syndromes, and the like, which all have a simple genetic etiology with wide-ranging cognitive consequences. In the light of the present model, one way to understand the relationship between complex genetic etiology and specific cognitive deficit is to speculate that in dyslexia and other specific disorders, certain genes are general risk factors for the occurrence of focal anomalies like ectopias, while other genes influence the precise location of such anomalies, for instance by generating molecular gradients interacting with ectopia risk factors. Yet other genes might be risk factors for the hormonal conditions leading to the sensorimotor syndrome. These hypotheses broadly predict that the genes implicated in all these specific cognitive disorders will be partly shared (those acting as general risk factors for cortical anomalies), and partly specific to each disorder (those influencing brain localization). The more specific predictions are potentially testable using current mouse models.

CLINICAL IMPLICATIONS

Current diagnostic categories are undermined by the heterogeneity within and the overlap between categories, as well as by the occasional focus on associated deficits as part of certain diagnostic procedures (e.g., clumsiness in dyslexia; Fawcett & Nicolson, 1996). They do not do justice to the variety of cognitive impairments that may arise and their different possible combinations. Although dyslexia, SLI, autism, and the like may remain convenient umbrella terms based on the most salient cognitive trait, a possibly more useful approach to learning disabilities would be in the form of a checklist enumerating all attested cognitive, sensory, and motor deficits, each child being characterized by his or her own combination of marks (and severity ratings) in the list. This would, in essence, replace ever-imperfect labels with a comprehensive, individual neurocognitive profile.

Attempts at remediation might also gain from such an approach. The present model suggests that there is little point proposing auditory, visual, or motor training schemes as general treatments for dyslexia and SLI since many of these children do not have sensory or motor impairments. The comprehensive diagnostic approach could, nevertheless, draw attention to sensorimotor impairments when present, which might justify treatment in their own right insofar as they are themselves a cause of trouble.

GENERAL DISCUSSION

It may be observed that the present model much resembles the traditional neuropsychological model for acquired brain lesions in that it postulates focal disruptions causing specific cognitive deficits, assuming a rather tight fit between brain area and function, even if the function is not yet developed at the time of the disruption. Some might argue that this makes the model highly implausible (Paterson, Brown, Gsödl, Johnson, & Karmiloff-Smith, 1999; Thomas & Karmiloff-Smith, 2002; Goswami, 2003). I would like to argue otherwise. The tight fit between brain area and function seems to be a basic fact about brain organization and development. Even for those functions that clearly have no evolutionary basis (e.g., orthographic processing), there seems to be one area of the brain that is more appropriate than others (e.g., orthographic representations reliably settle in a very specific subregion of the left fusiform gyrus: Cohen et al., 2002), presumably because not all areas of the brain have the optimal representational, computational, and connectional properties required for each particular function. And these properties of brain areas are largely genetically determined.

Certainly, when the optimal area for a particular function is disrupted, there can be a significant amount of compensation through brain plasticity, and more so in developmental than in acquired disorders. Indeed, it is well known that the right hemisphere can take over some linguistic functions from a dysfunctional or removed left hemisphere (Vargha-Khadem & Polkey, 1992; Bates et al., 1997; Frith & Vargha-Khadem, 2001). Functional brain imaging suggests that this does happen in dyslexics, too, as they show less activation than controls in their disordered left temporoparietal junction and inferior frontal gyrus, but more in the right counterpart areas (Shaywitz et al., 1998; Simos et al., 2002). But for all the hype about brain plasticity and reorganization, dyslexics, left-hemispherectomized children, as well as ectopic mice, remain significantly and specifically impaired, demonstrating that no other brain area does the job as well as the optimal one. What is known about brain development and plasticity is, therefore, entirely compatible with the idea that the congenital disruption of a limited brain area will lead to long-lasting disruption of the cognitive function that it would subserve under normal development.

Skeptics may further argue that it is unlikely that the effects of an early focal brain anomaly would remain circumscribed to that particular area and cognitive function, again because of plasticity (Karmiloff-Smith, 1998; Thomas & Karmiloff-Smith, 2002). But this again overlooks the fact that brain plasticity is far from total. Of course, development occurs and produces knock-on effects: in dyslexia, for instance, the phonological deficit alters the development of the orthographic system, and may also impact on the acquisition of vocabulary. Yet, there is no reason to expect that it should have consequences on *all* areas of the brain (after all, dyslexics are not overall mentally retarded). Indeed, this is not observed in the case of congenital focal brain lesions, which can also lead to relatively specific cognitive deficits in humans (Curtiss, de Bode, & Shields, 2000; Stromswold, 2000; Daigneault & Braun, 2002), just like in ectopic mice with focal cortical anomalies (Hyde, Sherman, Hoplight, and Denenberg, 2000; Hyde et al., 2001; Boehm et al., 1996; Hyde, Sherman, Stavnezer, & Denenberg, 2000; Hoplight, Sherman, Hyde, & Denenberg, 2001). The female rat model further demonstrates that disruption in one cortical area does not necessarily produce changes just one synapse away (Herman et al., 1997). The hypothesis of a specific cognitive deficit remaining specific throughout development, therefore, seems perfectly plausible and compatible with current knowledge in developmental neuroscience.

Within the framework of the present model, a sensory explanation of dyslexia, in order to be viable, has to make the following assumptions: (1) that a sensory dysfunction is present in all dyslexics at birth, but recovers in most of them to the point that it is detectable only in a minority by school age; (2) that in dyslexics who remain auditorily impaired, some factor also alters the relationship between the severity of the auditory deficit and that of the phonological deficit (as there is no reliable relationship at school age: Rosen 2003); (3) that the ectopias and concomitant brain anomalies observed in dyslexics' language areas *do not* by themselves cause any phonological deficit (since these anomalies exist before the sensory disruption); and (4) that the phonological deficit itself is not reflected by any additional physical disruption in those areas affected by the aforementioned anomalies, or, if it is, such disruption has so far gone unnoticed. Although such a conjunction of unlikely facts may appear implausible, it is, of course, possible that they will all turn out to be true. Further research should indeed aim to test these assumptions and more generally evaluate the respective predictions of the two competing frameworks; the sensorimotor one, and the domain-specific one.

The model outlined here opens up new avenues of research aiming to uncover the precise links between specific genes, brain anomalies, and cognitive deficits. But in order to meet that challenge, research on developmental disorders will have to complete a methodological revolution that has only recently begun: the production and analysis of reliable individual data at all levels of description. Indeed, the present model suggests that a number of genetic, neurological, and cognitive traits are consistently associated with dyslexia and other disorders, without actually *explaining* them. This implies that the usual studies focusing on group differences and correlations between measures are doomed to confuse core and associated deficits, cause, and correlation. The future belongs to longitudinal studies that will be able to trace causal pathways throughout development, across genetic, neurological, and cognitive measures, and within each individual subject.

Address correspondence to: Franck Ramus, Ecole Normale Supérieure, Laboratoire de Sciences Cognitives et Psycholinguistique, 46 rue d'Ulm, 75230 Paris Cedex 5, France; E-mail: franck.ramus@ens.fr

REFERENCES

Bailey, A., Luthert, P., Dean, A., Harding, B., Janota, I., Montgomery, M., Rutter, M., & Lantos, P. (1998). A clinicopathological study of autism. *Brain, 121*(Pt 5), 889–905.

Balogh, S. A., Sherman, G. F., Hyde, L. A., & Denenberg, V. H. (1998). Effects of neocortical ectopias upon the acquisition and retention of a non-spatial reference memory task in BXSB mice. *Brain Research. Developmental Brain Research, 111*(2), 291–293.

Bates, E., Thal, D., Trauner, D., Fenson, J., Aram, D., Eisele, J., & Nass, R. (1997). From first words to grammar in children with focal brain injury. *Developmental Neuropsychology, 13*(3), 275–343.

Binder, J. R., Frost, J. A., Hammeke, T. A., Bellgowan, P. S., Springer, J. A., Kaufman, J. N., & Possing, E. T. (2000). Human temporal lobe activation by speech and nonspeech sounds. *Cerebral Cortex, 10*(5), 512–528.

Bishop, D. V., Bishop, S. J., Bright, P., James, C., Delaney, T., & Tallal, P. (1999). Different origin of auditory and phonological processing problems in children with language impairment: Evidence from a twin study. *Journal of Speech, Language, and Hearing Research, 42*(1), 155–168.

Boehm, G. W., Sherman, G. F., Rosen, G. D., Galaburda, A. M., & Denenberg, V. H. (1996). Neocortical ectopias in BXSB mice: Effects upon reference and working memory systems. *Cerebral Cortex, 6*(5), 696–700.

Brown, W. E., Eliez, S., Menon, V., Rumsey, J. M., White, C. D., & Reiss, A. L. (2001). Preliminary evidence of widespread morphological variations of the brain in dyslexia. *Neurology, 56*(6), 781–783.

Castellanos, F. X., Lee, P. P., Sharp, W., Jeffries, N. O., Greenstein, D. K., Clasen, L. S., Blumenthal, J. D., James, R. S., Ebens, C. L., Walter, J. M., Zijdenbos, A., Evans, A. C., Giedd, J. N., & Rapoport, J. L. (2002). Developmental trajectories of brain volume abnormalities in children and adolescents with attention-deficit/hyperactivity disorder. *Journal of the American Medical Association, 288*(14), 1740–1748.

Cohen, L., Lehericy, S., Chochon, F., Lemer, C., Rivaud, S., & Dehaene, S. (2002). Language-specific tuning of visual cortex? Functional properties of the visual word form area. *Brain, 125*(Pt 5), 1054–1069.

Curtiss, S., de Bode, S., & Shields, S. (2000). Language after hemispherectomy. In J. Gilkerson, M. Becker, & N. Hyams (Eds.), *UCLA working papers in linguistics*. Los Angeles, CA: UCLA Department of Linguistics.

Daigneault, S., & Braun, C. M. (2002). Pure severe dyslexia after a perinatal focal lesion: Evidence of a specific module for acquisition of reading. *Journal of Developmental and Behavioral Pediatrics, 23*(4), 256–265.

Davis, C. J., Gayan, J., Knopik, V. S., Smith, S. D., Cardon, L. R., Pennington, B. F., Olson, R. K., & DeFries, J. C. (2001). Etiology of reading difficulties and rapid naming: The Colorado twin study of reading disability. *Behavior Genetics, 31*(6), 625–635.

Dehaene, S., Piazza, M., Pinel, P., & Cohen, L. (2003). Three parietal circuits for number processing. *Cognitive Neuropsychology, 20*(3/4/5/6), 487–506.

Denenberg, V. H., Sherman, G. F., Schrott, L. M., Rosen, G. D., & Galaburda, A. M. (1991). Spatial learning, discrimination learning, paw preference and neocortical ectopias in two autoimmune strains of mice. *Brain Research, 562*(1), 98–104.

Donnai, D., & Karmiloff-Smith, A. (2000). Williams syndrome: from genotype through to the cognitive phenotype. *American Journal of Medical Genetics, 97*(2), 164–171.

Eliez, S., Rumsey, J. M., Giedd, J. N., Schmitt, J. E., Patwardhan, A. J., & Reiss, A. L. (2000). Morphological alteration of temporal lobe gray matter in dyslexia: An MRI study. *Journal of Child Psychology and Psychiatry, and Allied Disciplines, 41*(5), 637–644.

Farmer, M. E., & Klein, R. M. (1995). The evidence for a temporal processing deficit linked to dyslexia: A review. *Psychonomic Bulletin & Review, 2*(4), 460–493.

Fawcett, A. J., & Nicolson, R. I. (1996). *The dyslexia screening test*. London: The Psychological Corporation.

Fawcett, A. J., Nicolson, R. I., & Dean, P. (1996). Impaired performance of children with dyslexia on a range of cerebellar tasks. *Annals of Dyslexia, 46*, 259–283.

Finch, A. J., Nicolson, R. I., & Fawcett, A. J. (2002). Evidence for a neuroanatomical difference within the olivo-cerebellar pathway of adults with dyslexia. *Cortex, 38*, 529–539.

Fisher, S. E., & DeFries, J. C. (2002). Developmental dyslexia: Genetic dissection of a complex cognitive trait. *Nature Reviews Neuroscience, 3*, 767–780.

Fitch, R. H., Brown, C. P., Tallal, P., & Rosen, G. D. (1997). Effects of sex and MK-801 on auditory-processing deficits associated with developmental microgyric lesions in rats. *Behavioral Neuroscience, 111*(2), 404–412.

Fitch, R. H., Tallal, P., Brown, C. P., Galaburda, A. M., & Rosen, G. D. (1994). Induced microgyria and auditory temporal processing in rats: A model for language impairment? *Cerebral Cortex, 4*(3), 260–270.

Flannery, K. A., Liederman, J., Daly, L., & Schultz, J. (2000). Male prevalence for reading disability is found in a large sample of black and white children free from ascertainment bias. *Journal of the International Neuropsychological Society, 6*(4), 433–442.

Frith, U. (2003). *Autism: Explaining the enigma* (2nd ed.). Oxford: Blackwell.

Frith, U., & Vargha-Khadem, F. (2001). Are there sex differences in the brain basis of literacy related skills? Evidence from reading and spelling impairments after early unilateral brain damage. *Neuropsychologia, 39*(13), 1485–1488.

Galaburda, A. M. (1999). Developmental dyslexia: A multilevel syndrome. *Dyslexia, 5*(4), 183–191.

Galaburda, A. M. (2001). Brain and sounds: Lessons from "dyslexic" rodents. In E. Dupoux. (Ed.), *Language, brain and cognitive development: Essays in honor of Jacques Mehler.* Cambridge, MA: MIT Press.

Galaburda, A. M., Corsiglia, J., Rosen, G. D., & Sherman, G. F. (1987). Planum temporale asymmetry: Reappraisal since Geschwind and Levitsky. *Neuropsychologia 25*, 853–868.

Galaburda, A. M., & Duchaine, B. C. (2003). Developmental disorders of vision. *Neurologic Clinics, 21*(3), 687–707.

Galaburda, A. M., & Kemper, T. L. (1979). Cytoarchitectonic abnormalities in developmental dyslexia: a case study. *Annals of Neurology, 6*(2), 94–100.

Galaburda, A. M., Menard, M. T., & Rosen, G. D. (1994). Evidence for aberrant auditory anatomy in developmental dyslexia. *Proceedings of the National Academy of Sciences of the United States of America, 91*(17), 8010–8013.

Galaburda, A. M., Sherman, G. F., Rosen, G. D., Aboitiz, & Geschwind, N. (1985). Developmental dyslexia: Four consecutive patients with cortical anomalies. *Annals of Neurology, 18*(2), 222–233.

Gauger, L. M., Lombardino, L. J., & Leonard, C. M. (1997). Brain morphology in children with specific language impairment. *Journal of Speech, Language, and Hearing Research, 40*(6), 1272–1284.

Gepner, B., & Mestre, D. (2002). Rapid visual-motion integration deficit in autism. *Trends in Cognitive Sciences, 6*(11), 455.

Geschwind, N., & Behan, P. (1982). Left-handedness: Association with immune disease, migraine, and developmental learning disorder. *Proceedings of the National Academy of Sciences of the United States of America, 79*(16), 5097–5100.

Geschwind, N., & Galaburda, A. M. (1985). Cerebral lateralization. Biological mechanisms, associations, and pathology: II. A hypothesis and a program for research. *Archives of Neurology, 42*(6), 521–552.

Gopnik, M. (1997). Language deficits and genetic factors. *Trends in Cognitive Sciences, 1*(1), 5–9.

Goswami, U. (2003). Why theories about developmental dyslexia require developmental designs. *Trends in Cognitive Sciences, 7*(12), 534–540.

Habib, M. (2000). The neurological basis of developmental dyslexia: An overview and working hypothesis. *Brain, 123*, 2373–2399.

Hall, E. D., Pazara, K. E., & Linseman, K. L. (1991). Sex differences in postischemic neuronal necrosis in gerbils. *Journal of Cerebral Blood Flow and Metabolism, 11*(2), 292–298.

Hari, R., Renvall, H., & Tanskanen, T. (2001). Left minineglect in dyslexic adults. *Brain, 124*(Pt 7), 1373–1380.

Herman, A. E., Galaburda, A. M., Fitch, R. H., Carter, A. R., & Rosen, G. D. (1997). Cerebral microgyria, thalamic cell size and auditory temporal processing in male and female rats. *Cerebral Cortex, 7*(5), 453–464.

Hill, E. L. (2001). Non-specific nature of specific language impairment: a review of the literature with regard to concomitant motor impairments. *International Journal of Language and Communication Disorders, 36*(2), 149–171.

Hoplight, B. J., Sherman, G. F., Hyde, L. A., & Denenberg, V. H. (2001). Effects of neocortical ectopias and environmental enrichment on Hebb-Williams maze learning in BXSB mice. *Neurobiology of Learning and Memory, 76*(1), 33–45.

Humphreys, P., Kaufmann, W. E., & Galaburda, A. M. 1990. Developmental dyslexia in women: Neuropathological findings in three patients. *Annals of Neurology, 28*(6), 727–738.

Hyde, L. A., Hoplight, B. J., Harding, S., Sherman, G. F., Mobraaten, L. E., & Denenberg, V. H. (2001). Effects of ectopias and their cortical location on several measures of learning in BXSB mice. *Developmental Psychobiology, 39*(4), 286–300.

Hyde, L. A., Sherman, G. F., Hoplight, B. J., & Denenberg, V. H. (2000). Working memory deficits in BXSB mice with neocortical ectopias. *Physiology & Behavior, 70*(1–2), 1–5.

Hyde, L. A., Sherman, G. F., Stavnezer, A. J., & Denenberg, V. H. (2000). The effects of neocortical ectopias on Lashley III water maze learning in New Zealand black mice. *Brain Research, 887*(2), 482–483.

Hyde, L. A., Stavnezer, A. J., Bimonte, H. A., Sherman, G. F., & Denenberg, V. H. (2002). Spatial and nonspatial Morris maze learning: Impaired behavioral flexibility in mice with ectopias located in the prefrontal cortex. *Behavioural Brain Research, 133*(2), 247–259.

Jacquemot, C., Pallier, C., LeBihan, D., Dehaene, S., & Dupoux, E. (2003). Phonological grammar shapes the auditory cortex: A functional magnetic resonance imaging study. *The Journal of Neuroscience, 23*(29), 9541–9546.

Jäncke, L., Wüstenberg, T., Scheich, H., & Heinze, H. J. (2002). Phonetic perception and the temporal cortex. *Neuroimage, 15*(4), 733–746.

Jernigan, T. L., Hesselink, J. R., Sowell, E., & Tallal, P. A. (1991). Cerebral structure on magnetic resonance imaging in language- and learning-impaired children. *Archives of Neurology, 48*(5), 539–545.

Kadesjö, B., & Gillberg, C. (2001). The comorbidity of ADHD in the general population of Swedish school-age children. *Journal of Child Psychology and Psychiatry, 42*(4), 487–492.

Kaplan, B. J., Wilson, B. N., Dewey, D., & Crawford, S. G. (1998). DCD may not be a discrete disorder. *Human Movement Science, 17*, 471–490.

Karmiloff-Smith, A. (1998). Development itself is the key to understanding developmental disorders. *Trends in Cognitive Sciences, 2*(10), 389–398.

Kaufmann, W. E., & Galaburda, A. M. (1989). Cerebrocortical microdysgenesis in neurologically normal subjects: A histopathologic study. *Neurology, 39*(2, Pt. 1), 238–244.

Kemper, T. L., & Bauman, M. L. (2002). Neuropathology of infantile autism. *Molecular Psychiatry, 7*(Suppl. 2), S12–S13.

Klingberg, T., Hedehus, M., Temple, E., Salz, T., Gabrieli, J. D., Moseley, M. E., & Poldrack, R. A. (2000). Microstructure of temporo-parietal white matter as a basis for reading ability: Evidence from diffusion tensor magnetic resonance imaging. *Neuron, 25*(2), 493–500.

Korenberg, J. R., Chen, X. N., Hirota, H., Lai, Z., Bellugi, U., Burian, D., Roe, B., & Matsuoka, R. (2000). Genome structure and cognitive map of Williams syndrome. *Journal of Cognitive Neuroscience, 12*(Suppl. 1), 89–107.

Krause, K. H., Dresel, S. H., Krause, J., la Fougere, C., & Ackenheil, M. (2003). The dopamine transporter and neuroimaging in attention deficit hyperactivity disorder. *Neuroscience and Biobehavioral Reviews, 27*(7), 605–613.

Larsen, J. P., Høien, T., Lundberg, I., & Ødegaard, H. (1990). MRI evaluation of the size and symmetry of the planum temporale in adolescents with developmental dyslexia. *Brain and Language, 39*(2), 289–301.

Leonard, C. M., Eckert, M. A., Lombardino, L. J., Oakland, T., Kranzler, J., Mohr, C. M., King, W. M., & Freeman, A. (2001). Anatomical risk factors for phonological dyslexia. *Cerebral Cortex, 11*(2), 148–157.

Leonard, C. M., Lombardino, L. J., Walsh, K., Eckert, M. A., Mockler, J. L., Rowe, L. A., Williams, S., & DeBose, C. B. (2002). Anatomical risk factors that distinguish dyslexia from SLI predict reading skill in normal children. *Journal of Communication Disorders, 35*(6), 501–531.

Levy, L. M., Reis, I. L., & Grafman, J. (1999). Metabolic abnormalities detected by 1H-MRS in dyscalculia and dysgraphia. *Neurology, 53*(3), 639–641.

Liégeois-Chauvel, C., de Graaf, J. B., Laguitton, V., & Chauvel, P. (1999). Specialization of left auditory cortex for speech perception in man depends on temporal coding. *Cerebral Cortex, 9*(5), 484–496.

Livingstone, M. S., Rosen, G. D., Drislane, F. W., & Galaburda, A. M. (1991). Physiological and anatomical evidence for a magnocellular defect in developmental dyslexia. *Proceedings of the National Academy of Sciences of the United States of America, 88*, 7943–7947.

Lovegrove, W. J., Bowling, A., Badcock, B., & Blackwood, M. (1980). Specific reading disability: Differences in contrast sensitivity as a function of spatial frequency. *Science, 210*(4468), 439–440.

Manning, J. T., Baron-Cohen, S., Wheelwright, S., & Sanders, G. (2001). The 2nd to 4th digit ratio and autism. *Developmental Medicine and Child Neurology, 43*(3), 160–164.

Manning, J. T., Scutt, D., Wilson, J., & Lewis-Jones, D. I. (1998). The ratio of 2nd to 4th digit length: A predictor of sperm numbers and concentrations of testosterone, luteinizing hormone and oestrogen. *Human Reproduction, 13*(11), 3000–3004.
McArthur, G. M., & Bishop, D. V. M. (2001). Auditory perceptual processing in people with reading and oral language impairments: Current issues and recommendations. *Dyslexia, 7*, 150–170.
McArthur, G. M., Hogben, J. H., Edwards, V. T., Heath, S. M., & Mengler, E. D. (2000). On the "specifics" of specific reading disability and specific language impairment. *Journal of Child Psychology and Psychiatry, 41*(7), 869–874.
Milne, E., Swettenham, J., Hansen, P., Campbell, R., Jeffries, H., & Plaisted, K. (2002). High motion coherence thresholds in children with autism. *Journal of Child Psychology and Psychiatry, 43*(2), 255–263.
Milne, E., White, S., Campbell, R., Swettenham, J., Hansen, P. C., & Ramus, F. (in press). Motion and form coherence detection in autistic spectrum disorder: Relationship to motor control and 2:4 digit ratio. *Journal of Autism and Developmental Disorders*.
Nicolson, R. I., & Fawcett, A. J. (1990). Automaticity: A new framework for dyslexia research? *Cognition, 35*(2), 159–182.
Nicolson, R. I., Fawcett, A. J., & Dean, P. (2001). Dyslexia, development and the cerebellum. *Trends in Neuroscience, 24*(9), 515–516.
O'Brien, J., Spencer, J., Atkinson, J., Braddick, O., & Wattam-Bell, J. (2002). Form and motion coherence processing in dyspraxia: Evidence of a global spatial processing deficit. *Neuroreport, 13*(11), 1399–1402.
Olson, R., & Datta, H. (2002). Visual-temporal processing in reading-disabled and normal twins. *Reading and Writing, 15*(1–2), 127–149.
Paterson, S. J., Brown, J. H., Gsödl, M. K., Johnson, M. H., & Karmiloff-Smith, A. (1999). Cognitive modularity and genetic disorders. *Science, 286*(5448), 2355–2358.
Paulesu, E., Démonet, J.-F., Fazio, F., McCrory, E., Chanoine, V., Brunswick, N., Cappa, S. F., Cossu, G., Habib, M., Frith, C. D., & Frith, U. (2001). Dyslexia: Cultural diversity and biological unity. *Science, 291*, 2165–2167.
Paulesu, E., Frith, U., Snowling, M., Gallagher, A., Morton, J., Frackowiak, R. S. J., & Frith, C. D. (1996). Is developmental dyslexia a disconnection syndrome? Evidence from PET scanning. *Brain, 119*, 143–157.
Peiffer, A. M., Dunleavy, C. K., Frenkel, M., Gabel, L. A., LoTurco, J. J., Rosen, G. D., & Fitch, R. H. (2001). Impaired detection of variable duration embedded tones in ectopic NZB/BINJ mice. *Neuroreport, 12*(13), 2875–2879.
Peiffer, A. M., Rosen, G. D., & Fitch, R. H. (2002a). Rapid auditory processing and MGN morphology in microgyric rats reared in varied acoustic environments. *Brain Research. Developmental Brain Research, 138*(2), 187–193.
Peiffer, A. M., Rosen, G. D., & Fitch, R. H. (2002b). Sex differences in rapid auditory processing deficits in ectopic BXSB/MpJ mice. *Neuroreport, 13*(17), 2277–2280.
Plante, E., Swisher, L., Vance, R., & Rapcsak, S. (1991). MRI findings in boys with specific language impairment. *Brain and Language, 41*(1), 52–66.

Poldrack, R. A., Wagner, A. D., Prull, M. W., Desmond, J. E., Glover, G. H., & Gabrieli, J. D. (1999). Functional specialization for semantic and phonological processing in the left inferior prefrontal cortex. *Neuroimage, 10*(1), 15–35.

Rae, C., Harasty, J. A., Dzendrowskyj, T. E., Talcott, J. B., Simpson, J. M., Blamire, A. M., Dixon, R. M., Lee, M. A., Thompson, C. H., Styles, P., Richardson, A. J., & Stein, J. F. (2002). Cerebellar morphology in developmental dyslexia. *Neuropsychologia, 40*(8), 1285–1292.

Rae, C., Lee, M. A., Dixon, R. M., Blamire, A. M., Thompson, C. H., Styles, P., Talcott, J., Richardson, A. J., & Stein, J. F. (1998). Metabolic abnormalities in developmental dyslexia detected by 1H magnetic resonance spectroscopy. *Lancet, 351*(9119), 1849–1852.

Ramus, F. (2003). Developmental dyslexia: Specific phonological deficit or general sensorimotor dysfunction? *Current Opinion in Neurobiology, 13*(2), 212–218.

Ramus, F., Rosen, S., Dakin, S. C., Day, B. L., Castellote, J. M., White, S., & Frith, U. (2003). Theories of developmental dyslexia: Insights from a multiple case study of dyslexic adults. *Brain, 126*(4), 841–865.

Robichon, F., & Habib, M. (1998). Abnormal callosal morphology in male adult dyslexics: Relationships to handedness and phonological abilities. *Brain and Language, 62*(1), 127–146.

Roof, R. L., Duvdevani, R., Braswell, L., & Stein, D. G. (1994). Progesterone facilitates cognitive recovery and reduces secondary neuronal loss caused by cortical contusion injury in male rats. *Experimental Neurology, 129*(1), 64–69.

Rosen, G. D., Herman, A. E., & Galaburda, A. M. (1999). Sex differences in the effects of early neocortical injury on neuronal size distribution of the medial geniculate nucleus in the rat are mediated by perinatal gonadal steroids. *Cerebral Cortex, 9*(1), 27–34.

Rosen, G. D., Sherman, G. F., Mehler, C., Emsbo, K., & Galaburda, A. M. (1989). The effect of developmental neuropathology on neocortical asymmetry in New Zealand black mice. *International Journal of Neuroscience, 45*(3–4), 247–254.

Rosen, G. D., Waters, N. S., Galaburda, A. M., & Denenberg, V. H. (1995). Behavioral consequences of neonatal injury of the neocortex. *Brain Research, 681*(1–2), 177–189.

Rosen, S. (2003). Auditory processing in dyslexia and specific language impairment: Is there a deficit? What is its nature? Does it explain anything? *Journal of Phonetics, 31*, 509–527.

Rumsey, J. M., Casanova, M., Mannheim, G. B., Patronas, N., De Vaughn, N., Hamburger, S. D., & Aquino, T. (1996). Corpus callosum morphology, as measured with MRI, in dyslexic men. *Biological Psychiatry, 39*(9), 769–775.

Schrott, L. M., Denenberg, V. H., Sherman, G. F., Waters, N. S., Rosen, G. D., & Galaburda, A. M. (1992). Environmental enrichment, neocortical ectopias, and behavior in the autoimmune NZB mouse. *Brain Research. Developmental Brain Research, 67*(1), 85–93.

Scott, S. K., & Johnsrude, I. S. (2003). The neuroanatomical and functional organization of speech perception. *Trends in Neuroscience, 26*(2), 100–107.

Shalev, R. S., & Gross-Tsur, V. (2001). Developmental dyscalculia. *Pediatric Neurology, 24*(5), 337–342.

Shaywitz, B. A., Shaywitz, S. E., Pugh, K. R., Mencl, W. E., Fulbright, R. K., Skudlarski, P., Constable, R. T., Marchione, K. E., Fletcher, J. M., Lyon, G. R., & Gore, J. C. (2002). Disruption of posterior brain systems for reading in children with developmental dyslexia. *Biological Psychiatry, 52*(2), 101–110.

Shaywitz, S. E., Shaywitz, B. A., Fletcher, J. M., & Escobar, M. D. (1990). Prevalence of reading disability in boys and girls. Results of the Connecticut longitudinal study. *Journal of the American Medical Association, 264*(8), 998–1002.

Shaywitz, S. E., Shaywitz, B. A., Pugh, K. R., Fulbright, R. K., Constable, R. T., Mencl, W. E., Shankweiler, D. P., Liberman, A. M., Skudlarski, P., Fletcher, J. M., Katz, L., Marchione, K. E., Lacadie, C., Gatenby, C., & Gore, J. C. (1998). Functional disruption in the organization of the brain for reading in dyslexia. *Proceedings of the National Academy of Sciences of the United States of America, 95*(5), 2636–2641.

Sherman, G. F., Morrison, L., Rosen, G. D., Behan, P. O., & Galaburda, A. M. (1990). Brain abnormalities in immune defective mice. *Brain Research, 532*(1–2), 25–33.

Sherman, G. F., Stone, L. V., Denenberg, V. H., & Beier, D. R. (1994). A genetic analysis of neocortical ectopias in New Zealand black autoimmune mice. *Neuroreport, 5*(6), 721–724.

Simos, P. G., Breier, J. I., Wheless, J. W., Maggio, W. W., Fletcher, J. M., Castillo, E. M., & Papanicolaou, A. C. (2000). Brain mechanisms for reading: The role of the superior temporal gyrus in word and pseudoword naming. *Neuroreport, 11*(11), 2443–2447.

Simos, P. G., Fletcher, J. M., Foorman, B. R., Francis, D. J., Castillo, E. M., Davis, R. N., Fitzgerald, M., Mathes, P. G., Denton, C., & Papanicolaou, A. C. (2002). Brain activation profiles during the early stages of reading acquisition. *Journal of Child Neurology, 17*(3), 159–163.

Snowling, M. J. (2000). *Dyslexia* (2nd ed.). Oxford: Blackwell.

Spencer, J., O'Brien, J., Riggs, K., Braddick, O., Atkinson, J., & Wattam-Bell, J. (2000). Motion processing in autism: Evidence for a dorsal stream deficiency. *Neuroreport, 11*(12), 2765–2767.

Stein, J. F. (2001). The magnocellular theory of developmental dyslexia. *Dyslexia, 7*(1), 12–36.

Stein, J. F., & Walsh, V. (1997). To see but not to read: The magnocellular theory of dyslexia. *Trends in Neuroscience, 20*(4), 147–152.

Stromswold, K. (2000). The cognitive neuroscience of language acquisition. In M. S. Gazzaniga (Ed.), *The new cognitive neurosciences*. Cambridge, MA: MIT Press.

Tallal, P. 1980. Auditory temporal perception, phonics, and reading disabilities in children. *Brain and Language, 9*(2), 182–198.

Temple, E. (2002). Brain mechanisms in normal and dyslexic readers. *Current Opinion in Neurobiology, 12*(2), 178–183.

Thomas, M. S. C., & Karmiloff-Smith, A. (2002). Are developmental disorders like cases of adult brain damage? Implications from connectionist modelling. *Behavioral and Brain Sciences, 25*(6), 727–788.

Tomblin, J. B., & Pandich, J. (1999). Lessons from children with specific language impairment. *Trends in Cognitive Science, 3*(8), 283–285.

van der Lely, H. K. J., Rosen, S., & McClelland, A. (1998). Evidence for a grammar-specific deficit in children. *Current Biology, 8*(23), 1253–1258.

van der Lely, H. K. J., & Stollwerk, L. (1997). Binding theory and grammatical specific language impairment in children. *Cognition, 62,* 245–290.

Vargha-Khadem, F., & Polkey, C. E. (1992). A review of cognitive outcome after hemidecortication in humans. In F. D. Rose & D. A. Johnson (Eds.), *Recovery from brain damage. Reflections and directions* (pp. 137–151). New York: Plenum Press.

Wang, Y., Paramasivam, M., Thomas, A., Bai, J., Rosen, G. D., Galaburda, A. M., & LoTurco, J. J. (submitted). Neuronal migration and the dyslexia susceptibility gene Dyx1c1.

Waters, N. S., Sherman, G. F., Galaburda, A. M., & Denenberg, V. H. (1997). Effects of cortical ectopias on spatial delayed-matching-to-sample performance in BXSB mice. *Behavioural Brain Research, 84*(1–2), 23–29.

Wolf, M., Goldberg-O'Rourke, A., Gidney, C., Lovett, M., Cirino, P., & Morris, R. (2002). The second deficit: An investigation of the independence of phonological and naming-speed deficits in developmental dyslexia. *Reading and Writing, 15*(1–2), 43–72.

Section • II

The Genetics of Dyslexia and Cortical Development

INTRODUCTION

Interest in the role of genetics in developmental dyslexia began in the mid 1980s with the first reports of linkage between dyslexia and chromosomal intervals. Over the years, there have been intervals on at least six chromosomes implicated. This provides us with a few interesting clues about developmental dyslexia in general and its genetic underpinnings in specific. The fact that there are at least six (and probably many more) genes is clearly indicative that developmental dyslexia is a very complex disorder. As has been demonstrated in the first section of this book, reading itself is a very complex task for the brain to accomplish, and there are likely to be many different ways to affect a brain that could result in difficulty in reading. Each of these changes in brain organization could be the result of one or more genes, so it is, therefore, not so surprising that nailing down the genetic basis of developmental dyslexia has proven to be difficult.

That being said, some candidate genes have been identified in the past few years. The first dyslexia susceptibility candidate gene, DYX1C1, which is located on Chromosome 15 and was identified in 2004 by Finnish researchers, is the subject of the first two chapters in this section. In the first, Cecilia Marino and Massimo Molteni present their careful work examining the genetics of dyslexia in their population of Italian developmental dyslexics. They report that they are unable to replicate the findings of the Finnish group, and suggest that, at least in their Italian population, DYX1C1 is not a dyslexia susceptibility gene. That there *is* a dyslexia susceptibility gene located on Chromosome 15 is without question, but at this point, Marino and Molteni (as well as others) have their doubts as to its specific identity.

In light of the data reported by Marino and Molteni, the chapter by Joe LoTurco and colleagues is intriguing. We know from previous work (see Fitch & Peiffer, and Galaburda, this volume) that small malformations of the cerebral cortex have been associated with developmental dyslexia. These anomalies are the result of problems during the process whereby neurons migrate from their place of origin (near the cerebral ventricle) to their final destination in the cerebral cortex. As it turns out, this process of cerebral cortex migration is quite complex, and is under the control of dozens of genes. In their chapter, LoTurco et al. report on their novel technique of using interference RNA (RNAi) to knock down the expression of genes in neurons at critical stages of development, in this case, right when these neurons are getting ready to leave the area around the ventricle and migrate to the cerebral cortex. Specifically, they transfect neurons with RNAi against DYX1C1 and monitor the movement of those neurons. As it turns out, those neurons that no longer express this purported dyslexia susceptibility gene do not complete their migration to the cerebral cortex. This is the first direct link between a dyslexia susceptibility gene and the type of cerebral cortical malformations seen in postmortem dyslexics.

Malformations of the cerebral cortex are not limited, of course, to selected cases of developmental dyslexia. In fact, there are many disorders of the nervous system that are characterized by problems with neuronal migration to the cerebral cortex, including epilepsy and lissencephaly. Joe Gleeson is one of the pioneers in the study of the genes that control neuronal migration, and in his chapter, he presents a review of some of his detailed work involving the basic cellular events and critical proteins involved in this complicated process. In addition, he reports his investigations of the intriguing Joubert syndrome, which is a defect in brain wiring in the cortico-spinal tract. What do these discussions have to do with developmental dyslexia? This chapter is a good demonstration of how synergy across various disciplines of neuroscience can occur. Although Gleeson's laboratory does not study dyslexia per se, his understanding of the process of neuronal migration can have a profound impact on how those of us who do study dyslexia view our own research. Something as seemingly far afield as Joubert syndrome may also prove useful to those of us curious as to how aberrant connections are formed in the developing brain (see Pugh et al., Galaburda, this volume).

Along these lines, the laboratory of Eduardo Soriano uses a different approach to examine the genes implicated in the development of the cerebral cortex. To do this, they have collected a library of genes that are expressed in the outermost layer of the cerebral cortex, which is where most of the signaling controlling cortical development takes place. They then compare these genes to those that are expressed in the lower layer of the cortex. By determining which of the genes in the upper layer are overexpressed compared to the lower layers, they believe they can get a handle on some novel genes that modulate cortical development. Their preliminary evidence on some of those genes are reported here, and there are undoubtedly more to be described in the future.

As mentioned before, developmental dyslexia is a complex disorder and attempts to dissect this trait using standard genetic techniques may prove quite difficult. One of the advantages of conducting research in today's climate is that we have access to a wealth of information concerning the genome that was not previously available. Moreoever, the easy access to statistical and bioinformatic tools allow us to begin to probe the genome for answers to complex questions. One of the leading practitioners of complex trait analysis (or the systems genetics approach) is Rob Williams, who, in the last chapter of this section, uses a suite of bioinformatic tools to begin to evaluate various candidates for dyslexia susceptibility genes. As these tools continue to mature, and as the databases underlying them continue to develop, one can easily envision the profound impact they will have on the study of complex traits like developmental dyslexia.

Chapter • 5

Chromosome 15 and Developmental Dyslexia

Cecilia Marino and Massimo Molteni

DEVELOPMENTAL DYSLEXIA

Developmental dyslexia (DD) is a specific learning disability diagnosed in children who fail to develop normal reading skills in spite of normal intelligence, adequate motivation, and schooling (DSM IV). It is a common condition, the estimated prevalence (5%–17.5%) depending on the cutoff imposed on the normal distribution of reading ability. The leading criterion to diagnose dyslexia remains that of a reading performance below the population mean (typically, a reading score 2 standard deviations below the general population mean). While reading performance is normally distributed in the population, the prevalence of dyslexia will vary enormously across different cultures because it depends on the specific complexity of the orthographic rules of the subject's given language. Accordingly, for a population like the Italians, exposed to a "shallow" (i.e., transparent) orthography, the prevalence of DD is half that of the U.S. population that is exposed to an orthography where the mapping between letters, speech sounds, and whole-word sounds is much more ambiguous and "deep."

THE GENETICS OF DEVELOPMENTAL DYSLEXIA

The focus of molecular genetics is to search for DNA variants that make probable the appearance of a certain phenotype. We may define a trait or a disease status as a phenotype only if genetic determinants have been demonstrated to play a significant role in the causation of it. Early description of developmental dyslexia referred to a familial aggregation of the disorder that appeared to be higher than chance among first-degree relatives of dyslexic probands. It was soon clear, however, that a disorder of reading could be influenced by cultural factors transmitted from parents to their offspring, or be the result of an inferior educational environment.

Whenever family studies are indicative of a higher morbidity risk among family members of an affected proband, twin studies have proven to be a powerful tool to help unravel the relative contribution of genetic and environmental factors. Twin studies confirmed significantly higher correlations of DD among monozygotic than dizygotic twins, which supports a substantial genetic contribution to the disease. Data from the Colorado Learning Disabilities Research Centre (CLDRC) provide evidence of significant genetic influences on deficits in some reading-related processes such as word recognition, orthographic coding, phonological decoding, and phonological awareness with estimates of heritability ranging from .45–.61 (DeFries, Fulker, & LaBuda, 1987; Gayan & Olson, 1999). Also, the normal variation on the distribution of common reading-related measures appears to be substantially determined by shared genetic factors.

Behavioral genetic analyses provided irrefutable evidence that we may treat both DD and its reading-related measures as phenotypes, thus allowing the search for causative genes. The question that arises instantly is, are we looking for genes that underlie a normal ability in the normal population whose variants are able to determine specifically a deficit in that ability? Or, are genetic variants that cause the deficit in the neuropsychological process not the same as those underlying the normal process? And still further, do genetic variants underlying the neuropsychological processes act together, and in what proportion, to determine the clinical entity of DD? Which genetic variants are necessary? Which are sufficient? Do they play in an additive manner with some sort of priority?

Segregation analyses of reading ability in the normal range produced evidence of a major gene with dominance; the putative dominant allele frequency is .35 with 57% of the population carrying at least one copy of this allele. This common allele, with low penetrance, accounts for 54% of the phenotypic variance in reading scores (Gilger, Borecki, DeFries, & Pennington, 1994). Segregation analyses of DD revealed a pattern of transmission of the disease consistent with Mendelian inheritance with evidence of a major gene transmission (Pennington et al., 1991). Another approach has been to estimate the number of quantitative trait loci (QTLs) and the most parsimonious patterns of inheritance contributing to the continuous reading-related phenotypes that have gained general consensus as the critical elements in DD. For example, evidence was found for one or two genes of at least modest effect contributing to phonological decoding-related phenotypes (i.e. "phonemic decoding" and "word attack"). Furthermore, a dominant major gene and a polygenic model, respectively, were found to best explain the transmission within families of the variation of these traits (Chapman, Raskind, Thomson, Berninger, & Wijsman, 2003).

What we have sidestepped until this point is that the genetic framework of DD is quite heterogeneous. Speaking metaphorically, when we apply molecular genetic strategies such as linkage or association analyses, in order to search for the underlying genes of DD, we must know that we are dealing with a kaleidoscope rather than a telescope.

The definition of the phenotype in linkage studies becomes, then, a crucial point. To summarize, three phenotypes appear to be comprehensive of the puzzling nature of the etiology of this disorder: (1) the normal variation of a reading phenotype in a randomly selected sample from general population, (2) the variation in the lower tail of the distribution of reading-related phenotypes, and (3) the discrete clinical entity of DD, with a standardized and shared criterion, which refers to a threshold on the quantitative normal distribution of the normal reading phenotype.

The neuropsychological component processes that showed a substantial heritability and a high correlation with the diagnosis of DD were mainly measures of phonological awareness, phonological decoding, orthographic coding, rapid automatic naming, word and nonwords spelling, and single-word reading. These measures have shown across studies a pattern of high inter-trait correlation, which raised the question of how to manage these phenotypes in linkage studies. In some cases, they have been collapsed into composite scores, with an evident statistical advantage but doubtful appropriateness. Recently, a number of twin studies addressed the ubiquitous need to obtain insights into the relationships between the effects that genetic factors have on each of these correlated phenotypes. Overall, these studies suggest that, given two correlated phenotypes, there may be genes shared by both phenotypes with additional genes uniquely influencing the variation of one of the two (Gayan & Olson, 2003). A detailed consideration of this literature throws lights on the issue of the genetic heterogeneity of DD and lays the foundations to plan more accurate linkage mapping studies through the identification of more homogenous phenotypes.

DYSLEXIA AND CHROMOSOME 15

Robust results have come from molecular genetic studies of DD on chromosome 15. These were prompted by an initial evidence of a 3.24 lod-score in a parametric linkage study of chromosome 15 in three-generation pedigrees segregating DD, which used heteromorphisms of the centromere region as markers (Smith, Kimberling, Pennington, & Lubs, 1983). These results, however, were not confirmed by two similar, successive studies (Bisgaard, Eiberg, Moller, Niebuhr, & Mohr, 1987; Rabin et al., 1993). In a more recent study, Smith, Kimberling, and Pennington (1991) replicated the earlier finding with markers within the 15q15-15qter region, using both a quantitative and qualitative phenotype definition of DD and a nonparametric approach (the Haseman-Elston regression model). Linkage within the 15q15-15qter region was further confirmed in a nonparametric analysis using the De Fries-Fulker regression approach and a quantitative definition of DD (Fulker, 1991).

Grigorenko et al. (1997) examined six multiplex families (n = 94) where probands were selected on the basis of childhood reading scores that placed them in the bottom 10% of the population. Four phenotypes have been described for each member of the families by two tests each: phonological awareness, phonological decoding, single-word reading, and rapid automatized naming. For each phenotype, an affected status was defined if scores were below the normative 10th percentile or 25th percentile on both tests used. A fifth phenotype was used; the discrepancy construct. Parametric and nonparametric linkage analyses were performed: a lod score of 3.15 was found in single-point linkage parametric analysis between the microsatellite D15S143 and "single-word reading" component of reading performance. For markers toward p-ter, the lod scores were generally positive. However, markers on the q-ter side of D15S143 were significantly negative. Multipoint analyses were positive but not significant. In the same study, nonparametric analyses yielded generally negative results although a significant result was obtained for D15S128 marker.

Schulte-Korne et al. (1998) examined seven multiplex families selected from a larger sample if they had an extended family history of spelling disability and at least a three-generation history of familial spelling problems. The affected status was defined based on a spelling achievement 1 SD below expected level or if they had a history of spelling disorder (on the basis of a questionnaire). Parametric and nonparametric linkage analyses were performed with 13 markers covering the whole chromosome 15 and a lod score of 1.26 (parametric) and of 2.19 (nonparametric multipoint) were found with marker D15S143. A multipoint lod score of 1.78 ($p = .0042$) was achieved at D15S132.

A two-stage, family-based association study was performed to investigate further this putative area of linkage (Morris et al., 2000). Single and multimarkers analyses were run between DD and six markers covering an area of 8 cM. Linkage disequilibrium was detected between DD and the haplotype D15S146/ D15S214/ D15S994, which includes an area of around 1cM within the putative region of linkage.

Recently, a lod score of 2.34 was identified within the same region of linkage peak with the phenotype "single-word reading" in a parametric linkage analyses of 111 families segregating dyslexia (Chapman et al., 2004).

DYX1C1: A Dyslexia Susceptibility Gene on Chromosome 15

Nopola-Hemmi et al. (2000) described a first two-generation family in which a translocation t(2;15) (q11;q21) cosegregates with reading problems in four members and a second family where a translocation t(2;15)(p13;q22) associates with dyslexia in one family member but not in three other translocation carriers. In the first pedigree, two females had dyslexia while one male suffered from an IQ below the normal range; the father was the latter carrier of the translocation for whom a history of profound difficulties in reading and writing had been described retrospectively. In the second pedigree, interestingly, one male carrying the translocation, with normal IQ and with no reading and writing problems, had two epileptic seizures and his EEG shows spike wave complexes over the right parietotemporal region. The FISH data suggest that both the independent translocation breakpoints on chromosome 15q map within 6-8 Mb of each other, residing in the region limited by the markers D15S143 and D15S1029.

The translocation breakpoint of the first pedigree has been further refined and the breakpoint was pinpointed to a region of 3229 bp. This interval includes exons 8 and 9 of a novel gene, DYX1C1, and there is also a 301-bp AT-rich region, known to occur at many chromosomal rearrangement sites. DYX1C1 contains 10 exons spanning about 78 kb of genomic DNA and it encodes for a predicted protein of 420 amino acids. The human DYX1C1 protein has three C-terminal tetratrico-peptide repeat (TPR) domains, a structural motif consisting of 34 amino acids residues that mediates protein-protein interactions (cell cycle regulation, transcriptional control, mitochondrial and peroxisomal protein transport, neurogenesis, and protein folding). Eight SNPs were identified by direct sequencing, five of which were in the coding region (4C>T, 270 G>A, 572 G>A, 1249 G>T, 1259 C>G), whereas three resided in the 5' untranslated region (-164C>T, -3G>A, -2G>A). An association was found between DD and alleles -3A and 1249T in a case-control sample (corrected p-values 0.016 and 0.048, respectively). Furthermore, the -3A/1249T haplotype was associated with DD in the case-control sample (p = 0.015) and in nine informative trios (transmission disequilibrium test, p = 0.025 (Taipale et al., 2003). The coding SNP, 1249C → T, truncates the protein by four amino acids while the -3G → A is located in the binding sequence of the transcription factors Elk-1, HSTF, and TFII-I, suggesting functional effects for the associated SNPs. For the first time, a candidate gene has been found to be associated with DD and the variants specifically associated with the disease probably code for a protein with altered function.

Questions about DYX1C1

The first question this amazing result raised was, does DYX1C1 lie within the region where the linkage peaks have been found (Smith et al., 1991; Grigorenko et al., 1997; Schulte-Korne et al., 1998)? Is it in linkage disequilibrium with markers previously found to be associated with DD? Within the boundaries of uncertainty of linkage maps, the breakpoint may be located about 7,8 Mb distally from the peaks of two linkage studies (D15S143) and around 15 Mb distally from the area covered by the haplotype D15S146/D15S214/D15S994, (about 500 kb) that was associated with DD (Morris et al., 2000). More studies are needed to better define the reciprocal distances between these markers/haplotypes and DYX1C1, but it seems that they do not share overlapping regions (Figure 1).

The finding of an involvement of the 15q15-15qter chromosomal region in DD was further investigated in an Italian-speaking population by a transmission/disequilibrium approach in 121 parent-offspring families (Marino et al., 2004). Probands' diagnosis of DD was based on the *Diagnostic and Statistical Manual of Mental Disorders, Fourth Edition* (*DSM–IV*) criteria, confirmed by an extensive clinical investigation that encompassed a careful medical as-

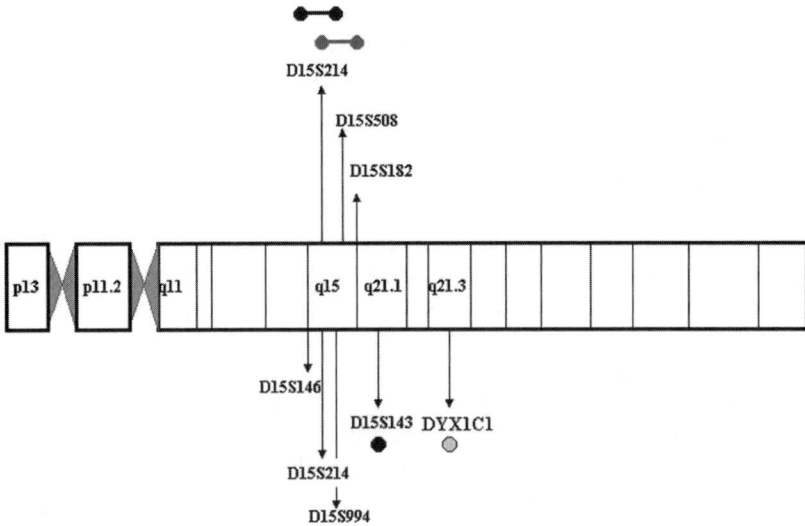

Figure 1. Schematic representation of the regions on chromosome 15q where the linkage and association signals were found. DYX1C1 (gray dot) lies around 7.8 Mb distally from the region where two linkage signals were found with D15S143 (black dot), and around 15 Mb distally from the haplotype associated with dyslexia in the English sample (black line) and 11 Mb from the area associated in the Italian sample (gray line).

sessment and a battery of reading relevant tests. Inclusion criteria were (1) performance on timed text-reading tests of a reading score 2 standard deviations below the general population mean in terms of accuracy and/or speed; (2) a reading score 1.5 standard deviation below the general population mean on at least one of the previous parameters, *and* an absolute score 2 standard deviations below the general population mean on accuracy or speed in reading single unrelated words or pronounceable nonwords; and (3) an IQ greater than 85. These criteria go beyond the *DSM–IV* criteria for dyslexia and emphasize the phonological disturbance as a core characteristic. This approach allows the detection of reading disability even in a "shallow" orthography such as Italian, which is more dyslexia-friendly and invites different word decoding strategies than deep orthographies like English.

It should be noted that because of transparent orthography, Italian words can generally be read both via the indirect, phonological route, and/or via the direct, lexical route, the latter probably being more involved in the case of highly familiar, high-frequency words. In contrast, word spelling requires more detailed orthographic knowledge, as phonologically plausible, but orthographically incorrect alternatives are sometimes possible in the written form. Therefore, only word spelling and sentence writing under dictation have been taken to represent the use of lexical, orthographic knowledge. Nonword reading and spelling, on the other hand, both require and measure, as it is usually assumed, access to phonological conversion rules (the phonological route).

The Transmission Disequilibrium Test (TDT) is a test of linkage in the presence of association, with greater power than other within-family association tests, and robustness against stratification bias (Spielman, McGinnis, & Ewens, 1993). It is based on the biased transmission of the risk allele (usually the variant allele) compared to the transmission of the nonrisk allele from the heterozygous parent to the affected child. The null hypothesis of no linkage and no association is that each allele has equal probability to be transmitted to the affected child from the heterozygous parent (random segregation). The alternative hypothesis of linkage and association between the marker and the disease alleles is that the probability that the risk allele is transmitted to the affected child is greater than 50% (for biallelic markers). The TDT was performed using the FBAT program <http://www.biostat.harvard.edu/~fbat/fbat.htm>, while for multiple markers' haplotype transmission, we used the program TRANSMIT version 2.5.4 < http://www.gene.cimr.cam.ac.uk/clayton/software/>.

Six microsatellite markers defining allelic variation across a 9 Mb region were chosen: D15S214, D15S994, D15S508, D15S182, D15S132, and D15S1028. In single-markers analyses, D15S214 was the only marker to approach significance for linkage disequilibrium with DD (p-value is 3.75 times above the corrected threshold). The results of TRANSMIT analyses with two-marker haplotypes indicate that the pattern of significance varies across the 15 possible combinations with mild trends toward linkage disequilibrium for combinations D15S214/D15S508, D15S214/D15S182 (p-values are 4.7 and 5.7 times above the corrected threshold, respectively).

We also examined the rate of transmission from parents to affected offspring of the 20 combinations of the three-marker haplotypes, the maximum number tolerated by TRANSMIT. Statistically significant evidence was obtained with the combination D15S214/D15S508/D15S182 (global χ^2= 25.451, df = 9, p = 0.0025; p-corrected for multiple tests = 0.05); haplotype 6-1-7 of the combination D15S214/D15S508/D15S182: showed a trend toward linkage disequilibrium (χ^2 = 6.99, df =1, p = 0.008, p corrected for nine tests = 0.07). This haplotype encompasses a region spanning around 4.3 Mb, approximately 4 cM, that partly overlaps the area where Morris et al. (2000) found a linkage disequilibrium in the English sample (Figure 1). Within the approximation of linkage maps, the area found to be associated with DD in the Italian sample maps about 11 Mb proximal from DYX1C1. The replication of the linkage signal in a population exposed to a shallow orthography such as Italian is of great importance to the field because it provides strength to the hypothesis that DD is a heritable disorder independent of linguistic differences. Until now, these findings had been reported for populations with deeper orthographies such as English and, to a less extent, German.

Support for DYX1C1 as contributing to DD was recently found in a sample of 148 families identified through a proband with reading difficulties (Wigg et al., 2004). Evidence for linkage disequilibrium with DD was found for the rs11629841 polymorphism in intron 4 and haplotypes of this polymorphism. However, quantitative analyses of reading and reading-related phenotypes were significant for the -3G allele, which contrasts with the original finding of Taipale et al. (2003) of an association with the alternative allele -3A of this polymorphism. Moreover, a linkage disequilibrium was found between DD and the most frequent and normal -3G/1249G haplotype, instead of the originally reported association with the more rare variant -3A/1249T haplotype.

Conversely, association between DYX1C1 and dyslexia was not replicated in a large sample of sibling pairs from UK (Scerri et al., 2004).

The relevance of DYX1C1 for DD was also investigated in 158 Italian nuclear families with 171 probands (Marino et al., 2005). Association studies are the appropriate statistical approach to detect genes with a small effect on the phenotypic variance. We adopted the within-family design to overcome spurious associations due to population stratification effects. The first aim of the study was to verify the association of the -3A and 1249 T alleles with DD found by Taipale et al. (2003). We also performed single and multimarker quantitative analyses with neuropsychological components of the dyslexic profile, since this strategy may improve the detection of the linkage signal and lead to a better understanding of the heterogeneity of DD.

Probands were administered a battery of reading relevant tests. Seven different phenotypic measures were then identified, including Phonological Decoding Accuracy and Speed, Orthographic Coding, Word Reading Accuracy and Speed, Word Spelling, and Nonword Spelling.

No single SNP showed significant association with either DD as a diagnostic category or the normalized quantitative phenotypes at the 0.017 (adjusted for three markers) and 0.002 (adjusted for three markers x seven phenotypes) significance levels, respectively. No haplotype showed significant association with either DD as a diagnostic category or the normalized measures of the neuropsychological phenotypes at the 0.013 (adjusted for four haplotypes) and 0.002 (adjusted for four haplotypes x seven phenotypes) significance levels, respectively.

We also examined the haplotype association of the combination -3G>A/1249G>T/1259C>G by TRANSMIT. Since data from all families can be used by TRANSMIT, 158 families were informative for this test, with no evidence of an association. We also ran the haplotype analyses for the combination -3G>A/1249 G>T with no evidence of an association. Thus, our association study did not confirm the importance of DYX1C1 in a sample of Italian dyslexics. According to our power calculations for disease status, the conditional power of our sample at a significance level of 5% is 80%, thereby lending support against false negative results.

CONCLUSIONS

Chromosome 15 is certainly involved in the etiology of DD. DYX1C1 has been identified as a causative gene, although it does not seem to be a necessary gene. The effect of DYX1C1 on DD is quite small and difficult to detect, but the association design is surely the most appropriate to detect such an effect in the population. The reason we failed to find it is probably due to the genetic heterogeneity of DD. DYX1C1 probably plays a role either within special population subgroups or within specific dyslexics' subtypes. More research is needed to clarify the relative relevance of this gene for DD along with the identification of the phenotypic framework associated with it.

On the other hand, it seems that there is another region on chromosome 15 with a clear linkage signal with DD that does not overlap with DYX1C1. This linked region seems to map within 15q15.1-15.3 while DYX1C1 lies within 15q21.3. The15q15.1-15.3 region probably contains one or more genes with a greater genetic effect than DYX1C1 but has yet to be identified. A great number of known genes lie within this area with functions that could possibly be related to DD. Nevertheless, only a precise a priori knowledge of the fine etiopathogenetic mechanisms of DD would allow the selection of the appropriate candidate genes for association studies. Searching for candidate genes within a smaller linkage disequilibrium peak area would certainly raise the chance that the selection hits directly the genes involved.

Future research efforts should converge toward increasing the markers' density within the region 15q15.1-15.3 and toward the construction here of a more densely refined linkage disequilibrium map for DD.

Address correspondence to: Ceclia Marino, M.D., Scientific Institute Eugenio Medea, Department of Child Psychopathology, Association "La Nostra Famiglia," 20 Don Luigi Monza Bossiso Parini Lecco 23842, Italy; E-mail: cmarino@bp.lnf.it

REFERENCES

Bisgaard, M. L., Eiberg, H., Moller, N., Niebuhr, E., & Mohr, J. (1987). Dyslexia and chromosome 15 heteromorphism: Negative LOD score in a Danish material. *Clinical Genetics, 32*, 118–119.

Chapman, N. H., Raskind, W. H., Thomson, J. B., Berninger, V. W., & Wijsman, E. M. (2003). Segregation analysis of phenotypic components of learning disabilities. II. Phonological decoding. *American Journal of Medical Genetics, 15*, 121B(1), 60–70.

Chapman, N. H., Igo, R. P., Thomson, J. B., Matsushita, M., Brkanac, Z., Holzman, T., Berninger, V. W., Wijsman, E. M., & Raskind, W. H. (2004). Linkage analyses of four regions previously implicated in dyslexia: Confirmation of a locus on chromosome 15q. *American Journal of Medical Genetics Part B, Neuropsychiatric Genetics, 15*, 131(1), 67–75.

DeFries, J. C., Fulker, D. W., & LaBuda, M. C. (1987). Evidence for a genetic aetiology in reading disability of twins. *Nature, 329*(6139), 537–539.

Fulker, D. W. (1991). Multiple regression of sib-pair data on reading to detect quantitative trait loci. *Reading and Writing, 3*, 299–313.

Gayan, J., & Olson, R. K. (1999). Reading disability: evidence for a genetic etiology. *European Child Adolescent Psychiatry, 8*(Suppl. 3), 52–55.

Gayan, J., & Olson, R. K. (2003). Genetic and environmental influences on individual differences in printed word recognition. *Journal of Experimental Child Psychology, 84*(2), 97–123.

Gilger, J. W., Borecki, I. B., DeFries, J. C., & Pennington, B. F. (1994). Commingling and segregation analysis of reading performance in families of normal reading probands. *Behaviour Genetics, 24*(4), 345–355.

Grigorenko, E. L., Wood, F. B., Meyer, S. B., Hart, L. A., Speed, W. C., & Shuster, A. (1997). Susceptibility loci for distinct components of developmental dyslexia on chromosome 6 and 15. *American Journal of Human Genetics, 60*, 27–39.

Marino, C., Giorda, R., Vanzin, L., Nobile, M., Lorusso, M. L., Baschirotto, C., Riva, L., Molteni, M., & Battaglia, M. (2004). A locus on 15q15-15qter influences dyslexia: Further support from a transmission/disequilibrium study in an Italian speaking population. *Journal of Medical Genetics, 41*, 42–46.

Marino, C., Giorda, R., Lorusso, M. L., Vanzin, L., Salandi, N., Nobile, M., Citterio, A., Beri, S., Crespi, V., Battaglia, M., & Molteni, M. (2005). A family-based association study of the DYX1C1 gene on 15q21.1 in

Developmental Dyslexia. *European Journal of Human Genetics, 13*(4), 491–499.

Morris, D. W., Robinson, L., Turic, D., Duke, M., Webb, V., & Milham, C. (2000). Family-based association mapping provides evidence for a gene for reading disability on chromosome 15q. *Human Molecular Genetics, 9*, 843–848.

Nopola-Hemmi, J., Taipale, M., Haltia, T., Lehesjoki, A. E., Voutilainen, A., & Kere, J. (2000). Two translocations of chromosome 15q associated with dyslexia. *Journal of Medical Genetics, 37*, 771–775.

Pennington, B. F., Gilger, J. W., Pauls, D., Smith, S. A., Smith, S. D., & De Fries, J. C. (1991). Evidence for major gene transmission of developmental dyslexia. *Journal of the American Medical Assosciation, 18*, 1527–1534.

Rabin, M., Wen, X. L., Hepburn, M., Lubs, H. A., Feldman, E., & Duara, R. (1993). Suggestive linkage of developmental dyslexia to chromosome 1p34-p36. *Lancet, 342*, 178.

Scerri, T. S., Fisher, S. E., Francks, C., MacPhie, I. L., Paracchini, S., Richardson, A. J., Stein, J. F., & Monaco, A. P. (2004). Putative functional alleles of DYX1C1 are not associated with dyslexia susceptibility in a large sample of sibling pairs from the UK. *Journal of Medical Genetics, 41*(11), 853–857.

Schulte-Korne, G., Grimm, T., Nothen, M. M., Muller-Myhsok, B., Cichon, S., & Vogt, I. R. (1998). Evidence for linkage of spelling disability to chromosome 15. *American Journal of Human Genetics, 63*, 279–282.

Smith, S. D., Kimberling, W. J., Pennington, B. F., & Lubs, H. A. (1983). Specific reading disability-identification of an inherited form through linkage analysis. *Science, 219*, 1345.

Smith, S. D., Kimberling, W. J., & Pennington, B. F. (1991). Screening for multiple genes influencing dyslexia. *Reading and Writing, 3*, 285–298.

Spielman, R. S., McGinnis, R. E., & Ewens, W. J. (1993). Transmission test for linkage disequilibrium, the insulin gene region and insulin-dependent diabetes mellitus (IDDM). *American Journal of Human Genetics, 52*, 506–516.

Taipale, M., Kaminen, N., Nopola-Hemmi, J., Haltia, T., Myllyluoma, B., Lyytinen, H., Muller, K., Karranen, M., Lindsberg, P. J., Hannula-Jouppi, K., & Kere, J. (2003). A candidate gene for developmental dyslexia encodes a nuclear tetratricopeptide repeat domain protein dynamically regulated in brain. *Proceedings of the National Academy of Science, 100*, 11553–11558.

Wigg, K. G., Couto, J. M., Feng, Y., Anderson, B., Cate-Carter, T. D., Macciardi, F., Tannock, R., Lovett, M. W., Humphries, T. W., & Barr, C. L. (2004). Support for EKN1 as the susceptibility locus for dyslexia on 15q21. *Molecular Psychiatry* (Jul 13); advance online publication.

Chapter • 6

Neuronal Migration and Dyslexia Susceptibility

Joseph J. LoTurco, Yu Wang, and Murugan Paramasivam

INTRODUCTION

Developmental dyslexia is the most common learning disorder in children, yet the underlying biological causes are not known. Several neurobiological correlates of dyslexia have now been identified, and current challenges become determining which, if any, of these correlates cause dyslexia. Dyslexia is clearly linked to genetic susceptibility. To date, a minimum of eight chromosomal loci have been implicated in dyslexia susceptibility through linkage studies (see Williams, this volume). As with any disorder with genetic influences, once single candidate genes are identified, then progress can be made in identifying the causes of susceptibility to the disorder. For example, if one or more mutations within the specified dyslexia genetic loci can be directly linked to a neurobiological correlates of dyslexia, then this would aid in determining a causal chain of events underlying at least some dyslexias.

The recent identification of the first single gene candidate for dyslexia susceptibility (Taipale et al., 2003; Wigg et al., 2004), EKN1/DYX1C1, now offers molecular and developmental neurobiologists the first opportunity to begin to study the cellular function of a protein implicated in dyslexia, and perhaps to link a potential genetic risk for dyslexia with neurobiological causes. Previous studies of the neuroanatomy and neurophysiology of dyslexia have indicated that early changes in brain structure, occurring before birth, may predispose the brain to latter difficulties in language processing. Among these early changes are alterations in the normal migration of neocortical neurons in the brains of dyslexic individuals (Galaburda, 1993; Galaburda, this volume; Galaburda & Kemper, 1979; Galaburda, Sherman, Rosen, Aboitiz, & Geschwind, 1985). In this chapter, we will describe recent studies in our laboratory in which we have defined a critical role for DYX1C1 in the development and migration of neurons in the cerebral neocortex. Interference of dyx1c1 protein expression interrupts normal neuronal migration in the developing cerebral cortex. While additional human genetic studies are still needed to support and confirm the role of DYX1C1 in dyslexia, the cellular and developmental studies indicate that the first candidate dyslexia susceptibility gene plays an important role in neuronal migration.

NEOCORTICAL MALFORMATION

Many different types of neocortical malformations associate with anomalous neurological function. The morphologies and severities of these malformations are diverse and correspondingly can have diverse neurological affects. Some malformations such as lissencephaly, polymicrogyria, or double cortex syndrome are extensive, easily detectable by MRI, and generally cause severe mental retardation and epilepsy. Other malformation types are subtle, small, and may only be detectable with postmortem neuropathological studies. The presence of small focal cortical anomalies have been linked to a variety of neurological and psychiatric conditions; however, a causal link between these small malformations and abnormal function has not been firmly established. Similarly, while genetic mutations have been identified in a number of genes that cause many of the more sever malformation types, the genetic underpinnings of small focal anomalies have not yet been ascertained. A challenge of current studies is to match different types and severities of neocortical malformation with different pathophysiologies. Although a comprehensive explanatory scheme has not yet been established, a general theme currently emerging is that malformations of neocortex increase neural circuit excitability in the developing brain (Gabel & LoTurco, 2002; Zsombok & Jacobs, this volume).

ECTOPIAS AND NEOCORTICAL FUNCTION

Small malformations in neocortex are one of the described neurobiological correlates of dyslexia, the most common of which were small aggregates of neurons and glia, heterotopias, which form on the surface of neocortex. These superficial cellular groupings or heterotopias, called "ectopias," are also associated with disturbances in the arrangements of neurons below them in the normal neuronal layers of neocortex (Galaburda & Kemper, 1979; Galaburda et al., 1985). Ectopias are too small to observe with current imaging technologies, and so studying their physiology has depended on the use of animal models that contain ectopias with remarkably similar morphologies to those present in human dyslexic brains (Sherman, Rosen, Stone, Press, & Galaburda, 1992; see Galaburda, this volume).

In a series of experiments conducted by Lisa Gabel (Gabel & LoTurco, 2001, 2002), the cellular pathophysiology of ectopias in inbred strains of mice was studied. These neocortical ectopias studied in mice were found to increase the excitability of neocortical circuits adjacent to the malformations. Interestingly, microsurgical removal of ectopias did not eliminate enhanced excitability, suggesting that altered function extends beyond local regions of the malformation. It should be noted that cortical circuits adjacent to the ectopias appeared physiologically normal until the circuits were perturbed with low concentrations of convulsant drugs. Therefore, circuits surrounding ectopias are not normally spontaneously epileptic, but rather have functional anomalies that reveal a pathophysiology under certain conditions. This may indicate that ectopias in neocortex create a vulnerability to acquiring an anomalous functional state. In addition to changes in cellular neurophysiology, ectopias in animal models have also been shown to be associated with alterations in learning and sensory processing in otherwise genetically identical mice (Frenkel, Sherman, Bashan, Galaburda, & LoTurco, 2000; Peiffer et al., 2001; Peiffer, Rosen, & Fitch, 2002; see Fitch & Peiffer, this volume). This indicates that the occurrence of ectopias, like dyslexia itself, may occur at a higher frequency given a certain genetic background, but are not fully determined by genetics.

OVERVIEW OF NEURONAL MIGRATION IN NEOCORTICAL DEVELOPMENT

To understand the cellular and molecular mechanisms that could be disrupted to create neocortical malformations such as ectopias, it is useful to review the cellular movements and migrations that occur during development of neocortex. All of the principal neurons of the cerebral neocortex are generated during embryonic and fetal development from a single layer of dividing progenitor cells that surround the lateral ventricles of the embryonic and fetal brain (Rakic, 2000). After new neurons are generated from this layer of progenitor cells, they migrate away and form seven neuronal layers. The migration away from their site of generation proceeds in an ordered and patterned fashion. The inner and outermost layers are formed first, and then the intervening layers are formed outermost first to innermost last. This ordered migration is largely guided by specialized cells—radial glial cells—that span the entire width of the developing cortex. Radial glial cells are the progenitor cells that give rise to new neurons through cell division, and form a scaffold and path for migration (Rakic, 2000). The termination of migration also depends upon the integrity of radial glia. Interruptions or breaches in the superficial branches of radial glial cells that form the glial limitans at the surface of the embryonic brain can result in the formation of ectopias (Choi & Matthias, 1987; Sherman et al., 1992). Loss of radial glial cell integrity can, therefore, cause aberrations in migration anywhere along the neuronal migration path from the deep sites of neuronal generation to the superficial sites of normal migration termination. Normal neuronal migration is also dependent on intracellular mechanisms within newly generated neuronal cells that allow for cellular motility. Disruptions in neuronal motility, in radial glia, or in the adhesion between radial glial and new neurons can alter the normal developmental patterning and migration in neocortex.

GENETIC DISRUPTION OF NEURONAL MIGRATION IN NEOCORTEX

Severe neocortical malformations have been directly related to mutations in a number of different genes. These genetically based neuronal migration disorders in humans are varied, and have been shown to cause a variety of malformation types and result from interference in multiple genes (e.g., Sheen & Walsh, 2003). Understanding how these migration genes control formation and migration in neocortex during embryonic development is revealing the specific cellular and molecular mechanisms that coordinate the key cellular mechanisms necessary for normal neuronal migration. For example, mutations in the doublecortin gene or DCX, causes epilepsy and severe mental retardation (des Portes et al., 1998; Gleeson et al., 1998; see Gleeson, this volume). DCX protein stabilizes tubulin within migrating neurons and is essential to cytoskeletal restructuring that must occur for normal neuronal motility. Mutation of DCX causes premature cessation of neuronal migration that results in double cortex syndrome and lisscencephaly, or smooth brain (Bai et al., 2003; des Portes et al., 1998; Gleeson et al., 1998). As reviewed in more detail elsewhere (Sheen & Walsh, 2003), mutations in several other genes including LIS1, ARX, FUKUTIN, and Filamin cause severe disruptions in neocortical development and neuronal migration, and correspondingly severe neurological impairment. More complex and heterogeneous disturbances of brain function such as dyslexia and specific language impairment may be related to more subtle changes in neocortical structure.

DYX1C1 AND NEURONAL MIGRATION

As mentioned above, microscopic anomalies within the cerebral neocortex of dyslexics suggest that dyslexia is associated with alterations in neuronal migration in the fetal brain (Galaburda, 1993; Galaburda, this volume). Consequently, we hypothesized that DYX1C1 plays a role in neuronal migration within developing neocortex. DYX1C1 is expressed in rat and human fetal neocortex during periods of neuronal migration. The first candidate dyslexia susceptibility gene is, therefore, expressed during prenatal periods of brain development and could, therefore, play a role in the early brain developmental changes associated with dyslexia.

In order to detemine the function of DYX1C1 in prenatal neuronal development, we used the method of RNAi interference (RNAi) by *in utero* electroporation (Bai et al., 2003). With this method, the activity and expression of a specific gene can be decreased in a subpopulation of neurons by targeting that gene with hairpin RNAi sequences that match the target gene. The targeted subpopulation of neurons can then be followed through development to determine the role played by a particular gene. As shown in Figure 1, when DYX1C1 was targeted, newly generated neurons failed to migrate normally from their site of generation at the surface of the ventricular zone (VZ) (see Figure 1 in the four-color section on page 222-A). Instead of migrating from the VZ up through the thickness and to the surface of the developing neocortex, cells treated with RNAi against DYX1C1 stalled with the intermediate zone and subventricular zone. The block in migration created by DYX1C1 RNAi demonstrates that DYX1C1 is essential to radial migration in developing neurons.

The genetic study that revealed DYX1C1 as a dyslexia susceptibility gene implicated the C-terminal portion of the gene in dyslexia susceptibility (Taipale et al., 2003). A large deletion of the C-terminus created by a balanced translocation of chromosome 15 and 2 was shown to segregate with dyslexia in a single family. The missing portion of this gene suggested that the C-terminus of DYX1C1 protein may be critical to its function in learning to read. To test whether the C-terminus of Dyx1c1 is also important to its function in neuronal migration, we performed rescue experiments with two constructs expressing two different pieces of DYX1C1. One construct, similar to the deletion in the dyslexic family reported by Taipale et al. (2003), was a truncation that lacked the final 77 amino acids that included the last two tetratricopeptide repeat (TPR) domains (aa 1-320). The second construct contained only the final 108 amino acids of the C-terminus and included all three TPR domains (aa 289-397) (Figure 2). Each construct was fused in frame with a green fluorescent tag (eGFP) so that we could trace the individual neurons that were successfully transfected with these constructs. The construct missing the C-terminus was not effective at rescuing migration arrest resulting from DYX1C1 RNAi, whereas the C-terminus alone was sufficient for full rescue (see Figure 2 in the four-color section on page 222-B). These results establish another link between dyslexia and altered neuronal migration, and indicate that the C-terminus of DYX1C1 is necessary and sufficient to its function in neuronal migration.

RELATIONSHIP BETWEEN DYX1C1 AND OTHER MIGRATION CONTROL GENES

In order to begin to understand the role of DYX1C1 relative to that of other genes controlling neuronal migration, we compared the cellular effects of DYX1C1 with that of RNAi directed against two other migration control genes: DCX and Dab1 (des Portes et al., 1998; Gleeson et al., 1998; Gleeson, this volume; Sheldon et al., 1997; Ware et al., 1997). RNAi directed against each of these genes resulted in interrupted migration to the cortical plate (CP), but resulted in distinct differences in the alterations in migration pattern, neuronal morphology, and neocortical architecture (Figure 3). Unlike either DCX or Dyx1c1 RNAi, Dab1 RNAi produced radial polarized cells in the IZ similar to control neurons; however, unlike controls, these cells had branched leading processes and failed to enter the CP (Figure 3A). As we previously reported (Bai et al., 2003), DCX RNAi resulted in multipolar cells that arrest within the IZ. The multipolar cells caused by DCX RNAi, however, were not as extensively branched as multipolar cells created by Dyx1c1 RNAi (see Figure 3 in the four-color section on page 222-C). Another difference between DCX and Dyx1c1 RNAi was seen by differing patterns of migration arrest. As shown in the cumulative probability plots in Figure 3B, Dyx1c1 RNAi resulted in cells migrating a shorter distance than cells treated with DCX RNAi. Furthermore, DCX RNAi showed a distinctly bimodal pattern of arrest, whereas Dyx1c1 RNAi led to a simpler unimodal pattern of arrest (see Figure 3B in the four-color section on page XXA). Taken together, these results demonstrate that Dyx1c1 plays a role in neuronal migration distinguishable from that of two other migration control genes. The different phenotypes also suggest a temporal order of function: Dyx1c1, followed by DCX and then Dab1. The general approach of comparing differences in morphology and migration patterns resulting from different RNAi treatments should aid future efforts in determining the relative roles and order of proteins that control neuronal migration in neocortex.

CELLULAR DYNAMICS OF DYX1C1 PROTEIN

Proteins that control migration in neocortical neurons belong to a variety of functional classes including kinases such as JNK-1 and CDK-5 (Reiner et al., 2004), cytoskeletal regulators such as DCX (Gleeson, Lin, Flanagan, & Walsh, 1999), signaling adaptors such as Dab1 (Sheldon et al., 1997), and proteins that associate with the cytoplasmic motor protein dynein such as Lis1 (Smith et al., 2000; Wynshaw-Boris & Gambello, 2001). Dyx1c1 lacks obvious sequence homologies that would place it in a particular functional class, so to explore its cellular role, we determined its localization and trafficking within migrating neurons. Dyx1c1-GFP localized throughout the cytoplasm as distinct particles within the soma and leading processes of migrating neurons (Figure 3C). Time-lapse videomicroscopy of cells within slices of embryonic neocortex indicated that these Dyx1c1 particles were highly dynamic. In the cytoplasm and leading process, Dyx1c1 moved rapidly (0.1-5 μm/sec) in all directions and also more slowly around the periphery of the nucleus (3-5 μm/minute) (Figure 3C). Within leading dendritic processes, Dyx1c1 moved bidirectionally at 0.1-1 μm/minute (Figure 3C). Multidirectional and rapid movements suggest that Dyx1c1 may interact with cytoplasmic motor proteins such as dynein. Consistent with such interaction, Dyx1c1 contains protein-protein interaction domains, three TPR domains, and a p23 homology domain, which indicate potential interaction with dynein protein complexes (Galigniana et al., 2002; Pratt, Galigniana, Harrell, & DeFranco, 2004; Silverstein et al., 1999). Future biochemical experiments will be necessary to determine whether Dyx1c1 interacts with dynein or other migration genes such as LIS1. Localization and trafficking support the hypothesis that Dyx1c1 functionally interacts with cytoplasmic motor proteins, and this may link it to other migration proteins such as LIS1.

CONCLUSIONS

The finding that DYX1C1 RNAi leads to primarily deep layer heterotopia and dyslexic brains were found to contain superficial layer ectopias, and laminar dysplasias suggests a possible mechanistic connection between these two different dysplasia types. Radial glial may provide a link. They span the entire width of developing cortex, closely interact with migrating neurons, and also form the external limiting barrier that normally restricts ectopic migration into the superficial layer. Without normal DYX1C1 function, neurons fail to polarize in the IZ and do not continue their migration along radial glia. The resultant reduction in direct interaction between migrating neurons and radial glia could cause a disruption in radial glial integrity at the pial surface (Gierdalski & Juliano, 2003; Hunter & Hatten, 1995; Schmid et al., 2003). Thus, the same disruption that causes some neurons to arrest could indirectly result in ectopias. Alternatively, DYX1C1 RNAi could directly affect radial glia.

More generally, our discovery that DYX1C1 is a neuronal migration gene supports the hypothesis that even very different neurological impairments may arise from disruptions in a common developmental pathway (Sheen & Walsh, 2003). Large disruptions in migration may create severe neurological impairment such as epilepsy or mental retardation, while smaller migration disruptions may create more subtle changes in neural processing and behavior (Frenkel et al., 2000; Peiffer et al., 2001). An emerging picture of dyslexia is that mutations in different susceptibility genes cause small abnormalities in neuronal migration, which in turn, lead to additional changes affecting neural processes important for reading.

Address correspondence to: Joseph J. LoTurco, Ph.D., Department of Physiology and Neurobiology, U-4156, University of Connecticut, Storrs, CT 06268; E-mail: loturco @oracle. pnb. uconn.edu

REFERENCES

Bai, J., Ramos, R. L., Ackman, J. B., Thomas, A. M., Lee, R. V., & LoTurco, J. J. (2003). RNAi reveals doublecortin is required for radial migration in rat neocortex. *Nature Neuroscience, 6*(12), 1277–1283.

Choi, B. H., & Matthias, S. C. (1987). Cortical dysplasia associated with massive ectopia of neurons and glial cells within the subarachnoid space. *Acta Neuropathologia (Berl), 73*(2), 105–109.
des Portes, V., Pinard, J. M., Billuart, P., Vinet, M. C., Koulakoff, A., Carrie, A., et al. (1998). A novel CNS gene required for neuronal migration and involved in X-linked subcortical laminar heterotopia and lissencephaly syndrome. *Cell, 92*(1), 51–61.
Frenkel, M., Sherman, G. F., Bashan, K. A., Galaburda, A. M., & LoTurco, J. J. (2000). Neocortical ectopias are associated with attenuated neurophysiological responses to rapidly changing auditory stimuli. *Neuroreport, 11*(3), 575–579.
Gabel, L. A., & LoTurco, J. J. (2001). Electrophysiological and morphological characterization of neurons within neocortical ectopias. *Journal of Neurophysiology, 85*(2), 495–505.
Gabel, L. A., & LoTurco, J. J. (2002). Layer I ectopias and increased excitability in murine neocortex. *Journal of Neurophysiology, 87*(5), 2471–2479.
Galaburda, A. M. (1993). Neuroanatomic basis of developmental dyslexia. *Neurology, 11*(1), 161–173.
Galaburda, A. M., & Kemper, T. L. (1979). Cytoarchitectonic abnormalities in developmental dyslexia: A case study. *Annals of Neurology, 6*(2), 94–100.
Galaburda, A. M., Sherman, G. F., Rosen, G. D., Aboitiz, F., & Geschwind, N. (1985). Developmental dyslexia: Four consecutive patients with cortical anomalies. *Annals of Neurology, 18*(2), 222–233.
Galigniana, M. D., Harrell, J. M., Murphy, P. J., Chinkers, M., Radanyi, C., Renoir, J. M., et al. (2002). Binding of hsp90-associated immunophilins to cytoplasmic dynein: Direct binding and in vivo evidence that the peptidylprolyl isomerase domain is a dynein interaction domain. *Biochemistry, 41*(46), 13602–13610.
Gierdalski, M., & Juliano, S. L. (2003). Factors affecting the morphology of radial glia. *Cerebral Cortex, 13*(6), 572–579.
Gleeson, J. G., Allen, K. M., Fox, J. W., Lamperti, E. D., Berkovic, S., Scheffer, I., et al. (1998). Doublecortin, a brain-specific gene mutated in human X-linked lissencephaly and double cortex syndrome, encodes a putative signaling protein. *Cell, 92*(1), 63–72.
Gleeson, J. G., Lin, P. T., Flanagan, L. A., & Walsh, C. A. (1999). Doublecortin is a microtubule-associated protein and is expressed widely by migrating neurons. *Neuron, 23*(2), 257–271.
Hunter, K. E., & Hatten, M. E. (1995). Radial glial cell transformation to astrocytes is bidirectional: Regulation by a diffusible factor in embryonic forebrain. *Proceedings of the National Academy of Sciences USA, 92*(6), 2061–2065.
Noctor, S. C., Martinez-Cerdeno, V., Ivic, L., & Kriegstein, A. R. (2004). Cortical neurons arise in symmetric and asymmetric division zones and migrate through specific phases. *Nature Neuroscience, 7*(2), 136–144.
Peiffer, A. M., Dunleavy, C. K., Frenkel, M., Gabel, L. A., LoTurco, J. J., Rosen, G. D., et al. (2001). Impaired detection of variable duration embedded tones in ectopic NZB/BINJ mice. *Neuroreport, 12*(13), 2875–2879.
Peiffer, A. M., Rosen, G. D., & Fitch, R. H. (2002). Sex differences in rapid auditory processing deficits in ectopic BXSB/MpJ mice. *Neuroreport, 13*(17), 2277–2280.

Pratt, W. B., Galigniana, M. D., Harrell, J. M., & DeFranco, D. B. (2004). Role of hsp90 and the hsp90-binding immunophilins in signalling protein movement. *Cell Signal, 16*(8), 857–872.

Rakic, P. (2000). Radial unit hypothesis of neocortical expansion. *Novartis Foundation Symposium, 228*, 30–42; discussion 42–52.

Reiner, O., Gdalyahu, A., Ghosh, I., Levy, T., Sapoznik, S., Nir, R., et al. (2004). DCX's phosphorylation by not Just aNother Kinase (JNK). *Cell Cycle, 3*(6), 747–751.

Schmid, R. S., McGrath, B., Berechid, B. E., Boyles, B., Marchionni, M., Sestan, N., et al. (2003). Neuregulin 1-erbB2 signaling is required for the establishment of radial glia and their transformation into astrocytes in cerebral cortex. *Proceedings of the National Academy of Sciences USA, 100*(7), 4251–4256.

Sheen, V. L., & Walsh, C. A. (2003). Developmental genetic malformations of the cerebral cortex. *Current Neurology Neurosciences Reports, 3*(5), 433–441.

Sheldon, M., Rice, D. S., D'Arcangelo, G., Yoneshima, H., Nakajima, K., Mikoshiba, K., et al. (1997). Scrambler and yotari disrupt the disabled gene and produce a reeler-like phenotype in mice. *Nature, 389*(6652), 730–733.

Sherman, G. F., Rosen, G. D., Stone, L. V., Press, D. M., & Galaburda, A. M. (1992). The organization of radial glial fibers in spontaneous neocortical ectopias of newborn New Zealand black mice. *Brain Research. Developmentl Brain Research, 67*(2), 279–283.

Silverstein, A. M., Galigniana, M. D., Kanelakis, K. C., Radanyi, C., Renoir, J. M., & Pratt, W. B. (1999). Different regions of the immunophilin FKBP52 determine its association with the glucocorticoid receptor, hsp90, and cytoplasmic dynein. *Journal of Biological Chemistry, 274*(52), 36980–36986.

Smith, D. S., Niethammer, M., Ayala, R., Zhou, Y., Gambello, M. J., Wynshaw-Boris, A., et al. (2000). Regulation of cytoplasmic dynein behaviour and microtubule organization by mammalian Lis1. *Nature Cell Biology, 2*(11), 767–775.

Taipale, M., Kaminen, N., Nopola-Hemmi, J., Haltia, T., Myllyluoma, B., Lyytinen, H., et al. (2003). A candidate gene for developmental dyslexia encodes a nuclear tetratricopeptide repeat domain protein dynamically regulated in brain. *Proceedings of the National Academy of Sciences USA, 100*(20), 11553–11558.

Ware, M. L., Fox, J. W., Gonzalez, J. L., Davis, N. M., Lambert de Rouvroit, C., Russo, C. J., et al. (1997). Aberrant splicing of a mouse disabled homolog, mdab1, in the scrambler mouse. *Neuron, 19*(2), 239–249.

Wigg, K. G., Couto, J. M., Feng, Y., Anderson, B., Cate-Carter, T. D., Macciardi, F., et al. (2004). Support for EKN1 as the susceptibility locus for dyslexia on 15q21. *Molecular Psychiatry, 9*(12), 1111–1121.

Wynshaw-Boris, A., & Gambello, M. J. (2001). LIS1 and dynein motor function in neuronal migration and development. *Genes and Development, 15*(6), 639–651.

Chapter • 7

Genetic Disorders of Neuronal Migration and Brain Wiring

Joseph Gleeson

The underlying basis for developmental dyslexia is not well understood, but there is mounting evidence that disordered brain development might be at least partly responsible. Landmark studies identified cortical abnormalities in several cases consisting of neuronal ectopias and architectonic dysplasias, both in males and females with developmental dyslexia (Galaburda, Sherman, Rosen, Aboitiz, & Geschwind, 1985; Humphreys, Kaufmann, & Galaburda, 1990). These abnormalities are likely due to disordered neuronal migration of newly generated neurons to the cortex, and such abnormalities were present in far fewer numbers in neurologically normal individuals than in individuals with dyslexia (Kaufmann & Galaburda, 1989), suggesting a possible link between developmental dyslexia and neuronal migration (Njiokiktjien, 1994).

The research on neuronal migration was performed by Dr. Teruyuki Tanaka and Finley Serneo in the Gleeson Laboratory. We obtained the Lis1 +/- mice from Dr. AnthonyWynshaw-Boris and Michael Gambello from UCSD. The work on brain wiring was performed by a collaborative group, by Drs. Alvaro Pascual-Leon, Masahito Kobayashi, and Gregor Thut from the Laboratory for Magnetic Brain Stimulation at Beth Israel Deaconess Medical Center and Harvard Medical School; by Drs. Susumu Mori, Lidia Nagae-Poetscher, Elaine Stashinko, and Alexander Hoon from the Division of MR Research at The Johns Hopkins University School of Medicine; by Drs. Melissa Henry, Susan Rivera, and Joseph Pinter at the University of California, Davis; and by Dr. Bernard Maria at the Medical University of South Carolina. Each of these collaborators is gratefully acknowledged for their involvement and hard work.

In addition to possible disorders of neuronal migration in the etiology of developmental dyslexia, alterations in brain wiring have also been hypothesized to play a role in this condition. Brain wiring refers to the connectivity of brain structures that can now be identified in living humans through the use of physiological and imaging techniques. For example, in a patient with alexia, a damaged fiber tract linking the left ventral occipito-temporal region to its right homolog across the lesioned area of corpus callosum was found (Molko et al., 2002). This is an extreme example of a wiring defect, in that there was frank destruction of a major tract. In another example, brain wiring was interrogated in a group of reading-impaired and control individuals. Left-sided temporo-parietal white matter diffusion anisotropy (i.e., white matter tract) differences were correlated with reading ability. These differences were noted in the microstructure of these white matter tracts, which may contribute to reading ability by determining the strength of communication between cortical areas involved in visual, auditory, and language processing (Klingberg et al., 2000). While these studies will need to be confirmed and extended, they suggest that abnormal brain wiring may be involved in the pathogenesis of developmental dyslexia.

The goal of the Gleeson laboratory is to understand the causes and mechanisms underlying human developmental brain abnormalities. While our laboratory does not have a focus on dyslexia, we are focused on two areas of research with relevance to the field of dyslexia. I have chosen to present two studies that were performed in my lab or collaboratively with other groups. The first section is focused on the basic mechanisms of neuronal migration. We are studying the fundamentals of how neurons move by studying cellular events and critical proteins that are mutated in individuals with migration disorders. I present evidence that the underlying defect in classical lissencephaly (smooth brain syndrome) due to mutations in the *LIS1* gene are caused by defective nuclear-centrosomal coupling during migration. This is a critical first step in understanding human disorders of migration. In the second, I present evidence of a human condition characterized by abnormal brain wiring. We have studied Joubert syndrome, a rare recessively inherited developmental brain disorder, and demonstrate a profound defect in the primary corticospinal feedback loop in these patients.

The goal of this chapter is to highlight recent advances in diseases with more straightforward bases that may help in our understanding of more complex disorders like dyslexia.

DEFECTS IN ONGOING NEURONAL MIGRATION ARE ASSOCIATED WITH MUTATIONS IN MICROTUBULE-ASSOCIATED PROTEINS

Mutations in microtubule-associated proteins (MAPs) are correlated with defects in ongoing neuronal migration. These conditions are seen in the human disorders of classical lissencephaly and in mouse migration disorders in which the cortex retains the proper inside-out configuration, but there is imprecise targeting of neurons to their correct cortical laminar position. The cellular basis underlying the cortical defect is still not completely understood, but probably is related to a cell-autonomous defect in migration speed.

As neurons exit the ventricular zone, they migrate long distances toward the cortical plate. It is the ongoing process of migration that appears to be defective in both type I lissencephaly (also called classical lissencephaly) and in double-cortex syndrome. In lissencephaly in humans, the normally six-layered cerebral cortex is replaced by a four-layered structure. These four layers have no obvious relationship to the normal six layers except for the marginal zone (the outermost layer), which is retained in lissencephaly. The majority of cortical plate neurons are found in the fourth layer.

Mutations in several genes lead to related forms of classical lissencephaly in human and in mouse. Mutations in *LIS1* (also known as *PAFAH1B1*) and *doublecortin* (*DCX*) were first identified as causative in humans. The protein products of these two genes are unrelated to one another structurally, although the two proteins can physically interact and cooperatively lead to microtubule polymerization (Caspi, Atlas, Kantor, Sapir, & Reiner, 2000). Heterozygous *LIS1* mutations are associated with lissencephaly, suggesting haploinsufficiency (decreased protein level) as the disease mechanism. The *DCX* gene is located on the X-chromosome. In families with *DCX* mutations, affected males show lissencephaly whereas affected females show a double cortex (DC) (Pinard et al., 1994). In DC, there is a normal six-layered outer cortex and an additional collection of neurons located in the subcortical white matter. The males have the more severe phenotype because they have a single X-chromosome, whereas females inherit two X-chromosomes with subsequent random X inactivation. Therefore, DC represents a mosaic phenotype. Whether the migration defect is strictly cell-autonomous, however, has remained unclear. Individuals with lissencephaly typically display severe mental retardation and intractable epilepsy, whereas individuals with DC typically display mild to moderate mental retardation and less severe epilepsy (Berg et al., 1998).

The cortex of *Lis1* heterozygous mice is better organized than might be expected from the human phenotype, yet neuronal birthdating studies indicate poor layer specificity, with neurons normally destined for the superficial layers tending to be positioned in deeper layers, abnormal radial glia and abnormal cortical plate splitting (Cahana et al., 2001; Hirotsune et al., 1998). Further reductions in the dosage of *Lis1* (for example, in compound heterozygotes carrying one null and one partial loss-of-function allele) result in even more severe migration defects, suggesting dosage-sensitive effects on migration (Gambello et al., 2003), in keeping with the haploinsufficiency model of the disease.

Surprisingly, the cortex of *Dcx* knockout male mice is morphologically normal, with proper cortical lamination as revealed by birthdating studies, and female heterozygous mice do not display a double-layered cortex. Nevertheless, there is a mild defect in hippocampal lamination and epilepsy in males, and nearly all male knockouts die just after birth for unclear reasons (Corbo et al., 2002). Given the absence of a strong cortical phenotype in the male knockouts, it was surprising that the acute inactivation of *Dcx* using small interfering RNA (siRNA) produced a significantly different phenotype (Bai et al., 2003; see LoTurco et al., this volume). In the cortex of mice injected with siRNA-producing plasmid, electroporated neurons had significantly delayed migration. Arrested cells were positioned within the subcortical white matter, whereas the majority of untransfected cells appeared to complete migration and were positioned within the cortical plate. In addition, some heterotopically localized neurons did not express the transgene marker, suggesting that the defect in migration was not completely cell-autonomous, or that some neurons might not have been electroporated with the reporter plasmid. The authors suggest that the reason a migration defect occurred after siRNA treatment but not with the traditional knockout was that siRNA produced an acute depletion, whereas the developing brain can compensate when the protein is completely absent, presumably through increased activity of other proteins. This idea will need to be tested further.

The role of LIS1 in migration has not yet been elucidated, but evidence is emerging that it functions on several pathways regulating both microtubule dynein motor function and actin signaling. Lis1 is highly conserved and seems to have similar functions in fungus, yeast, fly, and mouse (reviewed in Wynshaw-Boris & Gambello, 2001; Xiang, 2003). LIS1 belongs to the WD-40 superfamily of proteins that are involved in diverse protein-protein interactions. It interacts with cytoplasmic dynein and proteins of the centrosome (a.k.a. microtubule organizing center) including nuclear distribution-E (NudE) in fungus and its mammalian homologs mNudE and Nudel (NudE-like) (Feng et al., 2000; Kitagawa et al., 2000; Niethammer et al., 2000; Sasaki et al., 2000; Sweeney, Prokscha, & Eichele, 2001). In all species examined to date, LIS1 deficiency produces nuclear translocation defects, abnormal positioning of the centrosome, and altered distribution of the Golgi apparatus, consistent with the loss of cytoplasmic dynein function (Faulkner et al., 2000; Liu, Steward, & Luo, 2000; Sheeman et al., 2003; Smith et al., 2000). It is not clear whether LIS1 functions primarily at the minus or plus ends of microtubules, but converging evidence suggests an interaction with CLIP-170, a plus-end tracking protein. LIS1 and CLIP-170 may serve with dynein at sites involved in the loading of cargo onto microtubules, and/or in the control of microtubule dynamics (Coquelle et al., 2002; Tai, Dujardin, Faulkner, & Vallee, 2002).

LIS1 is also required for proper actin polymerization at the leading edge of migrating neurons (Kholmanskikh, Dobrin, Wynshaw-Boris, Letourneau, & Ross, 2003). LIS1 haploinsufficiency resulted in reduced filamentous actin at the leading edge, associated with an up-regulation of RhoA, and reduction in Rac1 and Cdc42 activities. Disruption of RhoA function increased Rac1/Cdc42 and rescued the motility defect in *Lis1+/-* neurons, suggesting a role in promoting actin polymerization through the regulation of Rho family GTPases.

The role of Doublecortin (DCX) in neuronal migration is still being elucidated. *Dcx* encodes a novel a MAP that is capable of polymerizing microtubules (Francis et al., 1999; Gleeson, Lin, Flanagan, & Walsh, 1999; Horesh et al., 1999). In human patients, essentially all of the missense mutations in DCX have been found in two microtubule-binding domains; at least some of these mutations appear to diminish interactions of DCX with microtubules (Sapir et al., 2000; Taylor, Holzer, Bazan, Walsh, & Gleeson, 2000). Regulation of the microtubule polymerizing activity of Dcx occurs through phosphorylation, and as with other MAPs, phosphorylation negatively regulates its affinity for microtubules. Several doublecortin kinases have been identified to date: protein kinase A (PKA) and the microtubule affinity regulatory kinase (MARK) (Schaar, Kinoshita, & McConnell, 2004), cyclin-dependent kinase-5 (Tanaka et al., 2004), and c-Jun N-terminal kinase (JNK) (Gdalyahu et al., 2004). These kinases act at different sites in Dcx and apparently in distinct subcellular compartments, but have similar effects in weakening the binding and localization of DCX to microtubules. Phosphorylation of DCX has been proposed to regulate the stability of a perinuclear "cage" of microtubules during migration (Rivas & Hatten, 1995) to regulate polarized growth at the leading edge and tips of neurites and to regulate cell movement.

To define subcellular mechanisms, we have combined in vitro neuronal migration assays with retroviral transduction. Retroviral transduction increases protein level approximately two-fold over baseline, indicating that the relatively weak retroviral promoter approximately doubles the amount of DCX or LIS1 in cells. This overexpression of wild-type DCX or LIS1, but not patient-related mutant versions, surprisingly increases migration rates by approximately 50% in neurons exiting from cerebellar granule neuron reaggregates. This allowed us to analyze whether DCX overexpression is sufficient to rescue the migration defect in *Lis1* knockout neurons. Retroviral transduction with LIS1 rescued the migration defect in *Lis1*+/- neurons, which is not surprising as LIS1 levels were restored to slightly above normal levels on average. Surprisingly, DCX overexpression largely restored migration in *Lis1*+/- neurons. This data suggest that LIS1 and DCX function on the same pathway to regulate migration.

The primary defect in migration of acutely dissociated *Lis1* +/- neurons appears to be in nuclear movement (Hirotsune et al., 1998). To understand the mechanism of this rescue and of the nuclear movement defect, the subcellular distribution of DCX and LIS1 were studied. LIS1 is localized predominantly to the centrosome in migrating neurons, and after disruption of microtubules, it redistributed to the perinuclear membrane region. DCX outlined microtubules extending from the perinuclear "cage" to the centrosome and into the leading process. This localization, together with the known interaction of LIS1 and dynein, immediately suggests a model for both proteins in migration. When dynein is positioned at the nuclear membrane, directional movement towards the minus end of the microtubule would move the nucleus towards the centrosome. This would suggest a role for LIS1 in nuclear-centrosome coupling (Figure 1). In order to test this, *Lis1*+/- were transduced with a virus expressing a centrosomal marker, and the distance between the nucleus and centrosome were measured in live migrating neurons. These neurons displayed increased separation between the nucleus and the preceding centrosome during migration, indicating defective nuclear-centrosome coupling (N-C coupling). Dynein inhibition resulted in similar defects in both nucleus-centrosome coupling and neuronal migration, indicating that recapitulation of the N-C coupling defect using a completely different method also results in defective migration. These N-C coupling defects were rescued by either LIS1 or

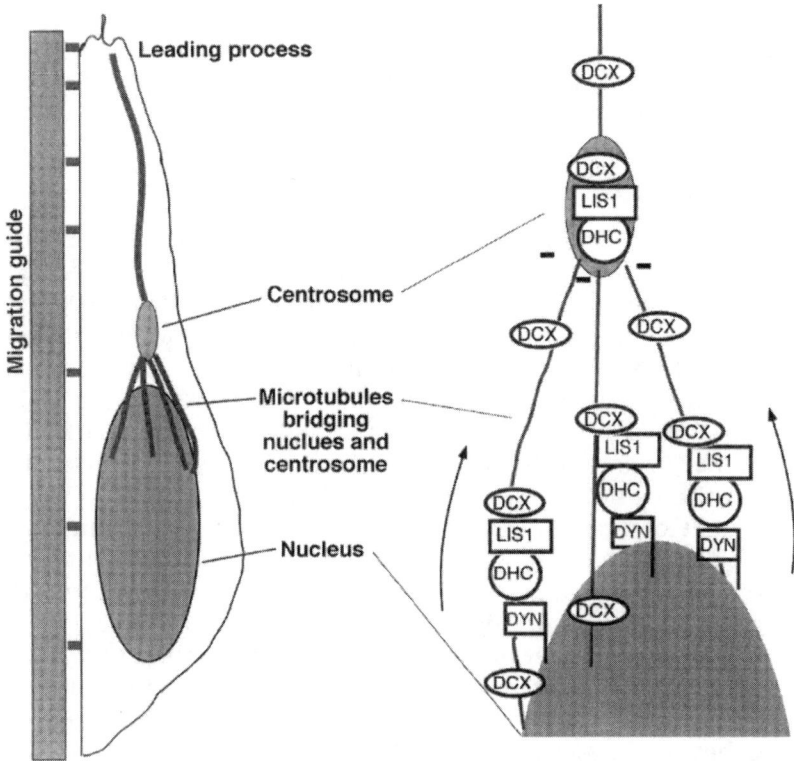

Figure 1. Model for the role of DCX and LIS1 in migration. Left: Schematic of a migrating neuron with the centrosome positioned ahead of the nucleus and coupled by bridging microtubules. Right: DCX co-localizes with these bridging microtubules. LIS1 is localized to the perinuclear membrane and the centrosome. Dynein (DHC), complexed with dynactin (DYN), may mediate movement of the nucleus towards the minus end of the microtubule at the centrosome. The model suggests DCX and LIS1 are required for nucleus-centrosome coupling during migration.

DCX transduction, which was expected as this transduction rescued the migration defect in these cells. These data together indicate LIS1 and DCX function with dynein to mediate N-C coupling during migration, and suggest defects in this coupling may contribute to migration defects in lissencephaly.

Future studies will focus on identifying other neuronal migration genes that lead to N-C coupling defects and how these coupling defects lead to altered migration. It will be critical to test whether the *Dcx-/y* mice display similar migration and N-C coupling defects, and whether these can be rescued by Lis1 overexpression. Another focus of this work is now centered on identifying how extracellular guidance molecules are transmitted to determine centrosome positioning and neuronal migration direction.

BRAIN WIRING DEFECTS IN JOUBERT SYNDROME

My laboratory, in collaboration with several other research groups, have defined a new type of neurological condition defined by a defect in brain wiring. Joubert syndrome (JS, OMIM213300) is a rare developmental brain disorder characterized radiographically by hypoplasia of the cerebellar midline, and clinically by ataxia, oculomotor apraxia, mental retardation (Boltshauser & Isler, 1977; Joubert, Eisenring, & Andermann, 1968), and a hallmark radiographic "molar-tooth sign" (MTS) in axial sections of the brainstem isthmus (Maria et al., 1997; Maria et al., 1999). The MTS is the result of a ventral and lateral indentation of the midbrain-hindbrain junction as well as a lengthening and horizontal displacement of the superior cerebellar peduncles, and now forms the diagnostic hallmark of this condition (Gleeson et al., 2003).

The development of neural circuits in invertebrate and vertebrate systems is regulated by molecules critical for proper neuronal circuitry, identified through various genetic and biochemical approaches. In *D. Melanogaster* and *C. elegans*, genetic screens have identified several classes of guidance molecules where mutations produce defects in axonal fasciculation, decussation, or projection (Kaprielian, Runko, & Imondi, 2001; Tayler & Garrity, 2003). In vertebrates, studies of determinates of axonal circuitry, largely using gene-targeting strategies in mouse, have revealed critical roles for *Unc5* and *DCC* in corticospinal tract (CST) development (Finger et al., 2002). Recently, gene-trapping technology has identified additional genes that are essential in CST development, including *EphA4* (Leighton et al., 2001). In these mutants, the CST, the main descending motor pathway from the cerebral cortex, is either misplaced dorsally in the brainstem and spinal cord or fails to decussate, resulting in a variety of neurological deficits.

We have evidence that profound defects in neuronal circuitry can also exist in humans with JS. Previous anatomic reports have suggested an absence of the pyramidal decussation, the cervicomedullary area of CST crossing (Friede & Boltshauser, 1978; ten Donkelaar, Hoevenaars, & Wesseling, 2000; Yachnis & Rorke, 1999), which is the locus of control of the hemibody by the contralateral cortical hemisphere. Existing literature does not mention any abnormalities of the ascending sensory spinocortical tract

(SCT), suggesting to us that patients with JS might have a wiring defect, resulting in the right cortical hemisphere controlling the right hemibody, but receiving sensory information from the left hemibody.

Detailed neuropathological analysis indicates that the CST fails to decussate at any level of the brainstem, suggesting that either it remains ipsilateral or that it crosses elsewhere along the neuroaxis. In JS, at least a subset of fascicles emanate from ascending sensory nuclei in their normal position where they cross the midline, suggesting that the SCT is at least partially decussated. Transcranial magnetic stimulation (TMS) analysis of either hemisphere shows predominantly ipsilateral evoked responses, indicating that the functional representation of the CST is ipsilateral. Somatosensory evoked potential (SEP) analysis of either median nerve shows predominantly contralateral cortical responses, indicating that the functional representation of the SCT is contralateral. Therefore, in this condition, one cortical hemisphere projects most motor output to the ipsilateral side of the body but receives fast-conducting tactile sensory input from the contralateral side. This wiring defect results in a striking mismatch between target of motor output and corresponding sensory information in each cerebral hemisphere (see Figure 2 in the four-color section on page 222-D), a discord that relates to the neurocognitive deficits in these individuals.

It would be ideal to identify the functional consequence of the defective brain wiring in JS, but the co-existent cerebellar malformation makes it difficult to establish which problems are due to the wiring defect versus the cerebellar malformation. Some of the deficits in JS are commonly associated with all forms of cerebellar and vermis malformations, including cerebellar ataxia, delayed motor development, and nystagmus (Illarioshkin et al., 1996; Kornberg & Shield, 1991; Rivier & Echenne, 1992). However, there are some specific deficits seen in JS that are not observed in patients with these other conditions. First, there is a very high incidence of mirror movements in JS. Second, a recent study identified bilateral fMRI cortical activation during unilateral finger tapping in JS (Parisi et al., 2004), and our preliminary data is consistent with this as well. The authors excluded mirror movement of the opposite hand as a trivial cause for bilateral cortical activation, suggesting that the cortical circuits may have rewired as a consequence of miswiring of the CST, or that there are altered interhemispheric interactions (Kobayashi, Hutchinson, Schlaug, & Pascual-Leone, 2003) to compensate for altered sensorimotor integration. Third, preliminary data indicate there is randomization of handedness in JS (roughly equal numbers of right- and left-handed predominance) despite a strong right-handed predominance among unaffected parents and siblings (Joubert Syndrome Foundation, unpublished observation). This suggests that the influence of genetic factors on handedness (Geschwind, Miller, DeCarli, & Carmelli, 2002) is relieved in these patients. Although there is a modest increase in left-handedness among children with developmental disabilities (Batheja & McManus, 1985), randomization in JS suggests that brain laterality fails to occur in these individuals. Thus, these specific functional deficits appear to relate to the miswiring of these circuits, but more work is needed to further elucidate these deficits.

Having motor outputs originate from a different hemisphere than the one that receives sensory information about body movement increases the length of neuronal circuitry and introduces a delay in sensory feedback into this information processing loop. Most individuals with JS display a variety of difficulties that fall under the rubric of "fine motor control," and are possibly related to the mismatches in sensory input and motor output that are demonstrated here. These deficits include difficulties in initiating pointing movements, finger tapping, matching eye movements with pointing movements (oculomotor apraxia), executing complex movements without visual guidance (such as dressing and walking), and executing precise movements in general (Fennell, Gitten, Dede, & Maria, 1999; Maria, Boltshauser, Palmer, & Tran, 1999). The altered wiring diagram in JS makes strong predictions about sensory-motor feedback loops that can be tested. For example, patient-initiated responses to being touched should be faster on the contralateral than the ipsilateral side, and patients should exhibit specific problems in taking into account the sensory consequences of their own movements. We plan to discern these predicted responses using a combination of sensory-motor paradigms to interrogate both the cortical and cerebellar pathways.

These results suggest that there may be a collection of neurodevelopmental disorders in humans in which abnormal wiring of the brain may account for a significant amount of the disability. With advanced *in vivo* imaging and physiology techniques, it might be possible to probe the wiring diagram of the brain in these individuals and to study how these structural abnormalities relate to function.

Address correspondence to: Joseph Gleeson, M.D., University of California at San Diego, Department of Neurosciences, Medical Teaching Facility 324, Medical School Campus, 9500 Gilman Drive, La Jolla, CA 92093-0624; E-mail: jogleeson@ucsd.edu

REFERENCES

Bai, J., Ramos, R. L., Ackman, J. B., Thomas, A. M., Lee, R. V., & LoTurco, J. J. (2003). RNAi reveals doublecortin is required for radial migration in rat neocortex. *Nature Neuroscience, 6*(12), 1277–1283.

Batheja, M., & McManus, I. C. (1985). Handedness in the mentally handicapped. *Dev Med Child Neurol, 27*(1), 63–68.

Berg, M. J., Schifitto, G., Powers, J. M., Martinez-Capolino, C., Fong, C. T., Myers, G. J., et al. (1998). X-linked female band heterotopia-male lissencephaly syndrome. *Neurology, 50*(4), 1143–1146.

Boltshauser, E., & Isler, W. (1977). Joubert syndrome: Episodic hyperpnea, abnormal eye movements, retardation and ataxia, associated with dysplasia of the cerebellar vermis. *Neuropadiatrie, 8*(1), 57–66.

Cahana, A., Escamez, T., Nowakowski, R. S., Hayes, N. L., Giacobini, M., von Holst, A., et al. (2001). Targeted mutagenesis of Lis1 disrupts cortical development and LIS1 homodimerization. *Proceedings of the National Academy of Sciences USA, 98*(11), 6429–6434.

Caspi, M., Atlas, R., Kantor, A., Sapir, T., & Reiner, O. (2000). Interaction between LIS1 and doublecortin, two lissencephaly gene products. *Human Moledular Genetics, 9*(15), 2205–2213.

Coquelle, F. M., Caspi, M., Cordelieres, F. P., Dompierre, J. P., Dujardin, D. L., Koifman, C., et al. (2002). LIS1, CLIP-170's key to the dynein/dynactin pathway. *Molecular Cell Biology, 22*(9), 3089–3102.

Corbo, J. C., Deuel, T. A., Long, J. M., LaPorte, P., Tsai, E., Wynshaw-Boris, A., et al. (2002). Doublecortin is required in mice for lamination of the hippocampus but not the neocortex. *The Journal of Neuroscience, 22*(17), 7548–7557.

Faulkner, N. E., Dujardin, D. L., Tai, C. Y., Vaughan, K. T., O'Connell, C. B., Wang, Y., et al. (2000). A role for the lissencephaly gene LIS1 in mitosis and cytoplasmic dynein function. *Nature Cell Biology, 2*(11), 784–791.

Feng, Y., Olson, E. C., Stukenberg, P. T., Flanagan, L. A., Kirschner, M. W., & Walsh, C. A. (2000). LIS1 regulates CNS lamination by interacting with mNudE, a central component of the centrosome. *Neuron, 28*(3), 665–679.

Fennell, E. B., Gitten, J. C., Dede, D. E., & Maria, B. L. (1999). Cognition, behavior, and development in Joubert syndrome. *Journal of Child Neurology, 14*(9), 592–596.

Finger, J. H., Bronson, R. T., Harris, B., Johnson, K., Przyborski, S. A., & Ackerman, S. L. (2002). The netrin 1 receptors Unc5h3 and Dcc are necessary at multiple choice points for the guidance of corticospinal tract axons. *The Journal of Neuroscience, 22*(23), 10346–10356.

Francis, F., Koulakoff, A., Boucher, D., Chafey, P., Schaar, B., Vinet, M. C., et al. (1999). Doublecortin is a developmentally regulated, microtubule-associated protein expressed in migrating and differentiating neurons. *Neuron, 23*(2), 247–256.

Friede, R. L., & Boltshauser, E. (1978). Uncommon syndromes of cerebellar vermis aplasia. I: Joubert syndrome. *Dev Med Child Neurol, 20*(6), 758–763.

Galaburda, A. M., Sherman, G. F., Rosen, G. D., Aboitiz, F., & Geschwind, N. (1985). Developmental dyslexia: Four consecutive cases with cortical anomalies. *Annals of Neurology, 18*, 222–233.

Gambello, M. J., Darling, D. L., Yingling, J., Tanaka, T., Gleeson, J. G., & Wynshaw-Boris, A. (2003). Multiple dose-dependent effects of Lis1 on cerebral cortical development. *The Journal of Neuroscience, 23*(5), 1719–1729.

Gdalyahu, A., Ghosh, I., Levy, T., Sapir, T., Sapoznik, S., Fishler, Y., et al. (2004). DCX, a new mediator of the JNK pathway. *Embo J. 23*(4), 823–832.

Geschwind, D. H., Miller, B. L., DeCarli, C., & Carmelli, D. (2002). Heritability of lobar brain volumes in twins supports genetic models of cerebral laterality and handedness. *Proceedings of the National Academy of Sciences USA, 99*(5), 3176–3181.

Gleeson, J. G., Keeler, L. C., Parisi, M. A., Marsh, S. E., Chance, P. F., Glass, I. A., et al. (2003). The molar tooth sign of the midbrain-hindbrain junction: Occurrence in multiple distinct syndromes. *American Journal of Medical Genetics, 25*(2), 125–134.

Gleeson, J. G., Lin, P. T., Flanagan, L. A., & Walsh, C. A. (1999). Doublecortin is a microtubule-associated protein and is expressed widely by migrating neurons. *Neuron, 23*(2), 257–271.

Hirotsune, S., Fleck, M. W., Gambello, M. J., Bix, G. J., Chen, A., Clark, G. D., et al. (1998). Graded reduction of Pafah1b1 (Lis1) activity results in neuronal migration defects and early embryonic lethality. *Nature and Genetics, 19*(4), 333–339.

Horesh, D., Sapir, T., Francis, F., Wolf, S. G., Caspi, M., Elbaum, M., et al. (1999). Doublecortin, a stabilizer of microtubules. *Human Molecular Genetics, 8*(9), 1599–1610.

Humphreys, P., Kaufmann, W. E., & Galaburda, A. M. (1990). Developmental dyslexia in women: Neuropathological findings in three cases. *Annals of Neurology, 28*, 727–738.

Illarioshkin, S. N., Tanaka, H., Markova, E. D., Nikolskaya, N. N., Ivanova-Smolenskaya, I. A., & Tsuji, S. (1996). X-linked nonprogressive congenital cerebellar hypoplasia: Clinical description and mapping to chromosome Xq. *Annals of Neurology, 40*(1), 75–83.

Joubert, M., Eisenring, J. J., & Andermann, F. (1968). Familial dysgenesis of the vermis: A syndrome of hyperventilation, abnormal eye movements and retardation. *Neurology, 18*(3), 302–303.

Kaprielian, Z., Runko, E., & Imondi, R. (2001). Axon guidance at the midline choice point. *Dev Dyn, 221*(2), 154–181.

Kaufmann, W. E., & Galaburda, A. M. (1989). Cerebrocortical microdysgenesis in neurologically normal subjects: A histopathologic study. *Neurology, 39*(2), 238–244.

Kholmanskikh, S. S., Dobrin, J. S., Wynshaw-Boris, A., Letourneau, P. C., & Ross, M. E. (2003). Disregulated RhoGTPases and actin cytoskeleton contribute to the migration defect in Lis1-deficient neurons. *The Journal of Neuroscience, 23*(25), 8673–8681.

Kitagawa, M., Umezu, M., Aoki, J., Koizumi, H., Arai, H., & Inoue, K. (2000). Direct association of LIS1, the lissencephaly gene product, with a mammalian homologue of a fungal nuclear distribution protein, rNUDE. *FEBS Lett, 479*(1–2), 57–62.

Klingberg, T., Hedehus, M., Temple, E., Salz, T., Gabrieli, J. D., Moseley, M. E., et al. (2000). Microstructure of temporo-parietal white matter as a basis for reading ability: Evidence from diffusion tensor magnetic resonance imaging. *Neuron, 25*(2), 493–500.

Kobayashi, M., Hutchinson, S., Schlaug, G., & Pascual-Leone, A. (2003). Ipsilateral motor cortex activation on functional magnetic resonance imaging during unilateral hand movements is related to interhemispheric interactions. *Neuroimage, 20*(4), 2259–2270.

Kornberg, A. J., & Shield, L. K. (1991). An extended phenotype of an early-onset inherited nonprogressive cerebellar ataxia syndrome. *Journal of Child Neurology, 6*(1), 20–23.

Leighton, P. A., Mitchell, K. J., Goodrich, L. V., Lu, X., Pinson, K., Scherz, P., et al. (2001). Defining brain wiring patterns and mechanisms through gene trapping in mice. *Nature, 410*(6825), 174–179.

Liu, Z., Steward, R., & Luo, L. (2000). Drosophila Lis1 is required for neuroblast proliferation, dendritic elaboration and axonal transport. *Nature and Cell Biolgy, 2*(11), 776–783.

Maria, B. L., Boltshauser, E., Palmer, S. C., & Tran, T. X. (1999). Clinical features and revised diagnostic criteria in Joubert syndrome. *Journal of Child Neurology, 14*(9), 583–590.

Maria, B. L., Hoang, K. B., Tusa, R. J., Mancuso, A. A., Hamed, L. M., Quisling, R. G., et al. (1997). "Joubert syndrome" revisited: Key ocular motor signs with magnetic resonance imaging correlation. *Journal of Child Neurology, 12*(7), 423–430.

Maria, B. L., Quisling, R. G., Rosainz, L. C., Yachnis, A. T., Gitten, J., Dede, D., et al. (1999). Molar tooth sign in Joubert syndrome: Clinical, radiologic, and pathologic significance. *Journal of Child Neurology, 14*(6), 368–376.

Molko, N., Cohen, L., Mangin, J. F., Chochon, F., Lehericy, S., Le Bihan, D., et al. (2002). Visualizing the neural bases of a disconnection syndrome with diffusion tensor imaging. *Journal of Cognitive Neuroscience, 14*(4), 629–636.

Niethammer, M., Smith, D. S., Ayala, R., Peng, J., Ko, J., Lee, M. S., et al. (2000). NUDEL is a novel Cdk5 substrate that associates with LIS1 and cytoplasmic dynein. *Neuron, 28*(3), 697–711.

Njiokiktjien, C. (1994). Dyslexia: A neuroscientific puzzle. *Acta Paedopsychiatry, 56*(3), 157–167.

Parisi, M. A., Pinter, J. D., Glass, I. A., Field, K., Maria, B. L., Chance, P. F., et al. (2004). Cerebral and cerebellar motor activation abnormalities in a subject with Joubert syndrome: Functional magnetic resonance imaging (MRI) study. *Journal of Child Neurology, 19*(3), 214–218.

Pinard, J. M., Motte, J., Chiron, C., Brian, R., Andermann, E., & Dulac, O. (1994). Subcortical laminar heterotopia and lissencephaly in two families: A single X linked dominant gene. *Journal of Neurology, Neurosurgery & Psychiatry, 57*(8), 914–920.

Rivas, R. J., & Hatten, M. E. (1995). Motility and cytoskeletal organization of migrating cerebellar granule neurons. *The Journal of Neuroscience, 15*(2), 981–989.

Rivier, F., & Echenne, B. (1992). Dominantly inherited hypoplasia of the vermis. *Neuropediatrics, 23*(4), 206–208.

Sapir, T., Horesh, D., Caspi, M., Atlas, R., Burgess, H. A., Wolf, S. G., et al. (2000). Doublecortin mutations cluster in evolutionarily conserved functional domains. *Human Molecular Genetics, 9*(5), 703–712.

Sasaki, S., Shionoya, A., Ishida, M., Gambello, M. J., Yingling, J., Wynshaw-Boris, A., et al. (2000). A LIS1/NUDEL/cytoplasmic dynein heavy chain complex in the developing and adult nervous system. *Neuron, 28*(3), 681–696.

Schaar, B. T., Kinoshita, K., & McConnell, S. K. (2004). Doublecortin microtubule affinity is regulated by a balance of kinase and phosphatase activity at the leading edge of migrating neurons. *Neuron, 41*(2), 203–213.

Sheeman, B., Carvalho, P., Sagot, I., Geiser, J., Kho, D., Hoyt, M. A., et al. (2003). Determinants of S. cerevisiae dynein localization and activation: Implications for the mechanism of spindle positioning. *Current Biology, 13*(5), 364–372.

Smith, D. S., Niethammer, M., Ayala, R., Zhou, Y., Gambello, M. J., Wynshaw-Boris, A., et al. (2000). Regulation of cytoplasmic dynein behaviour and microtubule organization by mammalian Lis1. *Nature and Cell Biology, 2*(11), 767–775.

Sweeney, K. J., Prokscha, A., & Eichele, G. (2001). NudE-L, a novel Lis1-interacting protein, belongs to a family of vertebrate coiled-coil proteins. *Mech Dev, 101*(1–2), 21–33.

Tai, C. Y., Dujardin, D. L., Faulkner, N. E., & Vallee, R. B. (2002). Role of dynein, dynactin, and CLIP-170 interactions in LIS1 kinetochore function. *Journal of Cell Biology, 156*(6), 959–968.

Tanaka, T., Serneo, F. F., Tseng, H. C., Kulkarni, A. B., Tsai, L. H., & Gleeson, J. G. (2004). Cdk5 phosphorylation of doublecortin ser297 regulates its effect on neuronal migration. *Neuron, 41*(2), 215–227.

Tayler, T. D., & Garrity, P. A. (2003). Axon targeting in the Drosophila visual system. *Current Opinions in Neurobiology, 13*(1), 90–95.

Taylor, K. R., Holzer, A. K., Bazan, J. F., Walsh, C. A., & Gleeson, J. G. (2000). Patient mutations in doublecortin define a repeated tubulin-binding domain. *J Biol Chem, 275*(44), 34442–34450.

ten Donkelaar, H. J., Hoevenaars, F., & Wesseling, P. (2000). A case of Joubert's syndrome with extensive cerebral malformations. *Clinical Neuropathology, 19*(2), 85–93.

Wynshaw-Boris, A., & Gambello, M. J. (2001). LIS1 and dynein motor function in neuronal migration and development. *Genes Development, 15*(6), 639–651.

Xiang, X. (2003). LIS1 at the microtubule plus end and its role in dynein-mediated nuclear migration. *Journal of Cell Biology, 160*(3), 289–290.

Yachnis, A. T., & Rorke, L. B. (1999). Neuropathology of Joubert syndrome. *Journal of Child Neurology, 14*(10), 655–659.

Chapter • 8

New Genes Involved in Cortical Development

Ferran Burgaya, Cristina Garcìa-Frigola, Rosa Andrés, Nathalia Vitureira, Guillermo López-Domènech, Luís de Lecea, and Eduardo Soriano

SUMMARY

In an attempt to elucidate the molecular basis of cortical development, we used a subtractive hybridization approach. A marginal zone-upper cortical plate target cDNA library was subtracted against a driver library obtained from the remaining lower layers. A 20-fold enrichment in target cDNAs was obtained in the subtracted population. Of the clones obtained, further studies are in progress on 3F3, a novel protein involved in RNA maturation, Podocalyxin, a sialoprotein characterized in renal glomerular epithelium, Alex3, a hinge protein related to b-catenin and Tetraspanin 5, a membrane coreceptor involved in signaling through integrins.

INTRODUCTION

Neuronal migration is an essential process for the development of the cerebral cortex. Abnormalities in migration processes that occur during cortical development are responsible for severe mental retardation, epilepsy, and learning disabilities in humans.

This study was supported by grants from the Ministry of Science to ES (SAF01-3290).

During the formation of the cerebral cortex, postmitotic neurons originated in the ventricular zone migrate toward the marginal zone following an "inside-out" progression, where newly generated neurons bypass previously positioned ones and settle in a more superficial location at the cortical plate. This process depends on a radial glial scaffold that neurons use for their movement (Angevine & Sidman, 1961; Marín-Padilla, 1971; Rakic, 1972; Supèr & Uylings, 2001). This radial migration is followed by pyramidal neurons, the main cell type of the neocortex. Interneurons, however, migrate tangentially following a distinct program (Anderson, Mione, Yun, & Rubenstein, 1999).

The development of the cerebral cortex depends on mechanisms such as cell recognition and adhesion, cell guidance through diffusible factors, signaling cascades, and cell motility (Anton, Cameron, & Rakic, 1996; Anton, Marchionni, Lee, & Rakic, 1997; Anton, Kreidberg, & Rakic, 1999; Cameron, Ruffin, Cho, Cameron, & Rakic, 1997; Alcántara, Ruiz, De Castro, Soriano, & Sotelo, 2000; Augsburger, Schuchardt, Hoskins, Dodd, & Butler, 1999; Dulabon et al., 2000). These events contribute to determine the final location of each neuron in the neocortex (Sidman & Rakic, 1973; Caviness & Sidman, 1973; Rakic, 1988). An intricate genetic program is responsible for the establishment of signaling cues and cell response. Several families of proteins that participate in cortical development have been characterized in recent years, including ligands and their corresponding receptors, signaling pathway components, transcription factors, and cytoskeletal elements.

SIGNALING AT THE CORTICAL PLATE

The marginal zone/layer I controls the migratory processes required for the histogenesis of the cerebral cortex (Marín-Padilla, 1984, 1988, 1998, 1999; Derer & Derer, 1990, 1992; Del Río, Martinez, Fonseca, Auladell, & Soriano, 1995). These findings were confirmed by the identification of Reelin, an extracellular matrix protein selectively expressed in the Marginal Zone by Cajal-Retzius cells, (Goffinet, 1995; D'Arcangelo et al., 1995, 1997; Hirotsune et al., 1995). The absence of Reelin and/or elements of its signaling pathway, including its receptors VLDLR and ApoER2 and the adaptor protein mDab1, alters neuronal migration patterns in the cerebral cortex (Howell, Gertler, & Cooper, 1997; Howell, Hawkes, Soriano, & Cooper, 1997; Howell, Herrick, & Cooper, 1999; Rice et al., 1998; D'Arcangelo et al., 1999; Hiesberger et al., 1999; Homayouni, Rice, Sheldon, & Curran, 1999; Trommsdorff, Borg, Margolis, & Herz, 1998; Trommsdorff et. al., 1999).

Additional molecules have been identified that participate in the control of several aspects of cortical migration such as cell locomotion, nucleokinesis, and adhesion: Dcx (Gleeson, Lin, Flanagan, & Walsh, 1999; Deconinck et al., 2003; Bai et al., 2003), 14-3-3e (YWHAE) (Cardoso et al., 2003), Pafah1b1 (Hirotsune et al., 1998; Cahana et al., 2001; Assadi et al., 2003), Filamin (Sheen et al., 2001), Cdk5 (Gilmore, Ohshima, Goffinet, Kulkarni, & Herrup, 1998; Homayouni & Curran, 2000; Kwon, Gupta, Zhou, Nikolic, & Tsai, 2000), p35 (Ohshima et al., 1996; Chae et al., 1997), integrins (Georges-Labouesse, Mark, Messaddeq, & Gansmuller, 1998; Anton et al., 1999; Dulabon et al., 2000; Graus-Porta et al., 2001), and Astrotactin (Adams, Tomoda, Cooper, Dietz, & Hatten, 2002).

Guidance molecules are also involved in cortical development including Semaphorins and their receptors, Neuropilins and Plexins (Marín, Yaron, Bagri, Tessier-Lavigne, & Rubenstein, 2001; He, Wang, Koprivica, Ming, & Song, 2002), Ephrins and Eph receptors (Wilkinson, 2001), Netrins and their corresponding receptors DCC, Neogenin and Unc-5 (Livesey, 1999), and the Slit-Robo system (Ghose & Van Vactor, 2002; see also Huber, Kolodkin, Ginty, & Cloutier, 2003, for review). Most guidance systems act through Rho GTPases and influence cytoskeletal dynamics, causing axonal repulsion, attraction and branching, neurite elongation, or neuronal migration. The signaling pathways between receptors and these proteins are poorly characterized.

The marginal zone orchestrates cortical development by controlling the processes that occur in the cortical plate (see references above). Therefore, we designed an experimental approach to identify genes selectively expressed by the most superficial layers of the developing cortex that could be responsible for some of the processes described above.

cDNA SUBTRACTION

We took advantage of a previously reported subtractive technique, "Directional tag PCR subtraction," which was designed and successfully applied for the identification of low abundant mRNAs with restricted expression patterns (Usui et al., 1994). This method renders mRNA clones enriched in a "target" tissue compared to a second tissue, the "driver."

We generated a subtractive cDNA library enriched in gene products from the most superficial layers of the developing mouse cortex by subtracting mRNAs from the marginal zone and upper cortical plate against mRNAs from the remaining cerebral cortex (see Figure 1). A process of differential screening allowed us to identify clones with exclusive or preferential expression in the marginal zone and/or the upper cortical plate (García-Frigola et al., 2004).

Generation of cDNA Libraries

To obtain the target tissue that included the marginal zone and upper cortical plate, cerebral cortices of E15-E16 mouse embryos were dissected and flat embedded in agar with the marginal zone side up. The tissue block was sectioned with a vibratome and the first 50 mm thick-section was used for cytoplasmic RNA isolation (Soriano, Alvarado-Mallart, Dumesnil, Del Rio, & Sotalo, 1997). The driver tissue, consisting of the cerebral cortex minus the upper cortical layers, was obtained by removing the most external layers of the cortical hemispheres through a sequential controlled treatment with collagenase A and trypsin. The remaining deep cortical structures were used for cytoplasmic RNA isolation as above. cDNA libraries were constructed for each tissue sample and

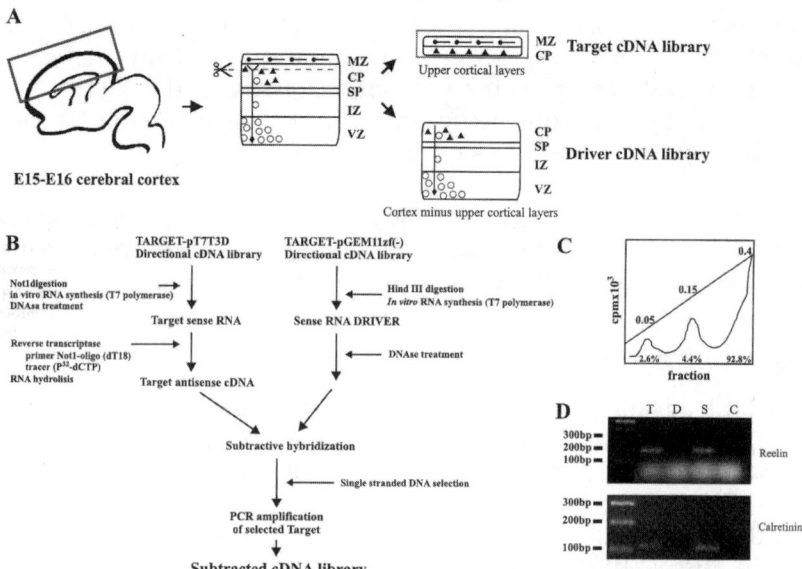

Figure 1. Schematic representation of the procedure followed to obtain the libraries used for this study. Taken from Garcìa-Frigola et al., 2004 with permission.

subtraction was performed as previously described (Usui et al., 1994). A scheme of the procedure is shown in Figure 1B.

Briefly, 1 mg of trace-labeled target cDNA was annealed with 30 mg of driver cRNA for 24h at 68°C. Tracer quantification after hydroxylapatite chromatography showed that the single-stranded cDNA fraction corresponded to 4% of the input material, representing a 20-fold enrichment in target products (Figure 1C). An aliquot of the single-stranded material was used as template in a 30-cycle PCR amplification step and the products were cloned into pBSK. The number of recombinant clones in this subtracted library was 5×10^5.

To validate the subtraction process, we performed a PCR assay to assess the presence of marginal zone specific genes (reelin and calretinin) in the libraries. Reelin and calretinin transcripts were cloned in the target and subtracted libraries, but were absent from the driver library (Figure 1D).

Library Screening

The subtracted library was electroporated into competent cells. Individual colonies were picked onto nylon filters from which replicas were made. Each filter was hybridized to target, driver, and subtracted cDNA probes, and exposed to sensitive films. Positive clones for the target and subtracted probes and negative for the driver probe were selected for further analysis.

A total of 120 subtracted clones were sequenced. Clones without polyA signal were considered subtraction artifacts and discarded. Eighty-five clone sequences were searched by BLAST analysis against the GenBank database and were confirmed to correspond to 76 genes. Reelin and calretinin, which were present in the subtracted library (Figure 2C), did not appear in the screening process, indicating that saturation had not been reached.

To better characterize the subtracted library, the expression pattern of 39 clones was analyzed by *in situ* hybridization or immunostaining on brain sections at three developmental stages: E16, P0, and adult. Most gene products were mainly expressed in the marginal zone and/or upper cortical plate. Interestingly, some showed enriched expression or were specific for the cortical layer V (see Table II). This can be attributed to the fact that cells that will give rise to adult layer V are located immediately below the marginal zone at E16, the developmental stage chosen for this study. A summary of the results obtained is presented in Tables I and II. When tools were available, further immunochemical studies were performed.

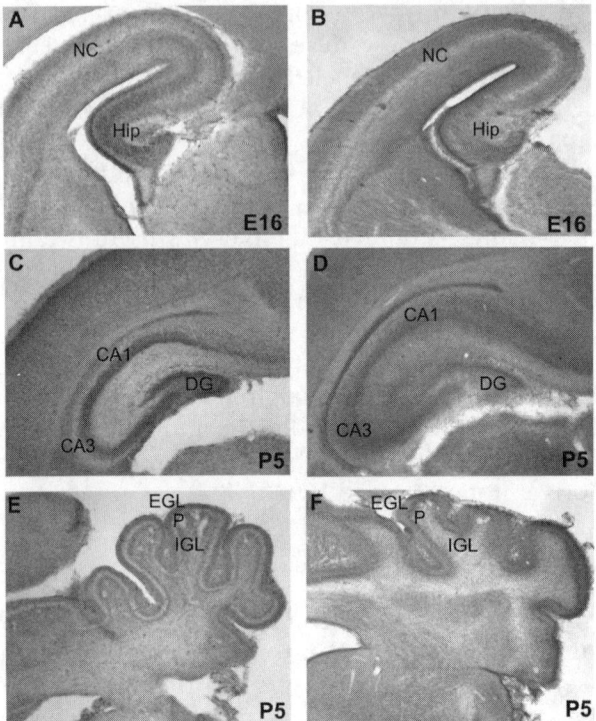

Figure 2. Pattern of Podocalyxin mRNA (A,C,E) and protein (B,D,F) expression in the developing cerebral cortex and in the cerebellum. Expression is prominent in the intermediate zone and cortical plate and hippocampal plates, as well as in the external granular layer and inner granular layer of the cerebellum. Abbreviations: Nc, neocortex; Hip, hippocampus; CAΣ, CA1, hippocampal subfields; DG, dentate gyrus; EGL and IGL, external and internal granular cell layer; P, Purkinje cell layer.

Clones corresponding to Tspan-5, Podocalyxin, and Alex3 showed interesting expression patterns, and were selected for further characterization. We obtained full-length cDNA sequences, raised antisera, and developed a variety of tools to perform the studies described below.

SUBTRACTED CLONES STUDIED

Table I summarizes the results from the sequencing analysis. The subtracted library contained products coding for proteins previously characterized, hypothetical genes of unknown function, EST sequences, and novel sequences.

Table I. Classification of the clones purified from the subtracted library.

Total Clones Screened	PolyA+	GENBANK Matching	Type of Product	Type of Protein	Examples
120	76	36 matched	25 proteins	signal and adhesion	FGF-1, HGF-like
				transcription factor and nuclear proteins (5)	CHOP-10, MMUSF
				transduction (2)	Flt3-int. pKCl
				catabolism (2)	DBA/2J, Gdx (ubiq.-like)
				cytoskeleton 1)	Peripherin
				synapse (1)	SAP102
				miscellaneous (7) (metabolism, adaptors, inhibitors)	Ferro-chelatase, Brain Glycogen phosphorylase
			11 unknown		
		40 unmatched	36 EST		
			4 novel		

Fourteen out of the 25 cDNAs that matched known gene products corresponded to proteins directly involved in cell signaling such as membrane proteins, growth factors, signal transduction components, transcription factors, and nuclear proteins. Five of the 25 matching species identified in the subtracted library corresponded to mRNAs whose products had not been previously reported in the CNS such as Podocalyxin, a membrane sialoprotein with cell adhesion functions (see below). Moreover, expression of 16 of the 25 clones had not been reported previously in the cerebral cortex including Peripherin (see below) and the transcription factor CHOP-10, involved in differentiation (Ron & Habener, 1992; Zinszner et al., 1998). We also detected the expression of rCGR11, an inhibitor of cell proliferation, which acts through interaction with p53 (Madden, Galella, Riley, Bertlsen, & Beaudry, 1996) and Fiz1, a zinc finger protein that binds to the membrane tyrosine kinase Flt3 (also expressed during brain development), which may transduce signals to the nucleus (Wolf &

Rohrschneider, 1999). We identified PKCI, an inhibitor of PKC involved in multiple signaling events, and SAP-102, a synaptic associated protein involved in the aggregation of neurotransmitter receptors, in the synapse, indicating that layer I has a relatively mature synaptic machinery by E16, as proposed elsewhere (Schwartz et al., 1998).

Secreted and membrane proteins are especially relevant for neuronal migration in the cerebral cortex. In this study, we found Neurexin II-?, a protein involved in interneuronal junctions and expressed in upper cortical layers in the adult rat (Ullrich, Ushkaryov, & Sudhof 1995). We also detected a clone encoding FGF-1, a member of the FGF family of secreted factors essential for neural development (Streit, Berliner, Papanayotou, Sirulnik, & Stern, 2000), and HGF-like, which belongs to the HGF family of factors implicated in cortical migration (Powell, Mars, & Levitt, 2001). Some of the subtracted cDNA clones encoded for transmembrane proteins involved in cell adhesion and migration processes outside the CNS such as Trophinin and Podocalyxin (see below).

Thirty-nine of the subtracted clones were analyzed by *in situ* hybridization on free-floating sections. The resulting expression patterns are shown in Table II. Twenty-eight of the 39 isolated clones were expressed in the upper cortical layers, comprising the marginal zone and the cortical plate. Moreover, 12 of these 28 clones were selectively expressed in the marginal zone and upper tier of the cortical plate (prospective layer V). Thirteen clones were widely expressed in all cortical layers, and two showed enriched expression in the ventricular zone and were considered false positive products of the subtraction. We analyzed the immunoreactivity patterns of the clones for which specific antibodies were available (Table III).

We conclude that all the clones tested are highly expressed in the cortex at E16, and most exhibit enriched expression in the upper cortical layers. The high expression of these clones at embryonic and postnatal stages and low or null levels in the adult indicates their role in cortical development. Furthermore, most

Table II. Patterns of expression followed by the clones enumerated in Table I.

Temporal Pattern	Cerebral Pattern	Cortical Pattern (embryo)
peak at E1 (24)	mainly cortical (9)	MZ + upper CP (13)
peak at P0 (6)	preferentially cortical (23)	MZ + main CP (14)
peak adult (1)	widespread (7)	pan-cortical (10)
constant with age (8)		ventricular (2)

Table III. Immunocytochemical patterns obtained when commercial antibodies were available.

Antigen	Temporal Pattern	Cerebral Pattern	Cortical Pattern (embryo)
PODOCALYXIN	postnatal peak	preferentially cortical	MZ + upper CP
PERIPHERIN	peak at P0	preferentially cortical	radial glia
TROPHININ	stable expression	preferentially cortical	CP + VZ

subtracted clones were not expressed in neurogenetic regions, indicating that they probably participate in processes other than proliferation.

Clone 3F3

The sequence of clone 3F3 is highly homologous to RRP5, a yeast protein involved in RNA maturation (Nagase, Seki, Ishikawa, Tanaka, & Nomura, 1996; Venema & Tollervey, 1996). Clone 3F3 hybridizes to a single transcript of 6 Kb in Northern blot assays. It is selectively expressed by layer V neurons and thalamic nuclei during brain development, suggesting a possible involvement in the establishment of thalamocortical projections. In the adult brain, expression was not detected. Low levels of 3F3 expression are found in several adult peripheral tissues (liver and testes) (García-Frigola et al., 2004). The theoretical protein encoded by 3F3 contains several S1 RNA-binding domains and several tetratricopeptide repeats, involved in RNA-protein interactions and the assembly of multiprotein complexes, respectively (Lamb, Tugendreich, & Hieter, 1995). These structural properties are consistent with the presumptive role of clone 3F3 in RNA maturation processes or its role as a splicing factor that is finely regulated during development.

Podocalyxin

Podocalyxin is a heavily sialyated and sulfated membrane protein expressed on the apical surface of the glomerular epithelial cells or podocytes and on vascular endothelia (Kershaw et al., 1997; Miettinen et al., 1999). Although first described as a marker of these tissues, Podocalyxin is also expressed in platelets, megakaryocites, and hematopoietic precursor cells (Miettinen et al., 1999). Biochemical analysis shows that Podocalyxin is a 140-160 kDa transmembrane protein composed of a highly glycosylated ectodomain, a unique transmembrane region, and a cytoplasmic tail with potential phosphorylation sites and a putative ligand (DTHL aminoacidic sequence) for a PDZ domain. However, Podocalyxin belongs to a family of sialomucins whose functions are poorly understood. Because of its high negative charge, Podocalyxin has been proposed to be an antiadhesin responsible for maintaining the filtration slits open (Dekan, Gabel, & Farquhar, 1991; Hilkens, Ligtenberg, Vos, & Litvinov, 1992; Orlando et al., 2001). Takeda, Go, Orlando, and Farquhar (2000) have shown direct evidence for a charge-repulsive effect of Podocalyxin on the surface of cultured cells, whereby expression of this protein inhibits cell-to-cell adhesion. On the other hand, Sassetti, Tangemann, Singer, Kershaw, and Rosen (1998) suggested a novel function for Podocalyxin as an adhesion molecule because in vascular endothelium, this protein binds to L-selectin and supports the L-selectin-dependent tethering and rolling of lymphocytes under flow.

The presence of Podocalyxin cDNA in our subtracted library led us to analyze the expression pattern of the transcript and protein in the developing brain. Higher levels of expression were detected, particularly in the cerebral cortex, hippocampus, and cerebellum, along development and in adult brain (see Figure 2). In these regions, the expression of Podocalyxin was particularly high at embryonic and early postnatal stages as P5. Labelling was considerable in the upper cortical layers (II-III), in the granule and pyramidal cell layers of the hippocampus, and in the external and internal granular layers of the cerebellum. Some proliferative regions, such as the rhombic lip (at E14) and the forebrain subventricular zone, were also stained along the development. The expression of Podocalyxin was also substantial in some axonal pathways such as the corpus callossum and the fimbria fornix between E16 and P15. Furthermore, we also detected expression in many neurons during axogenesis and synapse formation in hippocampal primary cultures.

In addition, Podocalyxin-deficient (podx1-/-) mice revealed changes in particular axonal pathways such as the olfactory tract, and in several neuronal migratory pathways, as it is the case for the genesis of cortical interneurons (subjected to tangential migration). Null mice exhibit profound defects in kidney development and die from anuric renal failure within 24 hours of birth (Doyonnas et al., 2001), thereby preventing the postnatal study of brain Podocalyxin.

Altogether, these results indicate that Podocalyxin is involved in the development of the CNS. In this regard, this membrane protein may regulate the adhesion processes necessary for migration and differentiation. In addition, it may play a permissive role in axon guidance, reducing the fasciculative interactions between axons and thereby allowing them to respond more effectively to a variety of extrinsic signals, including those from their targets. Moreover, many tissues that express polysialic acid (PSA) during development show a progressive loss of this carbohydrate as adult structures are formed. Thus, the maintained expression of Podocalyxin in adult tissues (hippocampus and cerebellum) points to a role in plasticity, and this possibility is supported by the observation that PSA is expressed in a variety of brain tissues that exhibit physiological plasticity (Bofanti, Olive, Poulain, & Theodosis, 1992).

Alex3

Alex3 is a protein of 379 amino acids with a molecular weight of about 40 Kda, which belongs to the recently described family of Alex proteins (Arm domain-proteins lost in epithelial cancers on chromosome X; see Kurochkin, Yonemitsu, Funahashi, & Nomura, 2001). The Alex family of proteins shows two armadillo/b-catenin-like repeats in its sequence. Proteins containing homologous motifs have been implicated in processes such as tumorigenesis, embryonic development, and maintenance of tissue integrity (Hatzfeld, 1999). Until now, proteins with less than six armadillo repeats had not been described; therefore, the Alex proteins might constitute a novel family. The other two members of the family, Alex1 and Alex 2, are expressed in almost all polarized tissues. It is speculated that these two proteins are involved in the suppression of tumours that originate from epithelial tissue because their expression is lost or significantly reduced in carcinomas or cell lines derived from carcinomas (Kurochkin et al., 2001).

In addition to its two completed armadillo repeats and three uncompleted ones, the amino acidic sequence of Alex3 presents a putative arginine-rich nuclear localization signal (NLS) and also various potential phosphorylation sites for Casein Kinase 2 (CK 2), Protein Kinase C (PK C), and cAMP-dependent Protein Kinase (PK A). Also, Alex3 contains other protein-protein interaction domains such as leucine-rich repeats. The SOSUI algorithm and the TMHMM program also predict a possible transmembrane domain at the N-terminus of these proteins (amino acids 5 to 27 or 7 to 29, depending on the source).

The coding sequences of all the Alex family members are constituted by a single exon, their corresponding genes being clustered in the human chromosome X. The mRNA expression of Alex3 is highly restricted to the CNS, in contrast with the other two members of the family that are widely distributed in almost all tissues. We performed *in situ* hybridizations to determine the distribution of the Alex3 transcript in the brain and in the whole embryo during development. The levels of the transcript were high in almost all the CNS and in the limb buds. Lower levels were detected by Northern blot in heart, liver, spleen, kidneys, and testes. The higher levels of Alex3 in murine brain were detected from developmental stage E10 until P0 or P5. From this stage, the expression levels were reduced but continued until adulthood. The expression was especially high in adult brain cortex, especially the pyramidal layer V (see Figure 3), the hippocampus, and cerebellum, and also some hypothalamic and mesencephalic nuclei (García-Frigola et al., 2004). In addition, an enriched expression of the Alex3 transcript was described in the initial segment of the epidydimis versus others segments (Hsia & Cornwall, 2003). These authors speculate that the enrichment of gene products like Alex3 and others in the epidydimis is one of the factors responsible for the rare appearance of cancer in such tissues.

b catenin is the critical point in the regulation of the Wnt signalling pathway. Its armadillo repeats are protein-protein interaction domains clearly related with processes such as tumorigenesis and embryonic development. b-catenin serves as a link between cadherins and the actin cytoskeleton in homotypic adhesion unions. Moreover, b-catenin plays a crucial role in the signalling of the Wnt pathway by acting as a transcription factor in the nucleus when it interacts with the Lef-1/Tcf transcription factors gene family. The armadillo domains present in Alex3, together with the technical approach followed for its isolation and the structural data of its sequence, allowed us to classify Alex3

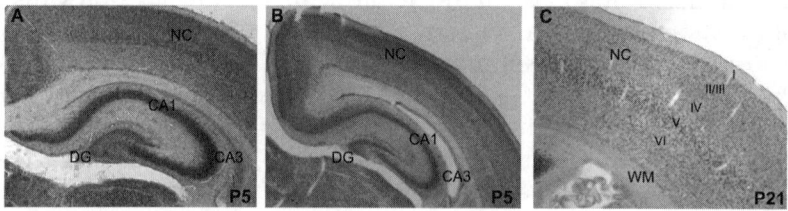

Figure 3. Pattern of Alex3 mRNA (A,C) and protein (B) expression at P5 and at P21. ALEX3 transcript and protein are widely distributed in the developing and adult hippocampus and cerebral cortex, being especially conspicuous at cortical layer V. Abbreviations as in Figure 2.

into important signalling pathways in several processes such as migration, axonal guide, neuritogenesis, and synaptogenesis in the development of laminar structures of the brain. The observation that Alex3 also contains a nuclear localization signal might explain its functional roles, although this must be confirmed.

Tspan5

The tetraspanin superfamily, also referred to as tetraspans or transmembrane 4 proteins (TM4SF), are 204-355 aminoacid cell-surface glycoproteins that span the membrane four times, forming two extracellular loops (EC; a small loop between the first and the second transmembrane domains, and a large loop between the third and fourth domain) and cytoplasmic N- and C- termini.

The human tetraspanin family comprises 28 highly homologous proteins. The tetraspanin family includes leucocyte antigens (CD9, CD37, CD53, CD63, CD81, CD82, and CD151), antigens first identified on tumors (TALLA-1, SAS), and although more distinct, the Uroplakins and the proteins encoded by the retinal dystrophy syndrome genes, RDS/peripherin and Rom-1 (Maecker, Todd, & Levy, 1997; Wright & Tomlinson, 1994).

With the exception of erythrocytes, all the cell types reported express several tetraspanins. Their tissue distribution and expression pattern is highly variable: some tetraspanins have a wide distribution (CD9, CD63, CD81, CD82), whereas others have a very restricted expression pattern (RDS/Peripherin and Rom-1) (Boucheix & Rubinstein, 2001).

One feature of tetraspanins is their capacity to form multimolecular complexes between them or with other types of membrane surface proteins. These interacting proteins range from membrane receptors (EGF-R, TGF-α), adhesion molecules ($\alpha\beta$ integrin dimmers) to signal transduction molecules (PKC, PI4 K) (Rubinstein et al., 1996; Hemler, Mannion, & Berditchevski, 1996; Stipp & Hemler, 2000; Shi, Fan, Shum, & Derynck, 2000; Berditchevski, Tolias, Wong, Carpenter, & Hemler,1997; Yauch Berditchevski, Harler, Reichner, & Hemler, 1998). The main region of tetraspanin interaction with other nontetraspanins proteins occurs through the large second extracellular loop (EC2), which appears to confer the specificity. The functional utility of these complexes is unknown but a model where tetraspanins may act as membrane microdomains organizers has been proposed (Yunta & Lazo, 2003).

The use of blocking antibodies against specific tetraspanins has clarified the involvement of these molecules in a number of cellular processes like proliferation, migration, and cellular adhesion (reviewed in Boucheix & Rubinstein, 2001; Shi et al., 2000; Yauch et al., 1998).

Although tetraspanins were initially identified as superficial antigens that are highly expressed in the immune system, recent data show the presence of these proteins in the embryonic and adult nervous system (Kopczynski, Davis, & Goodman, 1996; Zemni et al., 2000). A cDNA clone that codifies for mouse tetraspanin 5 (Tspan5) has been isolated (García-Frigola, Burgaya, Calbet, de Lecea, & Soriano, 2000; García-Frigola, Burgaya, de Lecea, & Soriano, 2001; Garcia-Frigola et al., 2004). mRNA expression studies using Northern blot have detected mTspan5 transcripts as early as E10 and as development progresses, the levels of Tspan5 increase to peak around the first postnatal week after which expression levels remain fairly constant until adulthood. In the CNS, its distribution and expression is highly variable. During development, mRNA transcripts have been detected by *in situ* hybridization in the telencephalon, the diencephalon, and the mesencephalon with high levels of mRNA expression in the cerebral cortex, hippocampus (Figure 4), and cerebellum (García-Frigola et al., 2001). The high expression observed in postmitotic neurons in the cortical plate and Purkinje cells points to a possible role of mTspan5 in neuronal differentiation and functional maturation. In addition, mTspan5 signal has also been detected in several migratory routes like the rostral migratory steam, migrating external granular layer, migrating Purkinje cells, rhombic lip, and the pontine migratory stream, indicating a possible role of this protein in migration during development (García-Frigola et al., 2001). The use of a rabbit polyclonal antibody generated in our laboratory, which specifically recognizes the variable region of the EC2 domain, has allowed us to study mTspan5 at the protein level. Thus, the data generated by immunohistochemistry correlate with the mRNA pattern expression observed by *in situ* hybridization (Figure 4).

To clarify the possible role of mTspan5 during development, we studied the interactions of mTspan5 with other molecules. Immunoprecipitation with rabbit mTspan5 Ab, followed by Western blotting for the $\alpha 3$ integrin subunit, demonstrated that both mTspan5 and $\alpha 3$ integrin interact (data not published). This observation indicates that mTspan5 may be involved in neurite outgrowth and adhesion, functions in which $\alpha 3$ integrin has largely been implicated. Furthermore, function blocking antibody to mTspan-5 *in vitro* significantly inhibited cell attachment to laminin substrate on E16 primary neuronal hippocampus and cerebral cortex cultures (data not published). This observation led

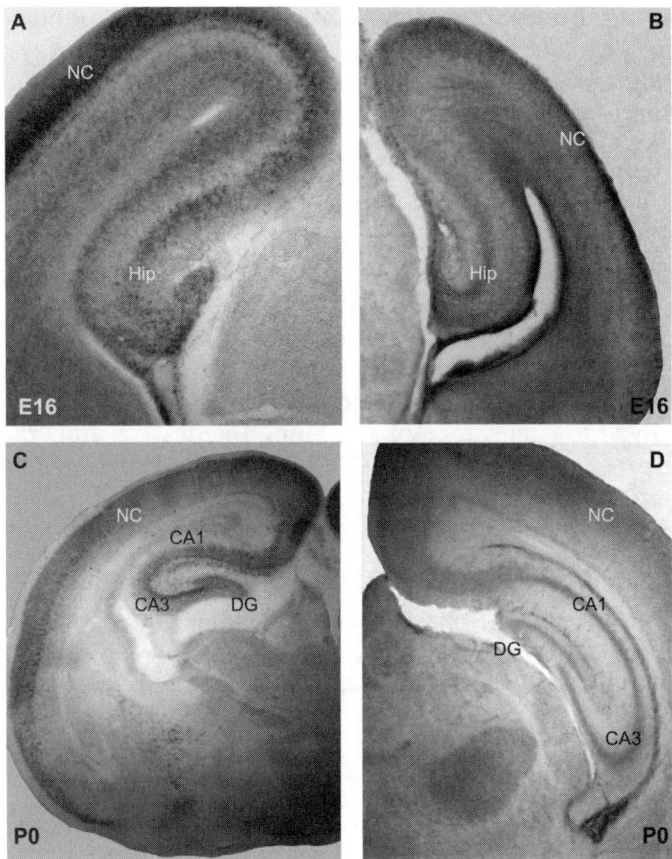

Figure 4. Pattern of Tspan5 mRNA (A,C) and protein (B,D) expression in the forebrain at E16 and P0. Note that transcripts and protein concentrate in the cortical and hippocampal plates and in the intermediate zone. Abbreviations as in Figure 2.

us to postulate that mTspan-5 contributes to support cell adhesion as well as to other functions such as cell migration. Whether mTspan5 modulates integrin-dependent cell adhesion or whether the effect observed is due to an independent integrin effect by mTspan5 remains to be elucidated.

FUTURE PROSPECTS

The fact that several hundreds of clones have been isolated from our library leads us to conclude that this study is far from being completed. Interestingly, many of the clones correspond to molecules involved in cell signalling through multiple pathways.

Some of these clones are puzzling because there is not much information available about them. The importance of neuronal RNA processing through 3F3 is unknown at present. There are not neural illnesses known to be related to the lack of Podocalyxin function; however, current analyses of podocalyxin KO mice show that a number of neuronal migration pathways are altered in the absence of this gene. Alex3 seems to play a protective role against some types of cancer, yet its transduction pathway is not characterized. Tspan5 is known to participate in migration and adhesion processes. The next steps in our studies correspond to the generation of transgenic Gain-of-function and Loss-of-function models to analyze the relevance of the cloned genes. Several transgenic overexpressing lines and knock-out mice have been generated already in our laboratory with the hope that they will provide some light on the functions of these genes for brain development.

Address correspondence to: Dr. Eduardo Soriano, Developmental Neurobiology and Regeneration Lab, Lab A1-S1, IRBB-PCB, Josep Samitier 5, Barcelona 08028, Spain; E-mail: esoriano@pcb.ub.es; phone: +34-93-4037117; fax: +34-93-4037116

REFERENCES

Adams, N. C., Tomoda, T., Cooper, M., Dietz. G., & Hatten, M. E. (2002). Mice that lack astrotactin have slowed neuronal migration. *Development, 129*, 965–972.

Alcántara, S., Ruiz, M., De Castro, F., Soriano, E., & Sotelo, C. (2000). Netrin 1 acts as an attractive or as a repulsive cue for distinct migrating neurons during the development of the cerebellar system. *Development, 127*, 1359–1372.

Anderson, S., Mione, M., Yun, K., & Rubenstein, J. L. (1999). Differential origins of neocortical projection and local circuit neurons: Role of Dlx genes in neocortical interneuronogenesis. *Cerebral Cortex, 9*(6), 646–654.

Angevine, J. B., & Sidman, R. L. (1961). Autoradiographic study of cell migration during histogenesis of cerebral cortex in the mouse. *Nature, 192*, 766–768.

Anton, E. S., Cameron, R. S., & Rakic, P. (1996). Role of neuron-glial junctional domain proteins in the maintenance and termination of neuronal migration across the embryonic cerebral wall. *The Journal of Neuroscience, 16*, 2283–2293.

Anton, E. S., Marchionni, M. A., Lee, K. F., & Rakic, P. (1997). Role of GGF/neuregulin signaling in interactions between migrating neurons and radial glia in the developing cerebral cortex. *Development, 124*, 3501–3510.

Anton, E. S., Kreidberg, J. A., & Rakic, P. (1999). Distinct functions of a3 and aV integrin receptors in neuronal migration and laminar organization of the cerebral cortex. *Neuron, 22,* 277–289.

Assadi, A. H., Zhang, G., Beffert, U., McNeil, R. S., Renfro, A. L., Niu, S., Quattrocchi, C. C., Antalffy, B. A., Sheldon, M., Armstrong, D. D., Wynshaw-Boris, A., Herz, J., D'Arcangelo, G., & Clark, G. D. (2003). Interaction of reelin signaling and Lis1 in brain development. *Nature Genetics, 35*(3), 270–276.

Augsburger, A., Schuchardt, A., Hoskins, S., Dodd, J., & Butler, S. (1999). BMPs as mediators of roof plate repulsion of commissural neurons. *Neuron, 24*(1), 127–141.

Bai, J., Ramos, R. L., Ackman, J. B., Thomas, A. M., Lee, R. V., & LoTurco, J. J. (2003). RNAi reveals doublecortin is required for radial migration in rat neocortex. *Nature Neuroscience, 6*(12), 1277–1283.

Berditchevski, F., Tolias, K. F., Wong, K., Carpenter, C. L., & Hemler, M. E. (1997). A novel link between integrins, transmembrane-4 superfamily proteins (CD63 and CD81), and phosphatidylinositol 4-kinase. *Journal of Biological Chemistry, 272*(5), 2595–2598.

Bofanti, L., Olive, S., Poulain, D. A., & Theodosis, D. T. (1992). Mapping of the distribution of polysialylated neural cell adhesion molecule throughout the central nervous system of the adult rat: An immunohistochemical study. *Neuroscience, 49,* 419.

Boucheix, C., & Rubinstein E. (2001). Tetraspanins. *Cell and Molecular Life Sciences, 58,* 1189–1205.

Cahana, A., Escamez, T., Nowakowski, R. S., Hayes, N. L., Giacobini, M., von Holst, A., Shmueli, O., Sapir, T., McConnell, S. K., Wurst, W., Martinez, S., & Reiner, O. (2001). Targeted mutagenesis of Lis1 disrupts cortical development and LIS1 homodimerization. *Proceedings of the National Academy of Sciences USA, 98*(11), 6429–6434.

Cameron, R. S., Ruffin, J. W., Cho, N. K., Cameron, P. L., & Rakic, P. (1997). Developmental expression, pattern of distribution, and effect on cell aggregation implicate a neuron-glial junctional domain protein in neuronal migration. *The Journal of Comparative Neurology, 387*(4), 467–488.

Cardoso, C., Leventer, R. J., Ward, H. L., Toyo-Oka, K., Chung, J., Gross, A., Martin, C. L., Allanson, J., Pilz, D. T., Olney, A. H., Mutchinick, O. M., Hirotsune, S., Wynshaw-Boris, A., Dobyns, W. B., & Ledbetter, D. H. (2003). Refinement of a 400-kb critical region allows genotypic differentiation between isolated lissencephaly, Miller-Dieker syndrome, and other phenotypes secondary to deletions of 17p13.3. *American Journal of Human Genetics, 72*(4), 918–930.

Caviness, V. S., Jr., & Sidman, R. L. (1973). Time of origin or corresponding cell classes in the cerebral cortex of normal and reeler mutant mice: An autoradiographic analysis. *The Journal of Comparative Neurology, 148*(2), 141–151.

Chae, T., Kwon, Y. T., Bronson, R., Dikkes, P., Li, E., & Tsai, L. H. (1997). Mice lacking p35, a neuronal specific activator of Cdk5, display cortical lamination defects, seizures, and adult lethality. *Neuron, 18*(1), 29–42.

D'Arcangelo, G., Miao, G., Chen, C., Soares, H., Morgan, I., & Curran, T. (1995). Protein related to extracellular -matrix proteins deleted—the mouse mutant reeler. *Nature, 374*(6524), 719–723.

D'Arcangelo, G., Nakajima, K., Miyata, T., Ogawa, M., Mikoshiba, K., & Curran, T. (1997). Reelin is a secreted glycoprotein recognized by the CR-50 monoclonal antibody. *The Journal of Neuroscience, 17*(1), 23–31.

D'Arcangelo, G., Homayouni, R., Keshvara, L., Rice, D. S., Sheldon, M., & Curran, T. (1999). Reelin is a ligand for lipoprotein receptors. *Neuron, 24*(2), 471–479.

Deconinck, N., Duprez, T., des Portes, V., Beldjord, C., Ghariani, S., Sindic, C. J., & Sebire, G. (2003). Familial bilateral medial parietooccipital band heterotopia not related to DCX or LIS1 gene defects. *Neuropediatrics, 34*, 146–148.

Dekan, G., Gabel, C., & Farquhar, M. G. (1991). Sulfate contributes to the negative charge of podocalyxin, the major sialoprotein of the glomerular filtration slits. *Proceedings of the National Academy of Sciences USA, 88*, 5398–5402.

del Rio, J. A., Martinez, A., Fonseca, M., Auladell, C., & Soriano, E. (1995). Glutamate-like immunoreactivity and fate of Cajal-Retzius cells in the murine cortex as identified with calretinin antibody. *Cerebral Cortex, 5*(1), 13–21.

Derer, P., & Derer, M. (1990). Cajal-Retzius cell ontogenesis and death in mouse brain visualized with horseradish peroxidase and electron microscopy. *Neuroscience, 36*(3), 839–856.

Derer, P., & Derer, M. (1992). Development and fate of Cajal-Retzius cells in vivo and in vitro. In S. C. Sharma & A. M. Goffinet (Eds.), *Development of the central nervous system in vertebrates* (pp. 113–127). New York: Plenum Press.

Doyonnas, R., Kershaw, D. B., Duhme, C., Merkens, H., Chelliah, S., Graf, T., & McNagny, K. M. (2001). Anuria, omphalocele, and perinatal lethality in mice lacking the CD34-related protein podocalyxin. *Journal of Experimental Medicine, 194*(1), 13–27.

Dulabon, L., Olson, E. C., Taglienti, M. G., Eisenhuth, S., McGrath, B., Walsh, C. A., Kreidberg, J. A., & Anton, E. S. (2000). Reelin binds alpha3beta1 integrin and inhibits neuronal migration. *Neuron, 27*(1), 33–44.

García-Frigola, C., Burgaya, F., Calbet, M., de Lecea, L., & Soriano, E. (2000). Mouse Tspan-5, a member of the tetraspanin superfamily, is highly expressed in brain cortical structures. *Neuroreport, 11*(14), 3181–3185.

García-Frigola, C., Burgaya, F., de Lecea, L., & Soriano, E. (2001). Pattern of expression of the tetraspanin Tspan-5 during brain development in the mouse. *Mechanics of Development, 106*(1–2), 207–212.

García-Frigola, C., Burgaya, F., Calbet, M., Lopez-Domenech, G., de Lecea, L., & Soriano, E. (2004). A collection of cDNAs enriched in upper cortical layers of the embryonic mouse brain. *Molecular Brain Research, 122*(2), 133–150.

Georges-Labouesse, E., Mark, M., Messaddeq, N., & Gansmuller, A. (1998). Essential role of alpha 6 integrins in cortical and retinal lamination. *Current Biology, 8*(17), 983–986.

Ghose, A., & Van Vactor, D. (2002). GAPs in Slit-Robo signaling. *Bioessays, 24*(5), 401–404.

Gilmore, E. C., Ohshima, T., Goffinet, A. M., Kulkarni, A. B., & Herrup, K. (1998). Cyclin-dependent kinase 5-deficient mice demonstrate novel developmental arrest in cerebral cortex. *The Journal of Neuroscience, 18*(16), 6370–6377.

Gleeson, J. G., Lin, P. T., Flanagan, L. A., & Walsh, C. A. (1999). Doublecortin is a microtubule-associated protein and is expressed widely by migrating neurons. *Neuron, 23*(2), 257–271.

Goffinet, A.M. (1995). A real gene for reeler. *Nature, 374,* 675–676.

Graus-Porta, D., Blaess, S., Senften, M., Littlewood-Evans, A., Damsky, C., Huang, Z., Orban, P., Klein, R., Schittny, J. C., & Muller, U. (2001). β1-class integrins regulate the development of laminae and folia in the cerebral and cerebellar cortex. *Neuron, 31*(3), 367–379.

Hatzfeld, M. (1999). The armadillo family of structural proteins. *International Review of Cytology, 186,* 179–224.

He, Z., Wang, K. C., Koprivica, V., Ming, G., & Song, H. J. (2002). Knowing how to navigate: Mechanisms of semaphorin signaling in the nervous system. *Science STKE, 2002*(119), RE1.

Hemler, M. E., Mannion, B. A., & Berditchevski, F. (1996). Association of TM4SF proteins with integrins: Relevance to cancer. *Biochemical and Biophysical Acta, 1287,* 67–71.

Hiesberger, T., Trommsdorff, M., Howell, B. W., Goffinet, A., Mumby, M. C., Cooper, J. A., & Herz, J. (1999). Direct binding of Reelin to VLDL receptor and ApoE receptor 2 induces tyrosine phosphorylation of disabled-1 and modulates tau phosphorylation. *Neuron, 24*(2), 481–489.

Hilkens, J., Ligtenberg, M. J., Vos, H. L., & Litvinov, S. V. (1992). Cell membrane-associated mucins and their adhesion-modulating property. *Trends in Biochemical Science, 17,* 359–363

Hirotsune, S., Takahara, T., Sasaki, N., Hirose, K., Yoshiki, A., Ohashi, T., Kusakabe, M., Murakami, Y., Muramatsu, M., Watanabe, S., Nakao K., Katsuki M., & Hayashizaki Y. (1995). The reeler gene encodes a protein with an EGF-like motif expressed by pioneer neurons. *Nature Genetics, 10*(1), 77–83.

Hirotsune, S., Fleck, M. W., Gambello, M. J., Bix, G. J., Chen, A., Clark, G. D., Ledbetter, D. H., McBain, C. J., & Wynshaw-Boris, A. (1998). Graded reduction of Pafah1b1 (Lis1) activity results in neuronal migration defects and early embryonic lethality. *Nature Genetics, 19*(4), 333–339.

Homayouni, R., Rice, D. S., Sheldon, M., & Curran, T. (1999). Dab1 binds to the cytoplasmic domain of amyloid precursor-like protein 1. *The Journal of Neuroscience, 19,* 7507–7515.

Homayouni, R., & Curran, T. (2000). Cortical development: Cdk5 gets into sticky situations. *Current Biology, 10,* 331–334.

Howell. B. W., Gertler, F. B., & Cooper, J. A. (1997). Mouse disabled (mDab1): A src binding protein implicated in neuronal development. *EMBO Journal, 16,* 121–132.

Howell, B. W., Hawkes, R., Soriano, P., & Cooper, J. A. (1997). Neuronal positioning in the developing brain is regulated by mouse disabled-1. *Nature, 389,* 733–737.

Howell, B. W., Herrick, T. M., & Cooper, J. A. (1999). Reelin-induced tyrosine phosphorylation of disabled 1 during neuronal positioning. *Genes and Development, 13,* 643–648.

Hsia, N., & Cornwall, G. A. (2003). DNA microarray analysis of region-specific gene expression in the mouse epididymis. *Biology of Reproduction, 70*(2), 448–457.

Huber, A. B., Kolodkin, A. L., Ginty, D. D., & Cloutier, J. F. (2003). Signaling at the growth cone: Ligand-receptor complexes and the control of axon growth and guidance. *Annual Review of Neuroscience, 26*, 509–563.

Kershaw, D. B., Beck, S. G., Wharram, B. L., Wiggins, J. E., Goyal, M., Thomas, P. E., & Wiggins, R. C. (1997). Molecular cloning and characterization of human podocalyxin-like protein. Orthologous relationship to rabbit PCLP1 and rat podocalyxin. *Journal of Biological Chemistry, 272*(25), 15708–15714.

Kopczynski, C. C., Davis, G. W., & Goodman, C. S. (1996). A neural tetraspanin, encoded by *late bloomer*, that facilitates synapse formation. *Science, 271*, 1867–1870.

Kurochkin, I. V., Yonemitsu, N., Funahashi, S. I., & Nomura, H. (2001). ALEX1, a novel human armadillo repeat protein that is expressed differentially in normal tissues and carcinomas. *Biochemical and Biophysical Research Community, 280*(1), 340–347.

Kwon, Y. T., Gupta, A., Zhou, Y., Nikolic, M., and Tsai, L. H. (2000). Regulation of N-cadherin-mediated adhesion by the p35-Cdk5 kinase. *Current Biology, 10*(7), 363–372.

Lamb, J. R., Tugendreich, S., & Hieter, P. (1995). Tetratrico peptide repeat interactions: To TPR or not to TPR? *Trends in Biochemical Science, 20*(7), 257–259.

Livesey, F. J. (1999). Netrins and netrin receptors. *Cell Molecular Life Sciences, 156*(1–2), 62–68.

Madden, S. L., Galella, E. A., Riley, D., Bertelsen, A. H., & Beaudry, G. A. (1996). Induction of cell growth regulatory genes by p53. *Cancer Research, 56*(23), 5384–5390.

Maecker, H. T., Todd, S. C., & Levy, S. (1997). The tetraspanin superfamily: Molecular facilitators. *FASEB Journal, 11*(6), 428–442.

Marín, O., Yaron, A., Bagri, A., Tessier-Lavigne, M., & Rubenstein, J. L. (2001). Sorting of striatal and cortical interneurons regulated by semaphorin-neuropilin interactions. *Science, 293*(5531), 872–875.

Marín-Padilla, M. (1971). Early prenatal ontogenesis of the cerebral cortex (neocortex) of the cat (Felis Domestica). A Golgi study. I. The primordial neocortical organization. *Zeitschrift fuer Anatomie und Entwicklungsgesch, 134*, 117–145.

Marín-Padilla, M. (1984). Neurons of layer I. In *Cerebral cortex, Vol. I* (pp. 447–478). New York: Plenum Press.

Marín-Padilla, M. (1988). Early ontogenesis of the human cerebral cortex. In A. Peters & E. G. Jones (Eds.), *Cerebral cortex, Vol. VII, Development and maturation of the cerebral cortex* (pp. 1–30). New York: Plenum Press.

Marín-Padilla, M. (1998). Cajal-Retzius cells and the development of the neocortex. *Trends in Neuroscience, 21*, 64–71.

Marín-Padilla, M. (1999). The development of the human cerebral cortex. A cytoarchitectonic theory. *Revista de Neurologia, 29*(3), 208–216.

Miettinen, A., Solin, M. L., Reivinen, J., Juvonen, E., Vaisanen, R., & Holthofer, H. (1999). Podocalyxin in rat platelets and megakaryocytes. *American Journal of Pathology, 154*(3), 813–822.

Nagase, T., Seki, N., Ishikawa, K., Tanaka, A., & Nomura, N. (1996). Prediction of the coding sequences of unidentified human genes. V. The coding sequences of 40 new genes (KIAA0161–KIAA0200) deduced by analysis of cDNA clones from human cell line KG-1. *DNA Ressearch, 3*(1), 17–24.

Ohshima, T., Kozak, C. A., Nagle, J. W., Pant, H. C., Brady, R. O., & Kulkarni, A. B. (1996). Molecular cloning and chromosomal mapping of the mouse gene encoding cyclin-dependent kinase 5 regulatory subunit p35. *Genomics, 35*(2), 372–375.

Orlando, R. A., Takeda, T., Zak, B., Schmieder, S., Benoit, V. M., McQuistan, T., Furthmayr, H., & Farquhar, M. G. (2001). The glomerular epithelial cell anti-adhesin podocalyxin associates with the actin cytoskeleton through interactions with ezrin. *Journal of the American Society of Nephrology, 12*(8), 1589–1598.

Powell, E. M., Mars, W. M., & Levitt, P. (2001). Hepatocyte growth factor/scatter factor is a motogen for interneurons migrating from the ventral to dorsal telencephalon. *Neuron, 30*(1), 79–89.

Rakic, P. (1972). Mode of migration to the superficial layers of fetal monkey neocortex. *The Journal of Comparative Neurology, 145*, 61–84.

Rakic, P. (1988). Specification of cerebral cortical areas. *Science, 241*, 170–176.

Rice, D. S., Sheldon, M., D'Arcangelo, G., Nakajima, K., Goldowitz, D., & Curran, T. (1998). Disabled-1 acts downstream of Reelin in a signaling pathway that controls laminar organization in the mammalian brain. *Development, 125*(18), 3719–3729.

Ron, D., & Habener, J. F. (1992). CHOP, a novel developmentally regulated nuclear protein that dimerizes with transcription factors C/EBP and LAP and functions as a dominant-negative inhibitor of gene transcription. *Genes and Development, 6*, 439–453.

Rubinstein, E., Le Naour, F., Lagaudriere-Gesbert, C., Billard, M., Conjeaud, H., & Boucheix, C. (1996). CD9, CD63, CD81, and CD82 are components of a surface tetraspan network connected to HLA-DR and VLA integrins. *European Journal of Immunology, 26*(11), 2657–2665.

Sassetti, C., Tangemann, K., Singer, M. S., Kershaw, D. B., & Rosen, S. D. (1998). Identification of podocalyxin-like protein as a high endothelial venule ligand for L-selectin: Parallels to CD34. *Journal of Experimental Medicine, 187*(12), 1965–1975.

Schwartz, T. H., Rabinowitz, D., Unni, V., Kumar, V. S., Smetters, D. K., Tsiola, A., & Yuste, R. (1998). Networks of coactive neurons in developing layer 1. *Neuron, 20*(3), 541–552.

Sheen, V. L., Dixon, P. H., Fox, J. W., Hong, S. E., Kinton, L., Sisodiya, S. M., Duncan, J. S., Dubeau, F., Scheffer, I. E., Schachter, S. C., Wilner, A., Henchy, R., Crino, P., Kamuro, K., DiMario, F., Berg, M., Kuzniecky, R., Cole, A. J., Bromfield, E., Biber, M., Schomer, D., Wheless, J., Silver, K., Mochida, G. H., Berkovic, S. F., Andermann, F., Andermann, E., Dobyns, W. B., Wood, N. W., & Walsh, C. A. (2001). Mutations in the X-linked filamin 1 gene cause periventricular nodular heterotopia in males as well as in females. *Human Molecular Genetics, 10*(17), 1775–1783.

Shi, W., Fan, H., Shum, L., & Derynck, R. (2000). The tetraspanin CD9 associates with transmembrane TGF-alpha and regulates TGF-alpha-induced EGF receptor activation and cell proliferation. *Journal of Cell Biology, 148*(3), 591–602.

Sidman, R. L., & Rakic, P. (1973). Neuronal migration, with special reference to developing human brain: A review. *Brain Research, 62*, 1–35.

Soriano, E., Alvarado-Mallart, R. M., Dumesnil, N., Del Rio, J. A., & Sotelo, C. (1997). Cajal-Retzius cells regulate the radial glia phenotype in the adult and developing cerebellum and alter granule cell migration. *Neuron, 18*(4), 563–577.

Stipp, C., & Hemler, M. E. (2000). Transmembrane-4-superfamily proteins CD151 and CD81 associate with alpha3 beta1 integrin, and selectively contribute to alpha3beta11-dependent neurite outgrowth. *Journal of Cell Science, 113*, 1871–1882.

Streit, A., Berliner, A. J., Papanayotou, C., Sirulnik, A., & Stern, C. D. (2000). Initiation of neural induction by FGF signalling before gastrulation. *Nature, 406*(6791), 74–78.

Supèr, H., and Uylings, H. B. (2001). The early differentiation of the neocortex: A hypothesis on neocortical evolution. *Cerebral Cortex, 11*(12), 1101–1109.

Takeda, T., Go, W. Y., Orlando, R. A., & Farquhar, M. G. (2000). Expression of podocalyxin inhibits cell-cell adhesion and modifies junctional properties in Madin-Darby canine kidney cells. *Molecular Biology of the Cell, 11*(9), 3219–3232.

Trommsdorff, M., Borg, J. P., Margolis, B., & Herz, J. (1998). Interaction of cytosolic adaptor proteins with neuronal apolipoprotein E receptors and the amyloid precursor protein. *Journal of Biological Chemistry, 273*(50), 33556–33560.

Trommsdorff, M., Gotthardt, M., Hiesberger, T., Shelton, J., Stockinger, W., Nimpf, J., Hammer, R. E., Richardson, J. A., & Herz, J. (1999). Reeler/Disabled-like disruption of neuronal migration in knockout mice lacking the VLDL receptor and ApoE receptor 2. *Cell, 97*(6), 689–701.

Ullrich, B., Ushkaryov, Y. A., & Sudhof, T. C. (1995). Cartography of neurexins: More than 1000 isoforms generated by alternative splicing and expressed in distinct subsets of neurons. *Neuron, 14*(3), 497–507.

Usui, H., Falk, J. D., Dopazo, A., de Lecea, L., Erlander, M. G., & Sutcliffe, J. G. (1994). Isolation of clones of rat striatum-specific mRNAs by directional tag PCR subtraction. *The Journal of Neuroscience, 14*(8), 4915–4926.

Venema, J., & Tollervey, D. (1996). RRP5 is required for formation of both 18S and 5.8S rRNA in yeast. *EMBO Journal, 15*, 5701–5714.

Wilkinson, D. G. (2001). Multiple roles of EPH receptors and ephrins in neural development. *Nature Reviews Neuroscience, 2*(3), 155–164.

Wolf, I., & Rohrschneider, L. R. (1999). Fiz1, a novel zinc finger protein interacting with the receptor tyrosine kinase Flt3. *Journal of Biological Chemistry, 274*, 21478–21484.

Wright, M. D., & Tomlinson, M. G. (1994). The ins and outs of the transmembrane 4 superfamily. *Immunology Today, 15*, 588–594.

Yauch, R. L., Berditchevski, F., Harler, M. B., Reichner, J., & Hemler, M. E. (1998). Highly stoichiometric, stable, and specific association of integrin alpha3beta1 with CD151 provides a major link to phosphatidylinositol 4-kinase, and may regulate cell migration. *Molecular Biology of the Cell, 9*(10), 2751–2765.

Yunta, M., & Lazo, P. A. (2003). Tetraspanin proteins as organisers of membrane microdomains and signalling complexes. *Cell Signalling, 15*, 559–564.

Zemni, R., Bienvenu, T., Vinet, M. C., Sefiani, A., Carrie, A., Billuart, P., McDonell, N., Couvert, P., Francis, F., Chafey, P., Fauchereau, F., Friocourt, G., des Portes, V., Cardona, A., Frints, S., Meindl, A., Brandau, O., Ronce, N., Moraine, C., van Bokhoven, H., Ropers, H. H., Sudbrak, R., Kahn, A., Fryns, J. P., Beldjord, C., & Chelly, J. (2000). A new gene involved in X-linked mental retardation identified by analysis of an X;2 balanced translocation. *Nature Genetics, 24*(2), 167–170.

Zinszner, H., Kuroda, M., Wang, X., Batchvarova, N., Lightfoot, R. T., Remotti, H., Stevens, J. L., & Ron, D. (1998). CHOP is implicated in programmed cell death in response to impaired function of the endoplasmic reticulum. *Genes and Development, 12*(7), 982–995.

Chapter • 9

Genomics and Dyslexia: Bridging the Gap

Robert W. Williams

Reading is a complex and highly variable skill that is strongly modulated by experience and the environment. But reading is also modulated by developmental, neuroanatomical, and functional characteristics that are themselves strongly influenced by gene variants (Fisher & DeFries, 2002). Heritability estimates for developmental dyslexia have a wide range (15% to 75% with a mean of about 35%) that are dependent on the particular groups that are studied, the specific tests, and the environmental context. Obviously, genetics is only part of the picture, but it is the part that is particularly amenable to direct molecular analysis. Advances in functional genomics are already having an impact, and the main purpose of this chapter is to illustrate a few

---

My thanks to many generous colleagues: to Kenneth F. Manly and Jintao Wang for building the Gene Network and WebQTL from the ground up; to Lu Lu, Yanhua Qu, and Jing Gu for providing key genetic and bioinformatic data sets; and to Elissa J. Chesler for her numerous innovative ideas, many of which have been incorporated into the Gene Network. WebQTL has also benefited greatly from the programming prowess of Stephen M. Pitts and Alexander G. Williams. Thanks also to a rapidly growing number of colleagues who have shared their data with the research community as part of the the Gene Network, usually well before publication of their key findings (please see the information pages associated with each data set and http://www.genenetwork.org/credit.html). Finally, I thank Glenn D. Rosen and Kathryn A. Graehl for their help in editing this article. Components of the Gene Network are supported by a Human Brain Project grant (P20 MH-62009) to RWW and Kenneth F. Manly (colony support, genotyping, and software development), by an NIAAA grant (U01AA13499 and U24AA13513) to RWW (microarray processing and DNA analysis), and by an NCI grant (U01CA105417) to KFM and RWW (bioinformatics and data integration).

of the new possibilities in exploiting novel genomics resources and tools to probe genetic and functional networks associated with developmental dyslexia.

THE COMPLEX GENETICS OF DYSLEXIA

Locus versus Gene. In principle, the heritable component of dyslexia can be subdivided into its constituent genetic factors. These factors are sometimes called gene loci, quantitative trait loci (QTL), or when the evidence is compelling, simply genes. A locus is defined as a chromosomal interval (e.g., chromosome band 15q21) that contains one or more variable (polymorphic) genes that affects a score, in this case, a measurement related to reading skill or a correlated behavioral characteristic. The term *locus* is used instead of *gene* to remind ourselves that we initially know only the general location of the relevant polymorphic gene or genes. The neighborhood in which the suspects live may be known, but there is still much detective work ahead. Discovering the correct genetic culprit in a locus that actually triggers differences in reading skill is a hard job sometimes referred to as *gene cloning*. A more appropriate phrase is just *gene identification*.

Genetic Complexity is the Norm. Variant versions of genes in a locus (also known as alleles) generate a fraction of the variation in reading skill. For a locus or gene to contribute to dyslexia, it has to come in at least two versions: a dyslexia susceptible form and one or more dyslexia resistant forms. When a locus has a particularly clear-cut effect in one or more families, it can appear to be a Mendelian locus with a pattern of inheritance sometimes labeled as dominant or recessive. However, this is exceptional. The gene variants that cause dyslexia do not act in isolation as do classical Mendelian mutations. It is a mistake to think that dyslexia is switched on or off depending on the state of a single gene. Associations between alleles and dyslexia are almost certainly complex. An allele that contributes to dyslexia in one family could, in principle, have effects that are completely neutralized or even positive in another family (Scerri et al., 2004). This masking can be caused by other sets of genes (sometimes called epistasis) or by environmental differences (sometimes called gene-by-environment effects). The consensus among geneticists is that dyslexia is generated by combinations of multiple gene variants (a multigenic trait) located on different chromosomes that interact in complex and still undefined ways among themselves and with subtle developmental and environmental factors (Fisher &

DeFries, 2002). This complexity explains why even monozygotic twins often perform differently on reading tasks.

A Summary of the *DYX* Loci

Over the past decade, mapping studies in humans have highlighted and progressively converged on a small number of chromosome intervals that contribute to different but overlapping measures of developmental dyslexia. There is now a concerted effort to exploit genomic tools in combination with large sets of dyslexic families to identify the gene variants that underlie these loci (*DYX1-DYX8*). Caution is in order, and the following quotation from Marlow et al. (2003) highlights the current challenge:

> Replication of linkage results for complex traits, such as developmental dyslexia, is exceedingly difficult, owing in part to the inability to measure the precise underlying phenotype, small sample sizes, genetic heterogeneity, and limitations of the statistical methods employed in analysis. Often, in any particular study, multiple correlated traits have been collected, yet these have been analyzed independently or, at most, in bivariate analyses. Theoretical arguments suggest that full multivariate analysis of all available traits should offer more power to detect linkage.

An efficient way to systematically review the current status of the family of *DYX* loci is to link to Online Mendelian Inheritance in Man (OMIM), the electronic version of Victor McKusick's classic text (McKusick, 1999). OMIM tends to be appropriately conservative in its annotation of *DYX* loci, and several loci are missing in action. A PubMed search using *DYX** and *dyslexia* as keywords returns 11 relevant articles (August 2004), many of which are listed in Table I, along with candidate genes that I have selected. Resources now make it practical to evaluate the merits of the genes situated in these *DYX* loci. This is the main focus of the second half of this review.

The Challenge. Initial successes in homing in on loci and even a few genes associated with the dyslexias have been reported in the last few years. For example, *TMOD2* and *DYX1C1* are now interesting—but far from definitive—candidates for *DYX1* (Cox & Zoghbi, 2000; Cox et al., 2003; Taipale et al., 2003; Scerri et al., 2004; Marino & Molteni, this volume). The expectation is that once specific dyslexia genes have been confidently identified, they will provide insights into causes, and perhaps even suggest additional treatments and training methods to overcome dyslexia. How warranted is enthusiasm at this point?

Huntington Disease as an Example. We already know that the effort involved in converting well-mapped loci into identified genes and the causal allelic variants is challenging, even in tightly controlled experimental mouse populations. It can be just as challenging to bridge the gap between a cloned gene and a mechanistic understanding of a complex behavior such as reading skill. The history of research on Huntington's disease provides a cautionary example of these steps: it took roughly a decade (1983 to 1993) to clone the key gene, now known as huntingtin (called the *HD* gene in humans and the *Hdh* gene in mice) that causes the autosomal dominant Huntington's disease. It has taken another decade to achieve even modest insight into the function of this ubiquitously expressed gene (see the thorough OMIM entry). The beta amyloid precursor protein (*APP*), apolipoprotein E (*APOE*), alpha synuclein, and the presenilins are other genes associated with neurodegenerative diseases, and again, knowing the gene is just a promising first step.

In contrast to most neurodegenerative diseases, dyslexia is a complex trait that is one result of activity patterns of millions of widely distributed neurons in numerous cortical and subcortical regions. We have good reasons to suspect comparatively subtle effects on timing and patterns of neuronal activity are the final common cause. There are no easy cellular markers (variable cortical ectopias are our best current anatomical markers). We already suspect that nearly a dozen QTLs may be involved (Table I). How bright are the prospects of identifying the *DYX* genes? Will we be able to bridge this gap between gene variants and a complex behavior? Will we be able to exploit animal models to study a skill that is uniquely human? The quick answer to each of these questions is *yes*; we should be optimistic.

Animal Models: Simple, not Simplistic. In this review, I provide some initial steps that illustrate how high throughput genomic methods coupled with advanced methods in complex trait analysis make it possible to explore causal and associative networks of molecules, cells, and circuits that influence complex behaviors. Although there are, by definition, no true animal models of dyslexia, there are, nonetheless, shared molecular networks that make mouse models extremely useful in understanding this cognitive problem. Optimism is justified, but it is equally important to be patient; 10 to 20 years is the right time frame. Dyslexia is a complex, higher-order cognitive problem, and pushing too fast will just push distracting chimeras to the front, not real solutions.

ANALYSIS OF THE *DYX1* CANDIDATE REGION

A direct way to bridge the gap between animal models and humans is to study the actions of genes in animals that are suspected to explain individual differences in reading ability among humans. Fundamental molecular roles of genes in brain development and neuronal function are generally closely matched in mice and humans. Mice provide experimental leverage.

As an example, consider the *DYX* loci and the set of candidate genes in these intervals, some of which are listed in Table I. What can we learn by exploring Web resources and genomic databases? Some questions that can be addressed include the following.

- What genes are located in each of the *DYX* intervals? In some cases there will be many genes in a *DYX* locus (*DYX1*), but in other cases such as *DYX3*, the locus contains very few candidates, making the analysis much easier.
- Which of these genes are expressed in brain during development or at maturity? Which are associated with synapse function or neuronal connectivity? What do we know about the functions of these genes from genetically engineered mice (knockout and transgenic lines) and from an analysis of recombinant inbred strains of mice?
- What are the relations between the set of candidate genes for a *DYX* locus and other gene products or other higher order traits (mRNA or proteins)? Do these sets or networks provide insight into the plausibility of candidate genes?
- Can we generate specific testable hypotheses about *DYX* candidate genes that can then be used in validation studies?

There are now a multitude of bioinformatic Web resources that we can use to begin answering these questions. I will rely on two large genomic databases, one called the Genome Browser (www.genome.ucsc.edu), the other called the Gene Network (www.genenetwork.org). Both sites incorporate numerous tools with which to explore chromosomal intervals and gene expression data (Table I). Neither of these resources provides definitive answers to questions about dyslexia. Instead, they should be considered powerful tools for exploratory analysis of *DYX* candidates and networks of interacting genes. We can provide functional annotation on the fly to many of the candidates listed in Table I to prioritize subsequent detailed studies of the type described in the companion article by LoTurco and colleagues (this volume). To come to firm conclusions about gene function and possible relations to reading skills, it will be necessarily to follow up with new

Table I: Summary of DYX loci

Locus	Chr	MB	Candidates	References
DYX1	15q21	42–57	TMOD2, RC3, DYX1C1, NEDD4, UNC13C, SUHW4, ONECUT1, MYO5A, SCG3, GNB5	Grigorenko et al., 1997; Schulte-Korne et al., 1998; Morris et al., 2000; Marino et al., 2004; and Morino & Molteni, this volume; Scerri et al., 2004
			Mouse Chr 2 (113.7–126.9 Mb); Chr 9 (57.0–76.0 Mb)	
DYX2	6p21.3	30–37	RXRB, NUDT3, MAPK14, SLC26A8	Cardon et al., 1994; Grigorenko et al., 1997; Fisher and DeFries, 2002; Fisher et al., 2002; Deffenbacher et al., 2004
			Mouse Chr 17 (26.0–36.0 Mb)	
DYX3	2p16	47–62	NRXN1, FBXO11, SPTBN1, BCL11A	Fagerheim et al., 1999; Petryshen et al., 2002
			Mouse Chr 17 (87.1, 90 Mb); Chr 11 (23.6–31.1)	
DYX4	6q11–q12	60–70	KHDRBS2, PTP4A1, GLULD1, BAI3	Petryshen et al., 2001
			Mouse Chr 1 (21.6–34.7 Mb)	
DYX5	3p12–q13	74–125	ROBO1, EPHA3, GAP43, LSAMP, DRD3	Nopola-Hemmi et al., 2001
			Mouse Chr 16 (34.8–74.9 Mb)	
DYX6	18p11.2	7.2–15.4	GNAL, ANKRD12, KIAA0802, MR5R, MC2R	Fisher et al., 2002
			Mouse Chr 17 (64.8–65.9 Mb); 18 (63.3–69.0)	
DYX7	11p15.5	1–3	not a true locus	Hsiung et al., 2004
DYX8	1p34–p36	15.5–47	~20 candidates	Tzenova et al., 2004
DYX?	7q32	125–132	SMO	Kaminen et al., 2003
DYX?	2p11	83–93	C2orf23	Kaminen et al., 2003

Based on an analysis of the Human May 2004 Genome Assembly. Candidates selected using expression data (Su et al., 2004) and WebQTL (Wang et al., 2003). Mouse homologous regions are provided for DYX1 to DYX6.

series of experiments, new bioinformatic resources, and most especially new families that suffer from dyslexias. A positive feature of both Genome Browser and the Gene Network is that they provide an open and agnostic way to evaluate the potential function and interactions of *DYX* candidate genes for which we currently do not have extensive functional data.

Criteria for the *DYX1* Candidates

The *DYX1* interval includes a long stretch of chromosome (Chr) 15 known as 15q21, a length of DNA that extends over about 15 million base pairs (42 to 57 Mb), and that is made up of three distinct subbands called 15q21.1, 15q21.2, and 15q21.3. Using the Genome Browser, it is simple to review the full complement of known genes in this entire region (Figure 1); link to the Genome

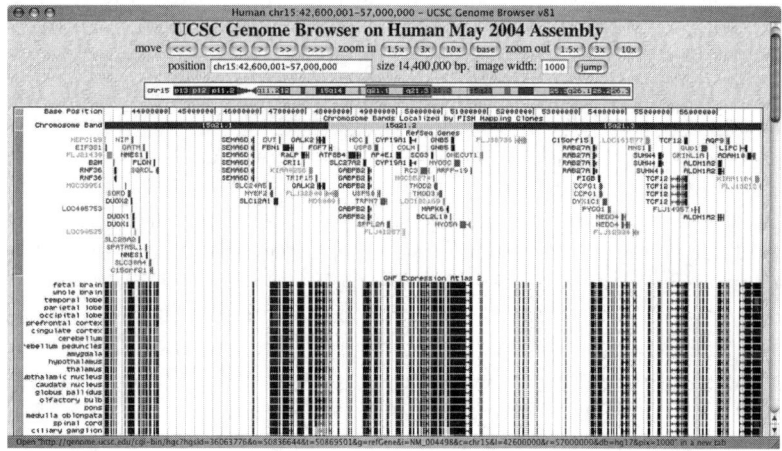

Figure 1. A view of the DYX1 locus region of the human genome from the Genome Browser listing the majority of known genes (upper half, blue font) and the expression level of a subset of these genes (lower third). Toward the top of the figure is a horizontal stick figure of the entire Chr 15 (left to right) with a box around the 15.4 Mb region (from 42.6 to 57 Mb) that is likely to contain the DYX1 gene (the 15q21 band). In order to list all of the genes in this interval, genes are staggered from top to bottom and left to right. The darker genes are well annotated; lighter fonts are poorly annotated genes. If a gene is highly expressed in a particular part of the brain, the gene block is colored red in the lower part of the figure. The candidate genes listed in Table I were extracted by reviewing similar figures for all DYX intervals. Link to <www.genome.ucsc.edu> to replicate this type of figure.

Browser and enter *15q21* as the *position* search field. The 15q21.1 region (about 5 Mb of DNA) contains roughly 45 genes, but few of these are yet known to have high expression levels in fetal or adult human brain (Su et al., 2004; http://symatlas.gnf.org). One exception is the myelin basic protein expression factor 2 repressor (*MYEF2*). While we should not discount this region entirely, we can put it on the back burner.

Chr* 15q21.2 *is a Hotbed of Synapse-related Genes. In contrast, the neighboring region, 15q21.2, contains a number of very strong candidates: *TMOD2, ONECUT1, RC3, MYO5A, GNB5,* and *SCG3*. These genes have high expression in human brain, and several of them are involved in synapse and vesicle function. Tropomodulin 2 (*TMOD2*) is a particularly interesting *DYX1* candidate because it is known to have an important role in learning, memory, and synaptic plasticity (Cox et al., 2003). Rabconnectin 3 (*RC3*) is a key player in *RAB3*-mediated calcium-dependent exocytosis of neurotransmitter (Kawabe et al., 2003). Secretogranin 3 (*SCG3*) is a highly expressed CNS gene of unknown function that is likely to be a component of dense core vesicles (Dopazo, Lovenberg, Danielson, Ottiger, & Sutcliffe, 1993). *GNB5* is a guanine nucleotide-binding protein subunit associated with the flailer neurological mouse mutant (Jones et al., 2000). *MYO5A* is a CNS myosin that binds to synaptic vesicles (Prekeris & Terrian, 1997) and that is associated with Griscelli syndrome retardation and hypotonia (Pastural et al., 1997). *ONECUT1* is a crucial coactivator of gene transcription that has a well-conserved role in neurogenesis in invertebrates, but it is best known in mammals for its key role in liver and pancreas development (Odom et al., 2004). It is also referred to as hepatocyte nuclear factor 6 (*HNF6*). We will return and review *ONECUT1/HNF6* in more detail below, but all of these genes are interesting biological and positional candidate for *DYX1*, and they deserve systematic scrutiny.

Finally, the 15q21.3 region contains *UNC13C, NEDD4* (a ubiquitin ligase also known as *neural precursor cell expressed developmentally 4*), *TCF12* (a basic helix-loop-helix transcription factor), *SUHW4* (suppressor of hairy wing 4, a zinc finger transcription factor), and *EKN1* (the latter is also known as *DYX1C1*). Most of these candidates are expressed in human fetal brain (*UNC13C, SUHW4, TCF12,* and *EKN1*), and all of them are reasonable *DYX1* candidates.

This synopsis of the set of strong candidates for *DYX1* highlights the risk of prematurely declaring victory in cloning a dyslexia locus (e.g., *EKN1 DYX1C1*). But this process also highlights the tremendous speed with which it is now possible to generate an extremely valuable list of vetted candidates once a *DYX* locus has mapped with sufficient precision. This same process can be systematically applied to all of the *DYX* loci (Table I).

The Gene Network

A logical step at this point is to take advantage of additional genomics resources to evaluate candidate genes associated with each of the *DYX* loci. Data on gene expression were exploited above in a simple way to confine our list to those candidates expressed at a reasonably high level in the central nervous system. This strategy is obviously not foolproof because a dyslexia gene could turn out to be a critical gene expressed transiently and at low levels even in the liver, but as part of the prioritizing process, we should first examine and test the most obvious candidates. Microarrays provide an extraordinary efficient tool with which to obtain very large numbers of assays of gene expression from CNS tissue samples. These assays, described in much more detail below, can be used to extend the analysis of the positional candidates highlighted in Step 1. This work tends to be experimental, and for that reason, we will now switch most attention to gene expression patterns in the mouse brain.

The *DYX1* candidate genes in humans have mouse homologs that are located primarily on mouse chromosome 9 between 75 and 80 Mb. Expression levels of these candidates have been measured using Affymetrix U74Av2 and M430 microarrays and entered into the Gene Network databases. For example, *Ekn1* is measured on the Affymetrix M430 microarray by probe set 1451605_at_A. *Tmod2* is measured on the same array by five different probe sets, although 1431325_a_at_A provides the highest signal. Finally, the expression of *Onecut1* in mouse forebrain is measured on the U74Av2 array by probe set 100737_at.[1]

The Gene Network now includes data sets for several Affymetrix data sets: forebrain (both U74Av2 and M430), cerebellum (M430 only), striatum (M430), and a hematopoietic stem cell (U74Av2). It is possible to explore and compare mRNA expression in any of these data sets, and to compare across data sets. It is also possible to extend the analysis up to the level of behavior. This is done comparing variation in expression with variation in behavior in the same strains of mice that have been collected into a

---

[1] Human genes symbols are written in all capital italic (e.g., *ONECUT1*), whereas those in mouse are written with only an initial capital letter (*Onecut1*).

database of classical phenotypes of the BXD strains. A multiscale biological analysis can be incredibly powerful (Chesler et al., 2003; Hitzemann et al., 2003).

The Gene Network and Recombinant Inbred Strains. Using the Gene Network, it is straightforward to evaluate the expression of *Onecut1*—or any of approximately 30,000 other genes—across a mapping panel that consists of as many as 80 different strains of recombinant inbred (RI) strains. RI strains are special types of mice that are made by intercrossing two parental strains of mice and then inbreeding the successive progeny of their second filial generation F2 progeny (Williams, Gu, Qi, & Lu, 2001), a process that takes about eight years. They are called "recombinant" because pieces of chromosomes of the two parental strains have been randomly and independently shuffled (or recombined) in each of the RI strains. The two parental strains of the RI strains that we have used are C57BL/6J (B or B6 for short) and DBA/2J (D or D2); the RI strains are, therefore, called the BXD set. About 80 BXD RI strains have now been made (Peirce Lu, Gu, Silver, & Williams, 2004). Because the genomes of the two parental strains—B6 and D2—have both been sequenced, we know in advance if any particular gene is polymorphic in the BXD RI set. *Onecut1* has approximately 25 single nucleotide polymorphisms (SNPs) that distinguish *B6* and *D2* alleles. These sequence differences may produce downstream effects that we will able to detect at many different levels. Downstream effects (phenotypes) that map back to the location of *Onecut1* (we treat *Onecut1* as a *DYX1* candidate gene) can potentially clarify the function of this gene in CNS development or function. The reason that it is useful to have data on many different RI strains may not be apparent and may appear to be overkill. It is not; in fact it would be extremely useful, but expensive, to have data on all 80 strains. The more strains we have, the more precise our mapping data and the more powerful our statistical inferences.

Affymetrix Arrays: Their Design and Analysis

It is worth understanding something about how these estimates of gene expression are generated. In the case of the Affymetrix U74Av2 array, the expression level of each mRNA is evaluated using 11 to 16 perfect match (PM) probes and 11 to 16 mismatch (MM) probes. All of the probes are approximately the same length as common PCR primers (25 nucleotides long). The PM probes are designed to exactly match the target mRNA, whereas their twin MM probes are essentially controls that contain a single sequence difference (essentially a SNP) in the middle at the position of the 13th nucleotide. The MM is sometimes helpful to evaluate non-specific binding of related mRNA sequences, but in our analysis, we typically rely solely on the PM signal. If the 16 PM probes are designed correctly, they should hybridize with high sensitivity and selectivity to a single complementary type of mRNA (Figure 2). Affymetrix arrays contain as many as 1.3 million of these probes that can be used to evaluate expression of up to about 45,000 mRNAs.

An obvious requirement is to make sure that the probes estimate the expression of the correct gene. Figure 2 illustrates shows how we can rapidly verify that the Affymetrix PM probes in principle hybridize specifically to *Onecut1* and not other genes with similar sequences. The Gene Network has a function called *Verify* (see the *Trait Data and Editing Form*) that automatically concatenates all of the PM probes and then uses the Genome Browser BLAT function to confirm that the probes target the correct part (usually the 3' end of the gene) of the correct gene.

mRNA Processing and Measurement. The original mRNA from the whole brain, a specific part of the brain, or even a single cell type is converted to its complementary sequence, amplified and labeled with digoxigenin, and sheared into short fragments (<100 nucleotides) that will bind to the DNA probes synthesized directly on the surface of the array. The amount of labeled complementary RNA (cRNA) that remains tightly bound to the probes is measured using a confocal laser scanner, and is expressed as a single brightness measure that varies from a low of about 10–40 (the background

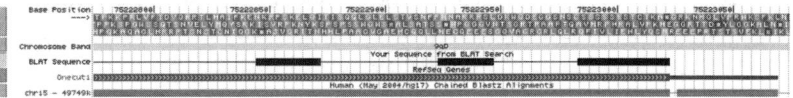

Figure 2. Verification that the probes designed to measure Onecut1 expression (probe set 100737_at) actually target the correct gene. The 16 PM probes on the Affymetrix U74Av2 array were aligned with the entire mouse genome and the single best match is (correctly) to the last exon of the Onecut1 gene. The top row gives the position of Onecut1 in the mouse genome on Chr 9-the region that corresponds to human 15q21.2. The broad grey region shows the three alternative reading frames (asterisk marks = stop codons, other letters = amino acid codes). From left to right, the middle row labeled Onecut1 highlights the last exon (thicker line with arrow heads), and the 3' untranslated region (medium-thick line to far right). The row labeled BLAT Sequence shows the probe sequence that is actually present on the U74Av2 microarray.

hybridization level) to about 100,000 (near the saturation point of the system). We take the log base 2 of these numbers so that the effective range for the array data is from 4 to 16 units (2^4 to 2^{16}). The average expression of all genes in a tissue is about 8. This log2 scale is convenient because a 1 unit difference represents approximately a two-fold difference in mRNA abundance in the tissue sample. Each array data set is actually scaled to the same mean expression value of 8 (this corrects for small differences in RNA concentration or labeling). The hybridization signal is, therefore, actually an estimate of the relative mRNA level in a tissue, not the true concentration.

Analysis of Array Data. Affymetrix hybridization signals should provide consistent and correlated estimates of expression across the set of PM probes that are supposed to measure the same mRNA. The 16 PM probes for *Onecut1* should provide a unanimous consensus. They do not. The hybridization of the set of probes to mRNA is surprisingly variable. For *Onecut1*, the signal for the probes varies from 6.46 ± 0.20 for probe 1 to 12.3 ± 0.30 for probe 7. That is about a 57-fold variation. Part of this striking or distressing variation is inevitable, given the physical chemistry of hybridization of short 25 nucleotide oligomer probes (Zhang, Miles, & Aldape, 2003). But much of the difference is probably due to cross-hybridizations with related sequences from nontarget mRNA types. A solution is to pool the PM data and devise a validated method to extract a single common expression estimate. We could, for instance, simply average the PM probes, giving each probe a single vote.

A more sophisticated method has been implemented in the Gene Network by Elissa Chesler and Jintao Wang. This method extracts the common signal of any subset of probes using a principal component analysis. The dominant signal (the first principal component) can then be used as a consensus estimate of gene expression. There are several other sophisticated methods to combine all of the probe values to a single consensus estimate. In the Gene Network, these methods are indicated by acronyms such as MAS5, RMA, PDNN, dCHIP, and HWT1PM that are appended as a suffix to the names of databases. *HWT1PM* stands for *Heritability Weighted Transform 1 Perfect Match*. This is a unique method developed by Kenneth Manly and colleagues that is also integrated into the Gene Network. Each probe is given a variable number of votes that is based on the consistency of its performance across a large array data set. *Consistency* in this context is evaluated using the heritability of the probe signal. This amounts to determining whether the probe gives approximately the same estimate in the same tissue and strain, while also detecting differences in expression between strains of mice (essentially a one-way ANOVA F score). If the probe signal is noisy and inconsistent, even within the same strain, then it will have a heritability that is close to zero and it will be discounted in subsequent analysis. In contrast, if a probe has a signal that is stable within strain and tissue, but that is consistently variable across strain and tissue, then that probe will have its vote weighted more heavily. To put this in slightly more formal statistical terms: probes are weighted by their intraclass correlations or F scores; in our case, the class or factor happens to be *strain*.

In the example that follows, using *Onecut1* as our *DYX1* candidate gene, I have relied on the HWT forebrain data set generated using the U74Av2 microarray (Figure 3; see www.genenetwork.org for more specific information on this data set). This is one of our best data sets and includes data from 100 arrays and 35 strains. Forebrain tissue from each strain was studied three times independently, and each independent sample included forebrain from three animals, usually from a single litter and always of the same

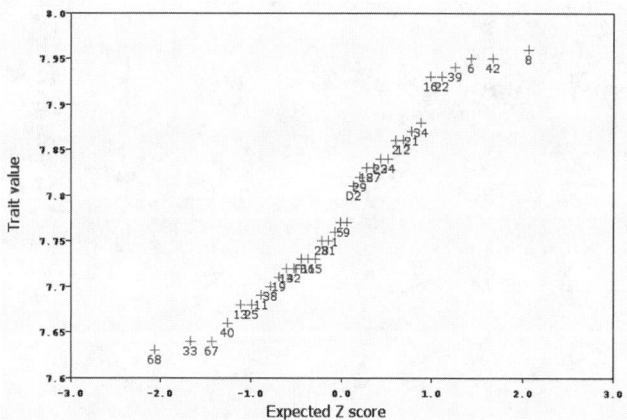

Figure 3. Onecut1 expression in the forebrain of adult BXD strains (heritability weighted transform). The numbers or letters associated with each point are strain abbreviations, from a low value in BXD68 to a high in BXD8. B6 = C57BL/6J, D2 = DBA/2J, F1 = the B6D2F1 hybrid. The y axis is an approximate estimate of the relative expression level on a log2 scale. The x axis lists the Z score that would be expected if the 35 values were selected from a normally distributed population. There are two rather pronounced breaks in the plot (at values of about 7.90 and 7.78). Breaks like this can be generated by gene variants or inadequately corrected batch effects.

sex. By the standards of current microarray studies, this is an unusually deep data set.

Genetic Covariance. Having data for *Onecut1* and up to 30,000 other genes in 32 RI strains already makes it possible to explore the genetic covariance, the tendency of set genes to be expressed as groups (Figures 4 and 5). We can use the natural variation in gene expression produced by polymorphisms in many genes. There are about 1.8 million SNPs that distinguish B6 and D2 strains. These polymorphisms have been recombined randomly among the 32 RI strains. This fact provides an excellent experimental design (a factorial design) that can be used to simultaneously study functional interactions among a huge variety of phenotypes. Variation in gene expression is just a molecular phenotype that we can treat in the same way that we treat reading ability scores. They can be correlated with other traits and the variation in traits can itself be "mapped." In other words, we can also look for the upstream sources of difference in the expression

	Trait1	Trait2	Trait3	Trait4	Trait5	Trait6	Trait7	Trait8	Trait9	Trait10	Trait11	Trait12
Trait1: Brain U74Av2 12/03 HWT1PM:100339_at	1.000	0.799 35	0.728 35	0.830 35	0.536 35	0.772 35	0.561 35	-0.797 35	0.607 35	-0.739 35	-0.778 35	0.799 35
Trait2: Brain U74Av2 12/03 HWT1PM:100391_at	0.820 35	1.000	0.767 35	0.804 35	0.669 35	0.872 35	0.557 35	-0.807 35	0.599 35	-0.717 35	-0.850 35	0.860 35
Trait3: Brain U74Av2 12/03 HWT1PM:100737_at	0.805 35	0.784 35	1.000	0.722 35	0.754 35	0.701 35	0.735 35	-0.820 35	0.772 35	-0.862 35	-0.836 35	0.785 35
Trait4: Brain U74Av2 12/03 HWT1PM:101136_at	0.840 35	0.839 35	0.805 35	1.000	0.614 35	0.814 35	0.642 35	-0.843 35	0.609 35	-0.718 35	-0.741 35	0.866 35
Trait5: Brain U74Av2 12/03 HWT1PM:101710_at	0.617 35	0.714 35	0.799 35	0.740 35	1.000	0.646 35	0.501 35	-0.573 35	0.536 35	-0.631 35	-0.692 35	0.610 35
Trait6: Brain U74Av2 12/03 HWT1PM:101814_at	0.817 35	0.897 35	0.787 35	0.894 35	0.718 35	1.000	0.575 35	-0.792 35	0.565 35	-0.616 35	-0.794 35	0.842 35
Trait7: Brain U74Av2 12/03 HWT1PM:102559_at	0.696 35	0.651 35	0.805 35	0.741 35	0.574 35	0.757 35	1.000	-0.645 35	0.744 35	-0.502 35	-0.544 35	0.651 35
Trait8: Brain U74Av2 12/03 HWT1PM:103423_at	-0.844 35	-0.828 35	-0.870 35	-0.863 35	-0.699 35	-0.855 35	-0.778 35	1.000	-0.641 35	0.850 35	0.858 35	-0.810 35
Trait9: Brain U74Av2 12/03 HWT1PM:103468_at	0.723 35	0.698 35	0.790 35	0.723 35	0.617 35	0.745 35	0.863 35	-0.756 35	1.000	-0.607 35	-0.627 35	0.655 35
Trait10: Brain U74Av2 12/03 HWT1PM:104071_at	-0.754 35	-0.725 35	-0.816 35	-0.716 35	-0.693 35	-0.679 35	-0.611 35	0.839 35	-0.695 35	1.000	0.850 35	-0.781 35
Trait11: Brain U74Av2 12/03 HWT1PM:104315_at	-0.791 35	-0.821 35	-0.824 35	-0.778 35	-0.745 35	-0.798 35	-0.638 35	0.858 35	-0.698 35	0.886 35	1.000	-0.825 35
Trait12: Brain U74Av2 12/03 HWT1PM:104430_at	0.810 35	0.849 35	0.817 35	0.857 35	0.654 35	0.887 35	0.821 35	-0.834 35	0.811 35	-0.779 35	-0.818 35	1.000

Figure 4. Correlation matrix of Onecut1 expression (Trait 3, highlighted to left) with a set of 11 other transcripts in the brain. The lower left values are Pearson product-moment correlations whereas the upper right values are Spearman rank order correlations. Each cell contains the correlation and the number of strains on which the correlation is based (n = 35 in all of these cells). As shown in figure 5, any one of these correlations can be selected to generate a scattergram. The identity of the traits in the matrix are as follows: Trait_1 = Slc10a1; 2 = Mapk8; 3 = Onecut1; 4 = Tnfsf8; 5 = Gria4; 6 = Gdf11; 7 = Bmp2; 8 = Cyb541; 9 = Mns1; 10 = Tnpo2; 11 = Arhgap1; 12 = Cd96.

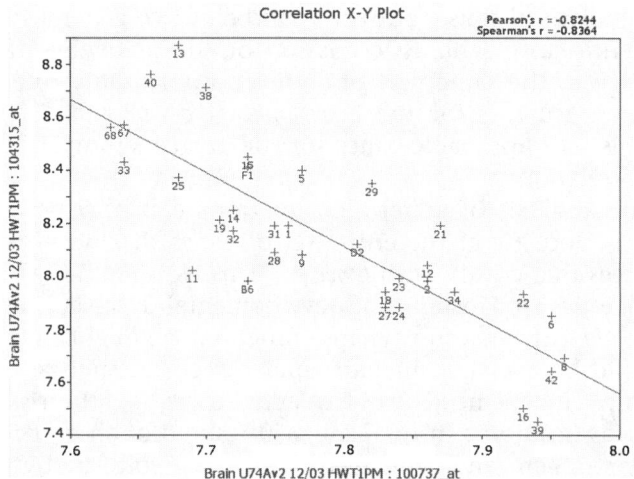

Figure 5. Genetic correlation between Onecut1 (x axis) and Rho GTPase activating protein 1 (Arhgap1). Each point represents the expression of both genes measured in triplicate in each strain (numbers are the strain abbreviations). Anyone of the correlations in Figure 4 can be converted into scattergrams of this sort by clicking on the appropriate data cell.

of *Onecut1*, just as we can look for the downstream consequences of variation in *Onecut1*.

The Gene Network can compute thousands of correlations between a reference trait (*Onecut1* expression) and thousands of other traits in databases that contain information on the same strains (Chesler et al., 2003; Chesler, Lu, Wang, Williams, & Manly 2004). As shown in Figure 4, *Onecut1* expression correlates well with expression differences in several genes involved in CNS function. For example, *Gria4* is a glutamate receptor located on Chr 9 at 4 Mb that is linked to human schizophrenia (Makino et al., 2003). *Onecut1* and *Gria4* have a correlation of 0.799. *Mapk8* ($r = 0.78$) is a kinase that modulates transcription activity in many tissues, including brain. *Gdf11* ($r = 0.79$), also known as *BMP11*, is a gene expressed in the brain that may regulate *Hox* expression. *Arhgap1* or RHOGAP ($r = -0.82$, Figure 5) is a GTPase activating protein and has important roles in cell signaling.

Significance of Genetic Correlations. Most of the correlations in Figure 4 have absolute values above $r = 0.75$, a highly significant correlation even with a correction for the large number of statistical tests the Gene Network has performed (point-wise p values <.0000001 but just over 10,000 tests). Genetic correlations have a biological cause, but they can be of two general types: one a conventional mechanistic relation or, alternatively, effects due to linkage to the same part of a chromosome. Only one of these covariates, *Mns1*, is located near *Onecut1* on Chr 9 at 77 Mb, so linkage is an improbable cause for the great majority of these genetic correlations.

The analysis of genetic correlations can now be easily extended by looking at the entire set of genes that have expression differences that covary with *Onecut1*. This list should have interesting properties. For instance, if developmental dyslexia is associated with subtle differences in synapse function, we might find that the list would be enriched in particular categories such as vesicular transport. The list needs to be selected to reduce the risk of false positive associations. In this case, a threshold of about 0.71 is reasonably stringent and generates a list of 500 correlated genes. The gene categories to which these 500 genes belong can then be compared to the expected distribution of a random list of 500 genes generate using the same array. Figure 6 is a graphic summary generated by the Gene Ontology Tree Machine in WebGestalt (Zhang, Schmoyer, Kirov, & Snoddy, 2004) that highlights enriched cate-

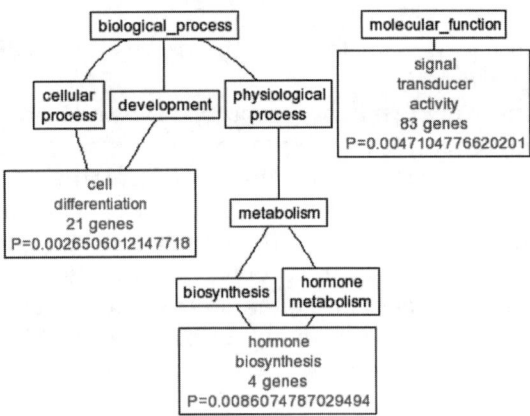

Figure 6. A gene ontology analysis of 500 transcripts that covary with strain differences in forebrain expression of Onecut1 of greater than 0.71. The WebGestalt output highlight those functional categories that are overrepresented in the list of 500 genes (see Zhang et al., 2004). WebGestalt and GOTM include 3535 different classification nodes arranged in 10 hierarchical levels. Only the top five levels are shown in this figure. Clicking on one of the categories such as cell differentiation provides the list of genes with correlations that have absolute values of >0.71 with Onecut1.

gories. In this case, the category *signal transducer activity* and cell differentiation are both relatively enriched categories.

Comparing across Scales

Onecut1 expression in adult forebrain can also be compared to over 800 classical phenotypes that have been collected for the BXD strains over a 25-year period (Chesler et al., 2003). For example, expression patterns of this gene have a moderate positive correlation with differences in dopamine transporter protein levels ($r = 0.60$, $n = 22$ strains; Janowsky et al., 2001) and a moderate negative correlation with the density of neurons in the spiral ganglion ($r = -0.61$, $n = 24$ strains; Willott & Erway, 1998). The nominal p values associated with these correlations are 0.0026 and 0.0011, respectively, values that are not actually significant given the large number of independent tests. But these values may be enough, given other prior data sets, to motivate a second comparative analysis of *Onecut1* expression with a larger sample of BXD strains. It is also important to consider that when data from a panel of RI strains are collected over a long period of time in different labs using different individuals at different ages, these genetic correlations will naturally tend to be degraded. Nonlinear interactions among nongenetic sources of variation and strain genotypes are particularly damaging to genetic correlations. Thus, a correlation of ~0.60 detected across two laboratories will tend to have a strong downward bias and will be lower than what we would obtain if the data had all been acquired in a single lab at a single time using a single set of animals.

The analysis of *Onecut1* summarized in the last several paragraphs and figures can be repeated for all of the *DYX* candidate genes in Table I. This is a time-consuming labor of love that we can hope will soon be semiautomated with a single click action: *Generate Report*. In the majority of cases, interesting inferences and hypotheses regarding functions and gene families will be generated. The utility of this bioinformatic data mining depends on the depth of the data and the sophistication of statistical and network analysis tools. It also depends on the original quality of the microarray data, and it is easy to chase chimeras. For example, expression data for *Ekn1/Dyx1c1* is not yet of high enough quality in the adult mouse brain to allow a useful analysis of its expression and coexpression. In the case of developmental dyslexia, it would be of tremendous value to have data sets on patterns of gene expression in the brains of the same BXD strains during several stages of development.

QTL ANALYSIS OF *DYX* CANDIDATES

The *DYX* loci listed in Table I were mapped using human families in which reading ability was highly variable. These same methods can also be applied to mapping variable expression of mRNAs such as *Onecut1* in the BXD RI strains. The BXD panel is essentially a large family that originates from two common strains. It is, therefore, possible to do much more than just study correlations among traits. It is possible to determine what upstream regions of the genome modulate the level of *Onecut1* expression or any other candidate gene. This is a causal connection rather than simply a statistical association. The reason we can claim causality for these relations is that we know that gene variants produce variation in phenotypes and not vice versa. Any upstream QTL that controls *Onecut1* expression may itself be an additional *DYX* candidate gene. It might be possible to uncover functions and networks of interacting genes that collectively contribute to dyslexia (Chesler et al., 2003). As an example of this approach, I will use the WebQTL of the Gene Network to search for such upstream controllers.

Interval Mapping of *DYX* Candidate Genes

The expression values listed in Figure 3 along the *y*-axis are precisely the data that we need to map loci that may be upstream sources of variation in *Onecut1* expression. A function labeled *Interval Mapping* in the WebQTL module of the Gene Network (see the *Trait Data and Editing Form*) systematically compares the continuous variation in expression with the two types of genotypes at each marker (B6 type or D2 type) across the whole genome, and plots the results as in Figure 7 in the four-color section on page 222-E. The *x*-axis is a schematic of 19 mouse autosomes and the X chromosome to the far right. In contrast, the left *y*-axis provides a statistical measure of chromosomal intervals that are linked with variance in *Onecut1*. If all of the variability in *Onecut1* were accounted for by a single Mendelian locus, then there would be a single very distinct peak. Instead, Figure 7 shows several modest upward deflections on chromosomes 5, 6, and 9. None of these regions in isolation provides much explanatory power, and none reaches the nominal criteria that we would want to definitively locate an upstream controller QTL for *Onecut1* expression.

However, all is not lost. So many other interesting transcripts covary with *Onecut1* (Figures 4 and 6), that we can ask whether these also share common QTLs with *Onecut1* on Chr 6 or Chr 9. The assumption is that common QTLs for covarying transcripts may provide some additional support. Ten of the 12 transcripts listed in Figure 4 also have modest LRS peaks at almost precisely the same Chr 6 locus as *Onecut1* (the exceptions are *Mapk8*, *Neurog3*, *Hey1*, *Ptprj*, and *Gria4*). These kinds of results can provide motivation to treat potential QTLs to more attention than they might appear to warrant based on stringent statistical criteria.

There is an even more effective tactic to extract signal from data sets that appear to have two or more weak QTLs. We ask this simple question: do pairs of loci collectively account for much of the variation in *Onecut1* expression? The next section describes the implementation and interpretation of these so-called pair scans.

Detecting Cooperating Pairs of QTLs that Modulate *DYX* Candidates

Looking for genetic linkage between all possible pairs of chromosomal regions and differences in a trait such as *Onecut1* expression is conceptually simple but computationally intensive. In the case of the BXD strains, we have genotypes for approximately 800 markers that would have to be tested in all possible pairs. It follows that there are about 320,000 explicit statistical tests (800 x 799/2) that we could perform. Fortunately, with a combination of a clever algorithm called DIRECT (Ljungberg, Holmgren, & Carlborg, 2004) and fast computers, it is now possible to perform a pair scan in seconds (Wang & Manly, implemented in WebQTL). Figure 8, shown in the four-color section on page 222-E, illustrates the graphic output of a pair scan. It is essentially a two-dimensional version of the QTL interval map of Figure 7 in which color is used to code the LRS. Red hotspots at the intersections of two chromosomes highlight combinations of loci that are linked to differences in *Onecut1* expression. In this case, the best combination involves a region on Chr 9 proximal to *Onecut1* near *Ddx25* and a region on Chr 16 near *Sod1* and the Down syndrome critical region. Of all 21 genes listed in Figure 6 (the Cell Differention set), *Onecut1* shares this pair of QTLs only with inositol trisphospate 3 kinase B (*Itpkb*), *Hey1*, and *Fancg*. These happen to be the three transcripts with which *Onecut1* has strong negative correlations.

A Synopsis on the Functional Genomics of **Onecut1.** The analysis of *Onecut1* leaves us with the following general conclusions and leads:

> 1. *Onecut1* has a plausible role in CNS development that could affect neuronal circuits. This inference is made

solely on the basis of adult gene expression patterns, and this hypothesis should be tested in the immature CNS. The hypothesis is supported strongly by extensive analysis of *Onecut1* function in invertebrates (Poustka et al., 2004). *Onecut1* also has expression that is coupled to many genes involved in signal transduction, providing additional indirect reasons to retain it as a *DYX1* candidate.

2. *Onecut1* is itself controlled by QTLs that map to Chr 9 and Chr 16; a pattern that it shares prominently with *Itpkb*, *Fancb*, and *Hey1*. It is logical to hypothesize that all four transcripts are jointly controlled by both QTLs. Given the known role of *Onecut1* as a master transcription factor, it is also reasonable to hypothesize that *Onecut1* inhibits the transcription of *Itpkb*, *Fancb*, and *Hey1*. If correct, this would be a reversal of the typical view of *Onecut1* as a transcriptional coactivator.

If in the near future we were to prove that the human *ONECUT1* was in fact the *DYX1* gene, then we would definitely be warranted in taking a close look at the human regions that are homologous to mouse Chr 9 and Chr 16 for additional *DYX* loci (human Chr 11 near 125 Mb and Chr 21 near 32 Mb). These other loci are not secondary. They are part of a network of interacting genes distributed on many chromosomes. Any member of the network may be polymorphic in different populations of humans, and with enough study and enough families, we will be able to define sets of functionally related *DYX* loci and genes that contribute to dyslexia.

CONCLUSION

Well over half of all genes are expressed in the human brain at some stage of development. Perhaps a quarter of these genes already have been studied in some detail, but in the great majority of cases, we still do not fully understand the intricate molecular networks in which they participate. Even the classical Mendelian diseases and genes such as Huntington's disease (*HD*), Lesh-Nyan disease (*HPRT*), and albinism (*TYR*) have puzzling effects on brain function that will take years to fully understand. Fortunately, the rate of progress is accelerating so rapidly that even optimists are occasionally surprised. Functional genomics and statistical techniques use to study complex traits such as dyslexia are just beginning to reach the point at which they are valuable and indispensable. We can now use these methods to describe and explain (1) the diverse and interwoven roles of genes and networks of gene products, (2) the consequences of abnormal gene expression or sequence, and (3) complex interactions with environmental factors. The Gene Network is a single example of a resource that can empower anyone with training and an Internet connection to explore gene function. In this chapter, I have provided a single example of how to mine bioinformatic resources to evaluate candidates genes that underlie the *DYX1* locus. The primarily catalyst and prerequisite is a set of well mapped *DYX* loci, and we are fortunate to already have a interesting set of these loci with which to work.

Address correspondence to: Robert W. Williams, Ph.D., University of Tennessee Health Science Center, Center for Genomics and Bioinformatics, 855 Monroe Avenue, Memphis, TN 38120; E-mail: rwilliam@nb.utmem.edu

REFERENCES

Cardon, L. R., Smith, S. D., Fulker, D. W., Kimberling, W. J., Pennington, B. F., & DeFries, J. C. (1994). Quantitative trait locus for reading disability on chromosome 6. *Science, 266*, 276–279.

Chesler, E. J., Wang, J., Lu, L., Qu, Y., Manly, K. F., & Williams, R. W. (2003). Genetic correlates of gene expression in recombinant inbred strains: A relational model system to explore neurobehavioral phenotypes. *Neuroinformatics, 1*, 343–357.

Chesler, E. J., Lu, L., Wang, J., Williams, R. W., & Manly, K. F. (2004). WebQTL: Rapid exploratory analysis of gene expression and genetic networks for brain and behavior. *Nature and Neuroscience, 7*, 485–486.

Cox, P. R., Fowler, V., Xu, B., Sweatt, J. D., Paylor, R., & Zoghbi, H. Y. (2003). Mice lacking Tropomodulin-2 show enhanced long-term potentiation, hyperactivity, and deficits in learning and memory. *Mol Cell Neurosci, 23*, 1–12.

Cox, P. R., & Zoghbi, H. Y. (2001). Sequencing, expression analysis, and mapping of three unique human tropomodulin genes and their mouse orthologs. *Genomics, 63*, 97–107.

Deffenbacher, K. E., Kenyon, J. B., Hoover, D. M., Olson, R. K., Pennington, B. F., DeFries, J. C., & Smith, S. D. (2004). Refinement of the 6p21.3 quantitative trait locus influencing dyslexia: Linkage and association analyses. *Human Genetics, 115*, 128–138.

Dopazo, A., Lovenberg, T. W., Danielson, P. E., Ottiger, H. P., & Sutcliffe, J. G. (1993). Primary structure of mouse secretogranin III and its absence from deficient mice. *Journal of Molecular Neuroscience, 4*, 225–233.

Fagerheim, T., Raeymaekers, P., Tonnessen, F. E., Pedersen, M., Tranebjaerg, L., & Lubs, H. A. (1999). A new gene (DYX3) for dyslexia is located on chromosome 2. *Journal of Medical Genetics, 36*, 664–669.

Fisher, S. E., & DeFries, J. C. (2002). Developmental dyslexia: Genetic dissection of a complex cognitive trait. *Nat Rev Neurosci, 3*, 767–780.

Fisher, S. E., Francks, C., Marlow, A. J., MacPhie, I. L., Newbury, D. F., Cardon, L. R., Ishikawa-Brush, Y., Richardson, A. J., Talcott, J. B., Gayan, J., Olson, R. K., Pennington, B. F., Smith, S. D., DeFries, J. C., Stein, J. F., & Monaco, A. P. (2000). Independent genome-wide scans identify a chromosome 18 quantitative-trait locus influencing dyslexia. *Nat Genet, 30,* 86–91.

Grigorenko, E. L., Wood, F. B., Meyer, M. S., Hart, L. A., Speed, W. C., Shuster, A., & Pauls, D. L. (1997). Susceptibility loci for distinct components of developmental dyslexia on chromosomes 6 and 15. *American Journal of Human Genetics, 60,* 27–39.

Hitzemann, R., Hitzemann, B., Rivera, S., Gatley, J., Thanos, P., Shou, L. L., & Williams, R. W. (2003). Dopamine D2 receptor binding, Drd2 expression and the number of dopamine neurons in the BXD recombinant inbred series: Genetic relationships to alcohol and other drug associated phenotypes. *Alcohol Clin Exp Res, 27,* 1–11.

Hsiung, G. Y., Kaplan, B. J., Petryshen, T. L., Lu, S., & Field, L. L. (2004). A dyslexia susceptibility locus (DYX7) linked to dopamine D4 receptor (DRD4) region on chromosome 11p15.5. *American Journal of Medical Genetics, 125B,* 112–119.

Janowsky, A., Mah, C., Johnson, R. A., Cunningham, C. L., Phillips, T. J., Crabbe, J. C., Eshleman, A. J., & Belknap, J. K. (2001). Mapping genes that regulate density of dopamine transporters and correlated behaviors in recombinant inbred mice. *J Pharmacol Exp Ther, 298,* 634–643.

Jones, J. M., Huang, J. D., Mermall, V., Hamilton, B. A., Mooseker, M. S., Escayg, A., Copeland, N. G., Jenkins, N. A., & Meisler, M. H. (2000). The mouse neurological mutant flailer expresses a novel hybrid gene derived by exon shuffling between Gnb5 and Myo5a. *Human Molecular Genetics, 9,* 821–828.

Kaminen, N., Hannula-Jouppi, K., Kestila, M., Lahermo, P., Muller, K., Kaaranen, M., Myllyluoma, B., Voutilainen, A., Lyytinen, H., Nopola-Hemmi, J., & Kere, J. (2003). A genome scan for developmental dyslexia confirms linkage to chromosome 2p11 and suggests a new locus on 7q32. *Journal of Medical Genetics, 40,* 340–345.

Kawabe, H., Sakisaka, T., Yasumi, M., Shingai, T., Izumi, G., Nagano, F., Deguchi-Tawarada, M., Takeuchi, M., Nakanishi, H., & Takai Y. (2003). A novel rabconnectin-3-binding protein that directly binds a GDP/GTP exchange protein for Rab3A small G protein implicated in Ca(2+)-dependent exocytosis of neurotransmitter. *Genes Cells, 8,* 537–546.

Ljungberg, K., Holmgren, S., & Carlborg, O. (2004). Simultaneous search for multiple QTL using the global optimization algorithm DIRECT. *Bioinformatics, 20,* 1887–1895.

Makino, C., Fujii, Y., Kikuta, R., Hirata, N., Tani, A., Shibata, A., Ninomiya, H., Tashiro, N., Shibata, H., & Fukumaki, Y. (2003) Positive association of the AMPA receptor subunit GluR4 gene (GRIA4) haplotype with schizophrenia: Linkage disequilibrium mapping using SNPs evenly distributed across the gene region. *American Journal of Medical Genetics, 116B,* 17–22.

Marino, C., Giorda, R., Vanzin, L., Nobile, M., Lorusso, M. L., Baschirotto, C., Riva, L., Molteni, M., & Battaglia, M. (2004). A locus on 15q15-15qter influences dyslexia: Further support from a transmission/disequilibrium study in an Italian speaking population. *Journal of Medical Genetics, 41,* 42–46.

Marlow, A. J., Fisher, S. E., Francks, C., MacPhie, I. L., Cherny, S. S., Richardson, A. J., Talcott, J. B., Stein, J. F., Monaco, A. P., & Cardon, L. R. (2003). Use of multivariate linkage analysis for dissection of a complex cognitive trait. *American Journal of Human Genetics, 72*, 561–570.

McKusick, V. (1999). *Mendelian inheritance in man: A catalog of human genes and genetic traits.* Baltimore: The Johns Hopkins University Press.

Morris, D. W., Robinson, L., Turic, D., Duke, M., Webb, V., Milham, C., Hopkin, E., Pound, K., Fernando, S., Easton, M., Hamshere, M., Williams, N., McGuffin, P., Stevenson, J., Krawczak, M., Owen, M. J., O'Donovan, M. C., & Williams, J. (2000). Family-based association mapping provides evidence for a gene for reading disability on chromosome 15q. *Human Molecular Genetics, 9*, 843–848.

Nopola-Hemmi, J., Myllyluoma, B., Haltia, T., Taipale, M., Ollikainen, V., Ahonen, T., Voutilainen, A., Kere, J., & Widen, E. (2001). A dominant gene for developmental dyslexia on chromosome 3. *Journal of Medical Genetics, 38*, 658–664.

Odom, D. T., Zizlsperger, N., Gordon, D. B., Bell, G. W., Rinaldi, N. J., Murray, H. L., Volkert, T. L., Schreiber, J., Rolfe, P. A., Gifford, D. K., Fraenkel, E., Bell, G. I., & Young, R. A. (2004). Control of pancreas and liver gene expression by HNF transcription factors. *Science, 303*, 1378–1381.

Pastural, E., Barrat, F. J., Dufourcq-Lagelouse, R., Certain, S., Sanal, O., Jabado, N., Seger, R., Griscelli, C., Fischer, A., & de Saint Basile, G. (1997). Griscelli disease maps to chromosome 15q21 and is associated with mutations in the myosin-Va gene. *Nature and Genetics, 16*, 289–292.

Peirce, J. L., Lu, L., Gu, J., Silver, L. M., & Williams, R. W. (2004). A new set of BXD recombinant inbred lines from advanced intercross populations in mice. *BMC Genet, 5*(1), 7.

Prekeris, R., & Terrian, D. M. (1997). Brain myosin V is a synaptic vesicle-associated motor protein: Evidence for a Ca2+-dependent interaction with the synaptobrevin-synaptophysin complex. *Journal of Cell Biology, 137*, 1589–1601.

Petryshen, T. L., Kaplan, B. J., Fu Liu, M., de French, N. S., Tobias, R., Hughes, M. L., & Field, L. L. (2001). Evidence for a susceptibility locus on chromosome 6q influencing phonological coding dyslexia. *American Journal of Medical Genetics, 105*, 507–517.

Petryshen, T. L., Kaplan, B. J., Hughes, M. L., Tzenova, J., & Field, L. L. (2002). Supportive evidence for the DYX3 dyslexia susceptibility gene in Canadian families. *Journal of Medical Genetics, 39*, 125–126.

Poustka, A. J., Kuhn, A., Radosavljevic, V., Wellenreuther, R., Lehrach, H., & Panopoulou, G. (2004). On the origin of the chordate central nervous system: Expression of onecut in the sea urchin embryo. *Evol Dev, 6*, 227–236.

Schulte-Korne, G., Grimm, T., Nothen, M. M., Muller-Myhsok, B., Cichon, S., Vogt, I. R., Propping, P., & Remschmidt, H. (1998). Evidence for linkage of spelling disability to chromosome 15. *American Journal of Human Genetics, 63*, 279–282.

Smith, E., Hargrave, M., Yamada, T., Begley, C. G., & Little, M. H. (2002). Coexpression of SCL and GATA3 in the V2 interneurons of the developing mouse spinal cord. *Dev Dyn, 224*, 231–237.

Scerri, T. S., Fisher, S. E., Francks, C., MacPhie, I. L., Paracchini, S., Richardson, A. J., Stein, J. F., & Monaco, A. P. (2004). Putative function allele of DYX1C1 are not associated with dyslexia susceptibility in a large sample of sibling pairs from the UK. *Journal of Medical Genetics, 10*(35), 21–32.

Su, A. I., Wiltshire, T., Batalov, S., Lapp, H., Ching, K. A., Block, D., Zhang, J., Soden, R., Hayakawa, M., Kreiman, G., Cooke, M. P., Walker, J. R., & Hogenesch, J. B. (2004). A gene atlas of the mouse and human protein-encoding transcriptomes. *Proceedings of the National Academy of Sciences USA, 101,* 6062–6067.

Taipale, M., Kaminen, N., Nopola-Hemmi, J., Haltia, T., Myllyluoma, B., Lyytinen, H., Muller, K., Kaaranen, M., Lindsberg, P. J., Hannula-Jouppi, K., & Kere, J. (2003). A candidate gene for developmental dyslexia encodes a nuclear tetratricopeptide repeat domain protein dynamically regulated in brain. *Proceedings of the National Academy of Sciences USA, 100,* 11553–11558.

Tzenova, J., Kaplan, B. J., Petryshen, T. L., & Field, L. L. (2004). Confirmation of a dyslexia susceptibility locus on chromosome 1p34–p36 in a set of 100 Canadian families. *American Journal of Medical Genetics, 127B,* 117–124.

Wang, J., Williams, R. W., & Manly, K. F. (2003). WebQTL: Web-based complex trait analysis. *Neuroinformatics, 1,* 299–308.

Williams, R. W. (2000). Mapping genes that modulate mouse brain development: A quantitative genetic approach. *Results Probl Cell Differ, 30,* 21–49. (www.nervenet.org/papers/brainrev99.html).

Williams, R. W., Gu, J., Qi, S., & Lu, L. (2001). The genetic structure of recombinant inbred mice: High-resolution consensus maps for complex trait analysis. *Genome Biol, 2*(11), 0046.

Willott, J. F., & Erway, L. C. (1998). Genetics of age-related hearing loss in mice. IV. Cochlear pathology and hearing loss in 25 BXD recombinant inbred mouse strains. *Hearing Research 119,* 27–36.

Zhang, B., Schmoyer, D., Kirov, S., & Snoddy, J. (2004). GOTree Machine (GOTM): A web-based platform for interpreting sets of interesting genes using Gene Ontology hierarchies. *BMC Bioinformatics, 5,* 16.

Zhang, L., Miles M. F., & Aldape, K. D. (2003). A model of molecular interactions on short oligonucleotide microarrays. *Nature and Biotechnology, 21,* 818–821.

Section • III

Animal Models of Cortical Development

INTRODUCTION

The chapters in this section are all concerned with animal models of cortical development. From the perspective of developmental dyslexia, our interest in this topic stems from the finding of malformations in the cerebral cortex of postmortem dyslexics. What is fascinating is that these five chapters approach the investigation of these malformations from completely different perspectives. Yet even though these laboratories approach the problem from disparate points of view, there is a commonality that emerges that all point to the profound impact that small malformations occurring during brain development can have on the organization of the brain and behavior. This impact can be directly related to the malformation itself, but as a number of authors suggest, it is the developing brain's *reaction* to these malformations that provide the underlying substrate for the subsequent cognitive and physiologic disturbances. In short, these chapters sharply bring into focus the notion that the developing brain is not like the adult brain, and that when one considers the brain basis of any developmental disorder (including dyslexia), one needs to take this seemingly self-evident fact into account.

It is appropriate that we begin this section with Peter Crino's chapter. He commences with a detailed review of some of the different types of malformations of the cerebral cortex that have been described in the human literature, as well as their consequences. This is followed by a discussion of the genes that have been associated with some of these malformations, and how the use of mouse models (knockouts and transgenics) has helped advance our understanding of how they operate. It is clear that single gene mutations may underlie several different types of malformations, and that understanding how these genes work may lead to new therapies, and perhaps treatments to ameliorate or even prevent their emergence.

The laboratory of Pierre Gressens has been interested in exploring some of the injuries that occur in both the pre- and postnatal period in humans. Using rats as their model system, they have found that injury (the introduction of toxins injurious to neurons) induces malformations in otherwise normal animals. What is particularly fascinating is that the *timing* of these "neurotoxic" insults is critical in determining the type of malformation that will occur. Thus, the same type of injury can cause disorders of neuronal migration or polymicrogyria or cystic periventricular leukomalacia or stroke-like lesions, depending on the stage of brain development at the time of the injury. This work also strongly implicates a number of external factors that modulate the effects of neurotoxins. Some of these agents can, on the one hand, exacerbate the effects of the injury, while others can be strongly protective and ameliorate their effects. As they point out in their chapter, these results have potentially intriguing implications for methods of intervention following early injury on the brain.

Much of the work in my own laboratory has centered on examining anatomic consequences of early injury to the developing cortical plate. This injury, which involves a short freeze lesion of the developing cortex, results in a cortical malformation resembling human polymicrogyria. My interest in this subject was spurred by the fact that this type of malformation has been seen in some postmortem dyslexic brains. It is noteworthy that there are a number of other laboratories that are using this identical model to study epilepsy. In their chapter, Zsombok and Jacobs detail the wealth of information that has been gained concerning the electrophysiologic properties of cortex in which a microgyria has been induced. Two findings are of particular note. First, it turns out that the source of the aberrant electrophysiologic activity is not the malformation itself, but rather the areas surrounding the microgyria. This suggests that this focal injury has widespread effects on the organization and circuitry of the brain, which will be a common thread in subsequent chapters. Second, the subtle differences in the timing of the injury has remarkable effects on the electrophysiologic activity. A freeze lesion placed on the day of birth in the rat results in much less epileptiform activity than the identical lesion performed one day later. This finding echoes that of the previous chapter, again demonstrating the changing vulnerabilities of the developing nervous system.

The "tish" (an acronym for "telencephalic internal structural heterotopias") rat was a fortuitous discovery of Kevin Lee and colleagues. This spontaneous mutation was originally identified by the presence of seizures. Subsequent investigations identified a malformation of development of the cerebral cortex consisting of subcortical band heterotopia. Lee and colleagues have done an extensive categorization of the anatomic, electrophysiologic, and behavioral consequences of these malformations. Similar to the induced malformations studied by Zsombok and Jacobs, the actual source of the electrophysiological disturbance that causes the seizures is not the malformation itself, but rather lies in areas just outside the malformation. Of particular interest is the finding that there are disturbances in behavior and anatomy in individuals that are heterozygous for the allele that causes the malformation. Lee et al. suggest that much of the behavioral and electrophysiologic effects may be independent of the direct effects of the malformation. Rather, it may well be the case that the subcortical band heterotopia are just the most obvious manifestations of a series of problems that occur during development. Importantly, they suggest that changes in circuitry that evolve as a consequence of the malformation may be the cause of much of the underlying difficulty associated with this disorder. This recapitulates the conclusions of the previous chapters, namely that the malformation itself may just be an obvious flag telling us that this brain is organized differently.

At some level, the suggestion of an animal model of developmental dyslexia may generate more than a little skepticism. After all, reading is most certainly a uniquely human characteristic. But as we've seen in the previous sections, there are other biological characteristics that seem to co-occur with developmental dyslexia. For the past decade, Holly Fitch and colleagues have investigated the link between malformations of the cerebral cortex (see Galaburda, this volume) to defects in rapid auditory processing (see Tallal, this volume). In the last chapter of this section, Fitch and Peiffer review their extensive collection of studies on this topic. They have found that rats and mice with malformations—some induced and some spontaneous—appear to have difficulties in the processing of rapid auditory information, and that these are more severe in younger animals. These difficulties appear more commonly in males as compared to females, which is fascinating when considered in light of evidence suggesting that males have a higher incidence of dyslexia. How exactly malformations of the cerebral cortex affect the low level processing of auditory signals is not known, but Fitch and Peiffer propose a testable model for how the system might operate.

Chapter • 10

Focal Malformations of Cortical Development: Epilepsy, Autism, and Dyslexia

Peter B. Crino

MALFORMATIONS OF CORTICAL DEVELOPMENT: OVERVIEW

Malformations of cortical development (MCD) are characterized by disruption of the normal cytoarchitecture of the cerebral cortex and altered cellular morphologies (for review see Walsh, 1999; Andermann, 2000; Crino, Miyata, & Vinters, 2002). MCD can affect broad regions of the cerebral cortex as in lissencephaly and hemimegalencephaly, or may be restricted to focal areas such as tubers in the tuberous sclerosis complex (TSC) or focal cortical dysplasia (FCD) with balloon cells. In lissencephaly and polymicrogyria, the normal six-layered organization of the cerebral cortex is replaced by a more primitive four-layered arrangement (Leventer, Mills, & Dobyns, 2000), whereas in FCD or tubers of TSC, there is a virtual loss of all lamination. Large collections of heterotopic neurons are identified in subcortical band heterotopia and periventricular nodular heterotopia. The morphology of individual neurons in many MCD subtypes is abnormal, suggesting a pervasive disruption of steps necessary for intact cortical development (Ferrer et al., 1992). Recent studies have

---

This work was supported by MH01658, NS39938, the Esther A. and Joseph Klingenstein Fund, the Tuberus Sclerosis Alliance/Center Without Walls, and Parents Against Childhood Epilepsy (PBC).

identified gene mutations responsible for select MCDs. However, the developmental pathogenesis of most MCD has not been defined. As a result of defining how gene mutations lead to abnormal cortical development, a recent scheme classifies MCD according to distinct neurodevelopmental stages including cell proliferation, migration, and cortical laminar organization (Barchovich & Kuziecky, 2000).

All MCD are highly associated with epilepsy (Andermann, 2000; Crino & Chou, 2000) in infants, (especially infantile spasms, IS), children, and adults. MCD is the most common neuropathologic abnormality encountered when cortical resection is performed to treat IS (Vinters et al., 1992, Vinters, De Rosa, & Farrell, 1993; Vinters, 2002; Prayson, 2000). MCD may account for 20% of all epilepsies (Brodtkorb, Nilsen, Smevik, & Rinck, 1992; Hauser, Annegers, & Kurland, 1993) and in some extensive MCD such as lissencephaly, hemimegalencephaly, and TSC, seizures may occur in 70%–90% of affected patients. More anatomically restricted malformations such as focal heterotopia or FCD with balloon cells are also associated with medically intractable seizures that persist into adulthood (Farrell et al., 1992). Estimates are that nearly 30% of cortical specimens resected as treatment for neocortical epilepsy contain some type of MCD (Vinters, 2000). Indeed, recent advances in neuroimaging have demonstrated that many cases of "cryptogenic" epilepsy actually result from subtle cytoarchitectural abnormalities (microdysgenesis). Finally, a subgroup of adult patients with temporal lobe epilepsy exhibit radiographic and histopathologic evidence of MCD, either alone or in combination with hippocampal sclerosis ("dual pathology;" Levesque, Nakasato, Vinters, & Babb, 1991; Ho, Kuzniecky, Gilliam, Faught, & Morawetz, 1998).

From a clinical perspective, virtually all seizure subtypes (e.g., generalized tonic-clonic, complex partial, atonic, myoclonic, atypical absence seizures, and infantile spasms) have been described in MCD. Anti-epileptic drug therapy in patents with MCD often fails and surgical therapy provides the only hope for seizure remission (Engel, 1996; Mathern et al., 1999; Peacock et al., 1996). Unfortunately, seizure cure following surgical resection of focal CDs is successful in less than 50% of patients. Even worse, a subgroup of patients may not be surgical candidates at all. The mechanisms of seizure initiation and epileptogenesis are unknown in MCD. Thus, the challenges to neurobiologists and neuropathologists who examine tissue from patients with MCDs are to explain the origin of the structural findings in the resected tissue, and to define precisely how and why these aberrations of the cerebral cortex produce intractable seizures.

MOLECULAR NEUROBIOLOGY OF FOCAL MCD

Recent studies have identified no fewer that 11 genes responsible for MCD associated with epilepsy. Subtle developmental malformations have been observed in a variety of neurological and psychiatric disorders without a definitive molecular correlate such as dyslexia, autism, and schizophrenia. The genes responsible for MCD have important functions in one or more stages of normal cortical development. All MCD result from loss of function gene mutations, and thus, the histopathologic features of each MCD yields a view of the role that the responsible gene plays in cortical development. In addition, the effect of each gene mutation also highlights the developmental epoch in which that gene is active in corticogenesis. These critical time-points provide a framework to understand the interface between gene mutations and abnormal neural development. For example, gene mutations that affect cell mitosis will disrupt the proliferative phases of cortical development but may have little effect on postmitotic neurons. Similarly, a gene mutation that alters cytoskeletal assembly during dynamic phases of neuronal migration will have distinct effects in an actively migrating neuron versus a neuron that has already achieved its laminar destination. In sum, a defined molecular event occurring within a specific developmental context results in a characteristic malformation (for review, see Crino, Miyata, and Vinters, 2002).

To better understand the function of the encoded gene products, the role of these genes in normal development is being studied experimentally in transgenic or knockout mouse strains. This chapter will discuss focal MCD in an attempt to highlight how the molecular pathogenesis of many MCD are becoming more clearly understood. FCD and small heterotopia are highly associated with seizures and also have implicated in a variety of neuropsychological disorders including dyslexia. FCD are characterized histologically by disorganized or absent cortical lamination and by the presence of cells exhibiting an abnormal morphology. Balloon cells ("BCs") specifically refer to cytomegalic cells in FCD that exhibit an aberrant cell morphology, short processes of indeterminate identity (e.g., axons versus dendrites, a laterally displaced nucleus, and phenotypic features suggestive of a mixed astrocytic and neural lineage). BCs are believed to be central in the pathogenesis of FCD. Intermingled with BCs are large, dysplastic neurons (cytomegalic neurons) that exhibit aberrant dendritic arbors and loss of radial orientation within the cortex in relation to the pial surface. These cells express protein markers more consistent with a neuronal phenotype. FCD may also exhibit excess numbers of astrocytes. The cytoarchitectural features of FCD suggest a cortical developmental abnormality affecting select steps during cell proliferative phase of cortical development (Barkovich & Kuzniecky, 2000). However, elucidating the molecular etiology of FCD has been problematic because they are sporadic disorders and no family pedigrees have been identified (Breillmann, Jackson, Torn-Broers, & Berkovic, 2001). In addition, there is currently no animal model of FCD with BCs, and thus, virtually all experimental analyses require human tissue resected during epilepsy surgery.

The precise developmental epoch in which FCD is generated is unknown and the search for candidate genes responsible for FCD is an area of intense research. An interesting recent study demonstrates discordant incidence of select FCD in monozygotic twins, suggesting that these lesions result from acquired factors such as prenatal insults and postfertilization genetic abnormalities (Briellmann ey al., 2001). There are two competing hypotheses regarding the formation of FCD. The first states these lesions result from an abnormality affecting a single neural precursor cell, which in turn, undergoes successive rounds of division to yield a clonal progeny that comprise the cellular constituents of the FCD. This scenario might develop if a somatic mutation were to occur in a single progenitor cell although it is not certain whether FCD reflects a regional or cell autonomous abnormality (i.e., a defect in neural precursors or radial glial cells). An intriguing possibility is that a mutation in one of the known MCD genes such as TSC1, TSC2, or PTEN, or even novel gene occurs as a somatic event in a neural precursor, that then gives rise to a clonal population of cells within the FCD (Hua & Crino, 2003). Interestingly, a recent study that evaluated TSC1 and TSC2 gene sequence in FCD did not identify deleterious gene mutations in FCD. While FCD does not exhibit a familial inheritance pattern, the histologic features of FCD suggest a consistent or uniform etiology (Mischel, Nguyen, & Vinters, 1995; Crino and Eberwine, 1997). The alternative hypothesis is that an external event affects the development of multiple precursor cells that yield multiple nonclonal cell types as progeny. Histologically, multiple cell types are present within FCD including dysplastic neurons, neurons within the subcortical white matter (heterotopic neurons), and BCs. Alternatively, some suggest that FCD is a late occurring event, possibly even a postnatal event (see Lombroso, 2000), resulting from external injury such as trauma or hypoxia-ischemia. Thus, a pivotal question is whether the central pathogenetic process affects laminar distribution and morphology, or whether there is a select cell type that is actually the abnormal cell type.

An interesting feature of BCs is the expression of a variety of cytoskeletal genes and proteins, many of which are expressed under normal circumstances only in neural precursor cells. These proteins are typically expressed on a regulated developmental schedule during corticogenesis and are necessary for appropriate neuronal differentiation, migration, or process outgrowth. For example, expression of select intermediate filament (IF) proteins such as nestin, α-internexin, and vimentin—proteins found in immature neurons—has been reported in subpopulations of balloon cells as well as dysplastic and heterotopic neurons within FCD (Crino, Trojanowski, & Eberwine, 1997; Yamanouchi et al., 1998). However, dysplastic neurons contain abnormal accumulations of highly- and nonphosphorylated neurofilament (NF) protein isoforms, which are normally expressed in more differentiated neurons (Duong, De Rosa, Poukens, Vinters, & Fisher, 1994). Thus, detection of select IFs in FCD that are normally expressed at either early or late stages of cortical development may yield clues to the maturational phenotype of dysplastic neurons, and supports the hypothesis that these cells may retain components of an immature developmental phenotype.

New functional insights shed light on how BCs form from neural progenitor cells. The tuberous sclerosis complex genes *TSC1* and *TSC2* encoded proteins hamartin and tuberin form a functional protein-protein complex that constitutively inhibits the mTOR (Target Of Rapamycin)/p70-S6-kinase/ribosomal S6 protein cascade (Arrazola et al., 2002). The mTOR/p70-S6-kinase/ribosomal S6 pathway contributes to ribosomal assembly and protein translation initiation, and serves as a regulator of cell growth and organogenesis (Potter, Huang, & Xu, 2001). Negative modulation of this cascade by hamartin-tuberin results in growth suppression and restricted cell size (Gao & Pan, 2001). Inactivation of hamartin-tuberin by Akt-mediated phosphorylation *in vitro* or by loss of function mutations in *TSC1* or *TSC2* leads to phosphorylation (activation) of mTOR, p70S6kinase, and ribosomal S6, and enhanced cell size and proliferation (Tee et al., 2002). Additional downstream proteins activated by p70S6kinase include STAT3 and 4EBP-1, which play roles in transcriptional and translational regulation (Onda et al., 2002). We have recently shown that BCs in FCD also express phosphorylated ribosomal S6 protein but not the upstream protein p70S6 kinase, suggesting that this cascade may be activated in FCD but by a mechanism that is distinct from loss of hamartin or tuberin function (Baybis et al., 2004).

Focal white matter heterotopia are common small cortical malformations that are often noted in resected epilepsy specimens

(Barkovich & Kuzniecky, 2000) as well as in patients with dyslexia (Marin-Padilla, 1999). These may be detected in any cortical region but may be enriched in the temporal lobes. Heterotopic neurons have been reported in normal brain autopsy series, and thus, further classification of these lesions as pathogenic is warranted. One hypothesis is that focal heterotopia reflect excessive proliferation of a small subset of cells that then fail to achieve their appropriate laminar destination. Alternatively, heterotopic cells may represent a small nidus of cells that failed to undergo cell death during development and thus remain. A third hypothesis is that heterotopic neurons may actually undergo local cell division akin to a small neoplasm.

How does cortical maldevelopment lead to neurological dysfunction? A pivotal question directly relevant to both clinical and laboratory investigations of MCD is why are cortical malformations so highly associated with epilepsy? An overriding hypothesis that has been supported by clinical studies is that in patients with focal types of dysplasias, the seizures emanate from the malformation rather than surrounding cortex (see Flint & Kriegstein, 1997). For example, in FCD with balloon cells, tubers, and polymicrogyria, intracranial grid recordings have clearly demonstrated that the ictal onset zone is either within the malformation or at the border zone with adjacent normal cortex (Palmini et al., 1995; Preul et al., 1997). An important recent study using human depth electrode recording showed that seizures in patients with another MCD, periventricular nodular heterotopia, may emanate directly from the heterotopia (Kothare et al., 1998).

Several theories have been proposed based on studies in human MCD and in animal models of MCD that include altered synaptic connectivity, aberrant expression of molecules that mediate synaptic transmission, and an imbalance between excitatory and inhibitory impulses associated with the dysplasia. Solid evidence has been provided in favor of each of these hypotheses and it is likely that, broadly speaking, epilepsy in MCD reflects contributions from multiple factors. However, it is unclear at this time whether the mechanisms of epileptogenesis in MCD will be similar or distinct across multiple MCD subtypes. In other words, epilepsy in MCD may be more akin to a final common electrophysiologic or clinical pathway for a variety of malformations. There may be important differences in epileptogenesis between individual MCD syndromes. As a corollary to this question, within each MCD, why are their distinct seizure phenotypes? For example, how can we mechanistically explain or investigate the occurrence of infantile spasms and complex partial epilepsy in tuberous sclerosis or in two distinct MCD subtypes such as tuberous sclerosis and lissencephaly? Implicit in this question is whether clinical epilepsy syndromes or semiologic subtypes are specific for each MCD subtype, or whether they reflect maturational contextual differences in cortical development. This point is critical since the clear failures in anti-epileptic drug treatment for many patients with MCD may imply an essential flaw in drug utility as a direct consequence of the pathoanatomic differences among these different brain lesions. Indeed, an inherent question in this idea is whether future anti-epileptic drug design may be predicated on individual cellular and molecular differences in epilptogenesis among different MCD subtypes. A final point is that it is often a tacit assumption that aberrant cortical cytoarchitecture alone is responsible for seizures in MCD. This is an especially important consideration since MCD have been well documented in patients with no history of epilepsy. Certainly, disorganized synaptic connectivity within MCD and between MCD and the surrounding cortex may enhance the likelihood of recurrent and propagated synchronous, paroxysmal discharges. However, an alternative hypothesis is that some of the genes responsible for individual MCD may, in fact, also serve as epilepsy susceptibility loci that confer hyperexcitability to neurons regardless of their laminar positioning.

The mechanisms of epileptogenesis in MCD have been investigated in human tissue and animal models of MCD (Baraban, 2001). Data addressing the physiological properties of neurons with MCD remains sparse, largely as a consequence of technical limitations of studying resected tissue *in vitro*, including limited viability of the tissue slice, the paucity of connections between the slice and surrounding cortex, and lack of true control tissue. Surprisingly little is known about mechanisms controlling excitatory and inhibitory tone in several important MCD syndromes including lissencephaly, band heterotopia, and nodular heterotopia. However, one MCD subtype that has been studied using cellular, electrophysiologic, and recently, molecular strategies, is Taylor type FCD since this MCD subtype is frequently identified in neocortical epilepsy surgical specimens as well as in temporal lobe resections. The cellular constituents of FCD may include a variable population of dysplastic neurons, heterotopic neurons, and large "balloon" neurons intermingled with neuronal subtypes of indeterminate laminar destiny. It is important to remember that it has yet to be defined whether all neurons within foci of FCD are, in fact, abnormal or within an incorrect laminar position, and thus, how we view the physiologic responses of these cells may depend on how we weight the contributions of each cell type. One hypothesis that has received experimental support is that there is decreased inhibitory and enhanced excitatory tone in FCD (Spreafico et al., 1998; Avoli, Bernasconi, Mattia, Olivier, & Hwa, 1999). The few studies that have addressed this hypothesis directly with field potential and intracellular recording within human FCD specimens have shown that dyslastic cortex is hyperexcitable (Mattia, Olivier, & Avoli, 1995; Mathern et al., 2000), and that a subset of dysplastic neurons generate repetitive ictal discharges in response to the K^+ channel blocker 4AP that can be blocked by NMDA receptor antagonists. (Avoli et al., 1999). These electrophysiological responses may result from several possible causes. First, several reports have demonstrated a reduction in the number of parvalbumin, somatostatin, and GAD65 immunolabeled inhibitory interneurons in FCD (Spreafico et al., 1998; Ferrer, Oliver, Russi, Casas, & Rivera, 1994; Spreafico et al., 2000). In cortical tubers, there are few GABAergic neurons identified by GAD65 immunolabeling and the expression of the vesicular GABA transporter (VGAT) mRNA, a marker for GABAergic neurons, is also reduced (White et al., 2001). Interestingly, using proton magnetic resonance spectroscopy to assay tuber samples, an increase in GABA was defined (Aasly et al., 1999), suggesting a possible compensatory response. Neurons within nodular subcortical heterotopias are largely calbindin immunoreactive, suggesting a GABAergic phenotype that has failed to migrate into cortex (Hannan et al., 1999). Taken together, these studies suggest that there is a paucity of GABAergic interneurons in MCD that represents reduction in the genesis of GABAergic cells, a selective failure of GABAergic cell migration from the median eminence during development, or enhanced death of GABAergic neurons. A second contributory factor to hyperexcitability in MCD is a selective reduction in $GABA_A$ receptor subunits in FCD, which argues that the synaptic machinery to modulate neural inhibition within FCD may be diminished. Reduced expression of $GABA_A$ $\alpha 1$, $\alpha 2$, $\beta 1$, and $\beta 2$ receptor subunit mRNAs is observed in human FCD (Crino, Duhaime, Baltuch, & White, 2001) and GABAergic terminals identified in close proximity to balloon neurons in FCD do not appear to make functional synapses (Garbelli et al., 1999). The reduction in GABAergic neurons and loss of GABAergic receptor subunits would alter critical inhibitory synaptic control, and render neurons in FCD more susceptible to sudden and prolonged excitability. A third factor related to hyperexcitability is that recent reports have demonstrated the expression of several glutamate receptor subunits is enhanced in FCD (Ying et al., 1998; Kerfoot, Vinters, & Mathern, 1999; Crino et al., 2001). For example, expression of the

NR2B site has been shown to be increased in FCD (Mikuni et al., 1999a; Crino et al., 2001). This site has been shown to modulate sustained calcium mediated depolarization and is an ideal candidate protein to account for recurrent hyperexcitability in FCD. The expression of the NR2B site was correlated with more widespread epileptiform abnormalities detected by surface grid electrodes (Najm et al., 2000). Increased NR2B mRNA and protein expression has been defined in tubers of the tuberous sclerosis complex by cDNA array and receptor ligand pharmacology (White et al., 2001). Increased expression of several other glutamate receptor subunits including GluR1, GluR2 have been defined in FCD (Crino et al., 2001; Kerfoot, Vinters, & Mathern, 1999). Diminished coupling of NR1 with calmodulin has been reported in three FCD specimens, an interaction that is essential for inactivation of the NR1 complex (Mikuni et al., 1999b). Two recent studies suggest that the number of excitatory neurons, as evidenced by expression of the neuronal glutamate transporter EAAT3/EAAC1, is increased in tubers (White et al., 2001) and in FCD (Crino, Miyata, & Vinters, 2002), suggesting that regional hyperexcitability in select MCD may result from enhanced numbers of excitatory neurons as well.

Corroborative studies in several animal models of MCD support the idea of an imbalance between excitatory and inhibitory tone in MCD (Jacobs, Kharazia, & Prince 1999; Zsombok & Jacobs, this volume). These models include the freeze induced microgyrus, *methylazoxymethanol* (*MAM*), *in utero* radiation, and several spontaneous and engineered rodent strains such as the flathead, OTX-1, p35, TISH, and NZB strains. The histologic features of these individual strains are quite distinct and only very few of them (e.g., the flathead strain) exhibit spontaneous seizures. Yet differential expression of select glutamate and GABA receptor subunits have been demonstrated nonetheless. For example, in the freeze microgyrus lesion model, selective upregulation of the NR2B site has been shown using patch clamp recordings (DeFazio & Hablitz, 2000) and there is a reduction in parvalbumin immunolabeled neurons within the microgyrus (Jacobs, Kharazia, & Prince, 1999). Interestingly, in a mouse model of cortical dysplasia generated by *in utero* irradiation, there is a reduction in the numbers of cortical parvalbumin and calbuindin immunoreactive neurons (Roper, Eisenschenk, & King, 1999). In rats treated with methylazoxymethanol (MAM), altered expression of GluR2, NR2A, and NR2B were reported within the heterotopic cell islands in the hippocampus and neocortex (Rafiki, Chevassus-au-Louis, Ben-Ari, Khrestchatisky, & Represa, 1998). In the mouse Lis1 mutant strain, hyperexcitability in the CA3 hippocampal sector reflected the cytoarchitectural disruption observed, including displaced somatostatin and parvalbumin immunoreactive neurons (Fleck, 2000). Disruption of ion channel function may also contribute to epileptogenesis of MCD although little data in expression of these channels in human brain tissue is available. In the freeze lesion model, loss of an inwardly rectifying potassium current as well as a reduction in gap junction coupling have been demonstrated (Bordey Lyons, Hablitz, & Sontheimer, 2001) although similar findings in humans are unknown. In the MAM model, selective reduction in Kv4.2 potassium channel was observed in heterotopia (Castro, Cooper, Lowenstein, & Baraban, 2001). These findings suggest that animal models of cortical malformations can provide important insights into epileptogenesis associated with MCD.

SUMMARY AND NEW DIRECTIONS: TARGETED THERAPY FOR EPILEPSY IN MCD

Prior to the 1990s, the molecular pathogenesis of MCD was largely the source of speculation. However, with the discovery of several genes responsible for MCD including *LIS1, doublecortin, FLN1, TSC1*, and *TSC2*, it is clear that single gene mutations may account for numerous subtypes of MCD (see Gleeson, this volume). The identification of MCD genes now permits in-depth analysis of the proteins encoded by these genes and may aid in designing new therapies targeted at these molecules. Thus, in the future, we may hope to modulate pathways in select MCD syndromes so that specific agents can be used to treat seizures in, for example, PH or TSC. Perhaps even more exciting is the potential to design therapeutic strategies to actually abolish or prevent the development of these malformations *in utero*.

Address correspondence to: Peter B. Crino, M.D., Ph.D., PENN Epilepsy Center and Department of Neurology, 3 West Gates Building, 3400 Spruce Street, University of Pennsylvania Medical Center, Philadelphia, PA 19104; phone: 215-349-5312

REFERENCES

Aasly J., Silfvenius H., Aas T. C., Sonnewald, U., Olivecrona, M., Juul, R., & White, L. R. (1999). Proton magnetic resonance spectroscopy of brain biopsies from patients with intractable epilepsy. *Epilepsy Research, 35*(3), 211–217.

Andermann, F. (2000). Cortical dysplasias and epilepsy: A review of the architectonic, clinical, and seizure patterns. *Advances in Neurology, 84,* 479–496.

Arrazola, P., Hino, O., Kobayashi, T., Yeung, R. S., Ru, B., & Pan, D. (2002). Tsc tumour suppressor proteins antagonize amino-acid-TOR signalling. *Nature Cell Biology, 4,* 699–704.

Avoli, M., Bernasconi, A., Mattia, D., Olivier, A., & Hwa, G. G. (1999). Epileptiform discharges in the human dysplastic neocortex: In vitro physiology and pharmacology. *Annals of Neurology, 46,* 816–826.

Baraban, S. (2001). Epileptogenesis in the dysplastic brain: A revival of familiar themes. *Epilepsy Currents 1,* 22–29.

Barkovich, A. J., & Kuzniecky, R. I. (2000). Gray matter heterotopia. *Neurology 55,* 1603–1608.

Baybis, M., Yu, J., Lee, A., Golden, J. A., Weiner, H., McKhann, G., 2nd, Aronica, E., & Crino, P. B. (2004). mTOR cascade activation distinguishes tubers from focal cortical dysplasia. *Annals of Neurology. 28;56*(4), 478–487.

Bordey, A., Lyons, S. A., Hablitz, J. J., & Sontheimer, H. (2001). Electrophysiological characteristics of reactive astrocytes in experimental cortical dysplasia. *Journal of Neurophysiology, 85*(4), 1719–1731.

Briellmann, R. S., Jackson, G. D., Torn-Broers, Y., & Berkovic, S. F. (2001). Causes of epilepsies: Insights from discordant monozygous twins. *Annals of Neurology, 49*(1), 45–52.

Brodtkorb, E., Nilsen, G., Smevik, O., & Rinck, P. A. (1992). Epilepsy and anomalies of neuronal migration: MRI and clinical aspects. *Acta Neurologica Scandinavica, 86*(1), 24–32.

Castro, P. A., Cooper, E. C., Lowenstein, D. H., & Baraban, S. C. (2001). Hippocampal heterotopia lack functional Kv4.2 potassium channels in the methylazoxymethanol model of cortical malformations and epilepsy. *The Journal of Neuroscience, 21,* 6626–6634.

Crino, P. B., Miyata, H., & Vinters, H. V. (2002). Neurodevelopmental disorders as a cause of seizures: Neuropathologic, genetic, and mechanistic considerations. *Brain Pathology, 12,* 212–233.

Crino, P. B., & Chou, K. (2000). Epilepsy and cortical dysplasias. *Current Treatment Options in Neurology, 2,* 543–552.

Crino, P. B., Duhaime, A. C., Baltuch, G., & White, R. (2001). Differential expression of glutamate and GABA-A receptor subunit mRNA in cortical dysplasia. *Neurology 56,* 906–913.

Crino, P. B., & Eberwine, J. (1997). Cellular and molecular basis of cerebral dysgenesis. *Journal of Neuroscience Research, 50,* 907–916.

Crino, P. B., Trojanowski, J. Q., & Eberwine, J. (1997). Internexin, MAP1B, and nestin in cortical dysplasia as markers of developmental maturity. *Acta Neuropathologica (Berlin), 93,* 619–627.

DeFazio, R. A., & Hablitz, J. J. (2000). Alterations in NMDA receptors in a rat model of cortical dysplasia. *Journal of Neurophysiology, 83,* 315–321.

Duong, T., Derosa, M. J., Poukens, V., Vinters, H. V., & Fisher, R. S. (1994). Neuronal cytoskeletal abnormalities in human cerebral cortical dysplasia. *Acta Neuropathologica (Berlin), 87*(5), 493–503.

Engel, J., Jr. (1996). Surgery for seizures. *New England Journal of Medicine, 334,* 647–652.

Farrell, M. A., Derosa, M. J., Curran, J. G., Secor, D. L., Cornford, M. E., Comair, Y. G., Peacock, W. J., Shields, W. D., & Vinters, H. V. (1992).

Neuropathologic findings in cortical resections (Including hemispherectomies) performed for the treatment of intractable childhood epilepsy. *Acta Neuropathologica (Berlin), 83*(3), 246–259.

Ferrer, I., Oliver, B., Russi, A., Casas, R., & Rivera, R. (1994). Parvalbumin and calbindin-D28k immunocytochemistry in human neocortical epileptic foci. *Journal of Neurological Sciences, 123*(1–2), 18–25.

Ferrer, I., Pineda, M., Tallada, M., Oliver, B., Russi, A., Oller, L., Noboa, R., Zújar, M. J., & Alcántara, S. (1992). Abnormal local-circuit neurons in epilepsia partialis continua associated with focal cortical dysplasia. *Acta Neuropathologica (Berlin), 83*(6), 647–652.

Fleck, M. W., Hirotsune, S., Gambello, M. J., Phillips-Tansey, E., Suares, G., Mervis, R. F., Wynshaw-Boris, A., & McBain, C. J. (2000, April). Hippocampal abnormalities and enhanced excitability in a murine model of human lissencephaly. *Journal of Neurocience, 20*(7), 2439–2450.

Flint, A. C., & Kriegstein, A. R. (1997). Mechanisms underlying neuronal migration disorders and epilepsy. *Current Opinions in Neurology, 10*(2), 92–97.

Gao, X., & Pan, D. (2001). TSC1 and TSC2 tumor suppressors antagonize insulin signaling in cell growth. *Genes and Development, 15*, 1383–1392.

Garbelli, R., Munari, C., De Biasi, S., Vitellaro-Zuccarello, L., Galli, C., Bramerio, M., Mai, R., Battaglia, G., & Spreafico, R. (1999). Taylor's cortical dysplasia: A confocal and ultrastructural immunohistochemical study. *Brain Pathology, 9*(3), 445–461.

Hannan, A. J., Servotte, S., Katsnelson, A., Sisodiya, S., Blakemore, C., Squier, M., & Molnar, Z. (1999). Characterization of nodular neuronal heterotopia in children. *Brain, 122*(pt. 2), 219–238.

Hauser, W. A., Annegers, J. F., & Kurland, L. T. (1993). Incidence of epilepsy and unprovoked seizures in Rochester, Minnesota: 1935–1984. *Epilepsia, 34*, 453–468.

Ho, S. S., Kuzniecky, R. I., Gilliam, F., Faught, E., & Morawetz, R. (1998). Temporal lobe developmental malformations and epilepsy: Dual pathology and bilateral hippocampal abnormalities. *Neurology, 50*(3), 748–754.

Hua, Y., & Crino, P. B. (2003). Single cell lineage analysis of focal cortical dysplasia. *Cerebral Cortex, 13*, 693–699.

Jacobs, K. M., Kharazia, V. N., & Prince, D. A. (1999, September). Mechanisms underlying epileptogenesis in cortical malformations. *Epilepsy Research, 36*(2–3), 165–188.

Kerfoot, C., Vinters, H. V., & Mathern, G. W. (1999). Cerebral cortical dysplasia: Giant neurons show potential for increased excitation and axonal plasticity. *Developmental Neuroscience, 21*, 260–270.

Kothare, S. V., VanLandingham, K., Armon, C., Luther, J. S., Friedman, A., & Radtke, R. A. (1998). Seizure onset from periventricular nodular heterotopias: Depth-electrode study. *Neurology, 51*(6), 1723–1727.

Leventer, R. J., Mills, P. L., & Dobyns, W. B. (2000). X-linked malformations of cortical development. *American Journal of Medical Genetics, 97*, 213–220.

Levesque, M. F., Nakasato, N., Vinters, H. V., & Babb, T. L. (1991). Surgical treatment of limbic epilepsy associated with extrahippocampal lesions: The problem of dual pathology. *Journal of Neurosurgery, 75*(3), 364–370.

Lombroso, C. T. (2000). Can early postnatal closed head injury induce cortical dysplasia? *Epilepsia, 41*, 245–253.

Marín-Padilla, M. (1999, May). Developmental neuropathology and impact of perinatal brain damage III: Gray matter lesions of the neocortex. *Journal of Neuropathology Experimental Neurology, 58*(5), 407–429.

Mathern, G. W., Cepeda, C., Hurst, R. S., Flores-Hernandez, J., Mendoza, D., & Levine, M. S. (2000). Neurons recorded from pediatric epilepsy surgery patients with cortical dysplasia. *Epilepsia, 41*(Suppl. 6), S162–S167.

Mathern, G. W., Giza, C. C., Yudovin, S., Vinters, H. V., Peacock, W. J., Shewmon, D. A., & Shields, W. D. (1999). Postoperative seizure control and antiepileptic drug use in pediatric epilepsy surgery patients: the UCLA experience, 1986–1997. *Epilepsia, 40*(12), 1740–1749.

Mattia, D., Olivier, A., & Avoli, M. (1995). Seizure-like discharges recorded in human dysplastic neocortex maintained in vitro. *Neurology, 45,* 1391–1395.

Mikuni, N., Babb, T. L., Ying, Z., Najm, I., Nishiyama, K., Wylie, C., Yacubova, K., Okamoto, T., & Bingaman, W. (1999a). NMDA-receptors 1 and 2A/B coassembly increased in human epileptic focal cortical dysplasia. *Epilepsia, 40*(12), 1683–1687.

Mikuni, N., Nishiyama, K., Babb, T. L., Ying, Z., Najm, I., Okamoto, T., Luders, H. O., & Wylie, C. (1999b). Decreased calmodulin-NR1 coassembly as a mechanism for focal epilepsy in cortical dysplasia. *Neuroreport, 10*(7), 1609–1612.

Mischel, P. S., Nguyen, L. P., & Vinters, H. V. (1995). Cerebral cortical dysplasia associated with pediatric epilepsy: Review of neuropathologic features and proposal for a grading system. Journal of Neuropathlgy and Experimental *Neurology, 54,* 137–153.

Najm, I. M., Ying, Z., Babb, T., Mohamed, A., Hadam, J., LaPresto, E., Wyllie, E., Kotagal, P., Bingaman, W., Foldvary, N., Morris, H., & Luders, H. O. (2000). Epileptogenicity correlated with increased N-methyl-D-aspartate receptor subunit NR2A/B in human focal cortical dysplasia. *Epilepsia, 41*(8), 971–976.

Onda, H., Crino, P. B., Zhang, H., Murphey, R., Rastelli, L., Rothberg, B., & Kwiatkowski, D. (2002). Tsc2 null murine neuronal epithelial cells are a model for human tuber giant cells, & show activation of an mTOR pathway. *Molecular Cell Neuroscience, 21,* 561–574.

Palmini, A., Gambardella, A., Andermann, F., Dubeau, F., Dacosta, J. C., Olivier, A., Tampieri, D., Gloor, P., Quesney, F., Andermann, E., Paglioli, E., Pagliolineto, E., Coutinho, L., Leblanc, R., & Kim, H. I. (1995). Intrinsic epileptogenicity of human dysplastic cortex as suggested by corticography and surgical results. *Annals of Neurology, 37*(4), 476–487.

Peacock, W. J., Wehby-Grant, M. C., Shields, W. D., Shewmon, D. A., Chugani, H. T., Sankar, R., & Vinters, H. V. (1996). Hemispherectomy for intractable seizures in children: A report of 58 cases. *Childs Nervous System, 12*(7), 376–384.

Potter, C. J., Huang, H., & Xu, T. (2001). Drosophila Tsc1 functions with Tsc2 to antagonize insulin signaling in regulating cell growth, cell proliferation, & organ size. *Cell 105,* 357–368.

Prayson, R. A. (2000). Clinicopathological findings in patients who have undergone epilepsy surgery in the first year of life. *Pathology International, 50,* 620–625.

Preul, M. C., Leblanc, R., Cendes, F., Dubeau, F., Reutens, D., Spreafico, R., Battaglia, G., Avoli, M., Langevin, P., Arnold, D. L., & Villemure, J. G. (1997). Function and organization in dysgenic cortex. Case report. *Journal of Neurosurgery, 87*(1), 113–121.

Rafiki, A., Chevassus-au-Louis, N., Ben-Ari, Y., Khrestchatisky, M., & Represa, A. (1998). Glutamate receptors in dysplasic cortex: An in situ hybridization and immunohistochemistry study in rats with prenatal treatment with methylazoxymethanol. *Brain Research, 782*(1–2), 142–152.

Roper, S. N., Eisenschenk, S., & King, M. A. (1999). Reduced density of parvalbumin- and calbindin D28-immunoreactive neurons in experimental cortical dysplasia. *Epilepsy Research, 37*(1), 63–71.

Spreafico, R., Battaglia, G., Arcelli, P., &ermann, F., Dubeau, F., Palmini, A., Olivier, A., Villemure, J. G., Tampieri, D., Avanzini, G., & Avoli, M. (1998). Cortical dysplasia: An immunocytochemical study of three patients. *Neurology, 50*(1), 27–36.

Spreafico, R., Tassi, L., Colombo, N., Bramerio, M., Galli, C., Garbelli, R., Ferrario, A., Lo Russo, G., & Munari, C. (2000). Inhibitory circuits in human dysplastic tissue. *Epilepsia, 41*(Suppl. 6), S168–S173.

Tee, A. R., Fingar, D. C., Manning, B. D., Kwiatkowski, D. J., Cantley, L. C., & Blenis, J. (2002). Tuberous sclerosis complex-1 and -2 gene products function together to inhibit mammalian target of rapamycin (mTOR)-mediated downstream signaling. *Proceedings of the National Academy of Sciences USA, 99*, 13571–13576.

Vinters, H. V. (2000). Surgical pathologic findings of extratemporal-based intractable epilepsy. A study of 133 consecutive cases. *Archives of Pathology and Laboratory Medicine, 124*, 1111–1112.

Vinters, H. V. (2002). Histopathology of brain tissue from patients with infantile spasms. *International Review of Neurobiology, 49*, 63–76.

Vinters, H. V., De Rosa, M. J., & Farrell, M. A. (1993). Neuropathologic study of resected cerebral tissue from patients with infantile spasms. *Epilepsia, 34*, 772–779.

Vinters, H. V., Fisher, R. S., Cornford, M. E., Mah, V., Secor, D. L., De Rosa, M. J., Comair, Y. G., Peacock, W. J., & Shields, W. D. (1992). Morphological substrates of infantile spasms: studies based on surgically resected cerebral tissue. *Childs Nervous System, 8*(1), 8–17.

Walsh, C. A. (1999). Genetic malformations of the human cerebral cortex. *Neuron, 23*(1), 19–29.

White, R., Hua, Y., Scheithauer, B., Lynch, D. R., Henske, E. P., & Crino, P. B. (2001). Selective alterations in glutamate and GABA receptor subunit mRNA expression in dysplastic neurons and giant cells of cortical tubers. *Annals of Neurology, 49*(1), 67–78.

Yamanouchi, H., Jay, V., Otsubo, H., Kaga, M., Becker, L. E., & Takashima, S. (1998). Early forms of microtubule-associated protein are strongly expressed in cortical dysplasia. *Acta Neuropathologica (Berlin), 95*(5), 466–470.

Ying, Z., Babb, T. L., Comair, Y. G., Bingaman, W., Bushey, M., & Touhalisky, K. (1998). Induced expression of NMDAR2 proteins and differential expression of NMDAR1 splice variants in dysplastic neurons of human epileptic neocortex. *Journal of Neuropathology and Experimental Neurology, 57*(1), 47–62.

Chapter • 11

Excitotoxic Lesions of the Developing Brain

Frank Plaisant, Romain H. Fontaine, Bettina Mesplès, and Pierre Gressens

During the last 15 years, the etiology of brain injury in human fetuses and neonates has been considered by many to be multifactorial rather than only linked to cardiovascular instability and hypoxia-ischemia (Nelson & Ellenberg, 1996; Evrard, Miladi, Bonnier, & Gressens, 1992; Dammann & Leviton, 1997). Several preconceptional, prenatal, and perinatal factors (like hypoxic-ischemic insults, endocrine imbalances, genetic factors of susceptibility, growth factor deficiency, abnormal competition for growth factors, excess free reactive oxygen species production, maternal infection yielding excess cytokines and other pro-inflammatory agents, exposure to toxins, maternal stress, and so on) have been implicated in the pathophysiology of brain lesions associated with cerebral palsy (Figure 1). Although some of the potentially noxious factors are present *in utero* and by themselves may cause permanent injury to the developing brain prior to neonatal life, several groups hypothesized that some of these factors act as predisposing factors ("prodamage conditions"), increasing the susceptibility to injury when there is a second unfavorable event (Nelson & Grether, 1998; Dommergues, Patkai, Renauld, Evrard, & Gressens, (2000); Gressens, Rogido, Paindaveine, & Sola, 2002; Dammann, Kuban, & Leviton, 2002; Eklind et al., 2001).

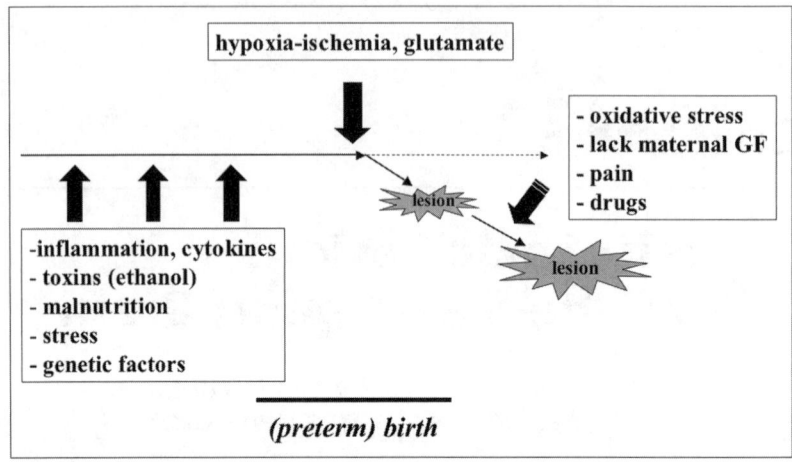

Figure 1. Schematic representation of the multiple-hit hypothesis where a combination of environmental and/or genetic factors (boxes give examples of such factors) occurring during the prenatal, perinatal, and/or postnatal periods (the horizontal arrow indicates normal brain development) induce brain lesions or modulate their severity (the oblique arrow, when compared to horizontal dotted arrow, points to disruption of normal brain development and formation of brain lesion). GF, growth factors.

EXCITOTOXIC LESIONS AT SUCCESSIVE STEPS OF BRAIN DEVELOPMENT

Excess release of glutamate could represent a molecular mechanism common to some of the risk factors for brain lesions in the foetus and neonate. Glutamate can act on several types of receptors including N-methyl-D-aspartate (NMDA), alpha-3-amino-hydroxy-5-methyl-4-isoxazole propionic acid (AMPA), kainate, and metabotropic receptors. To test this hypothesis, we used different glutamate agonists, including ibotenate (NMDA and metabotropic receptor agonist), NMDA, or S-bromowillardiine (AMPA and kainate receptor agonist) at different stages of rodent brain development, from neural tube closure to the end of the second postnatal week (Marret, Mukendi, Gadisseux, Gressens, & Evrard, 1995; Marret, Gressens, & Evrard, 1996; Gressens, Marret, & Evrard, 1996; Redecker et al., 1998). The results showed a pattern of brain damage that was dependant on the stage of brain maturation (Figure 2) and which mimicked several brain lesions observed in human fetuses and neonates.

1. Whole mouse embryo cultures were cultured at the 7-somite stage for 24 hours in the presence of ibotenate.

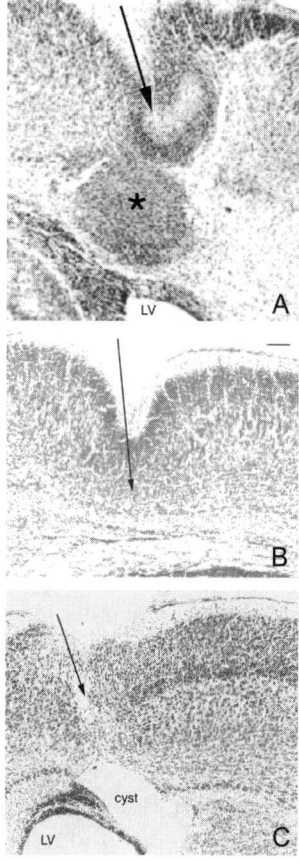

Figure 2. Pattern of lesions induced by ibotenate according to the stage of brain maturation. A. Periventricular heterotopia (*) and cortical defect (arrow) following ibotenate injection to a P0 hamster (stage of migration of granular and supragranular layer neurons). B. Selective destruction of layers V-VI neurons (arrow) following ibotenate injection to a P0 mouse (immediately after completion of neuronal migration). C. Neuronal loss in all cortical layers (arrow) following ibotenate injection to a P5 mouse (after completion of neuronal migration). LV, lateral ventricle. Bar = 80 μm.

During this developmental period of neural tube closure and early premigratory differentiation of the neuroepithelium, no macroscopic or light-microscopic effect of ibotenate was detected.

2. During maturation of neuronal layer V and during migration of neurons destined to granular and supragranular layers, postnatal day (P) 0 hamsters intracerebrally

injected at birth with ibotenate display arrests of migrating neurons at different distances from the germinative zones. The resulting cytoarchitectonic patterns include periventricular nodular heterotopias, subcortical band heterotopias, and intracortical halts of migrating neurons. These migratory disturbances are isolated or associated with microgyria (see below). The radial glial fibers and the extracellular matrix are exempt of any detectable damage, which could suggest a defect of their guiding role. The periventricular heterotopias induced by ibotenate are similar to the neuronal ectopic nodules encountered in Aicardi's and in other human syndromes including the X-linked periventricular heterotopias. The subcortical band heterotopias mimic some aspects of the human double cortex and lissencephalies.
3. After completion of neuronal layer V and during the full settlement of supragranular layers, P0 mice injected with ibotenate disclose a laminar neuronal depopulation of layer V-VIa, sharply mimicking human microgyria and a overlying sulcus in a normally lissencephalic brain.
4. Injected after completion of migration (P5-P10 in mouse or P7 in rat), ibotenate, NMDA, or S-bromowillardiine produce a severe neuronal loss in all neocortical layers (II, III, IV, V, and VI). This developmental lesional pattern mimics remarkably well neocortical lesions occurring in the full term human newborns. Furthermore, at this developmental stage, glutamate agonists induce the formation of periventricular white matter cysts, mimicking some aspects of the periventricular leukomalacia, which is frequent in the premature newborn. This white matter cyst evolves over weeks toward a glial scar as in human preterms.

All the lesions produced by ibotenate or NMDA are antagonized by DL-2-amino-7-phosphonoheptanoic acid, a competitive NMDA receptor antagonist, or MK-801, a noncompetitive NMDA receptor antagonist, but not by L(+)-2-amino-3-phosphonopropionic acid, a metabotropic receptor antagonist. On the other hand, lesions produced by S-bromowillardiine are blocked by NBQX, a selective AMPA-kainate receptor antagonist.

These studies emphasize the dramatic developmental role of glutamate through NMDA or AMPA-kainate receptors in the occurrence of neuronal migration disorders, and gray and white matter damage.

The asynchronism of the ontogenic windows between the ibotenate-induced cortical plate damage (P0 to adult) and the cystic white matter lesions (P2 to P10) strongly suggests that white matter lesions are not secondary to cortical plate lesions. The fact that melatonin (Husson et al. 2002), vasoactive intestinal peptide (Gressens et al., 1997), and nociceptin antagonists (Laudenbach et al., 2001) protect the white matter, but not the cortical plate, against ibotenate, combined with the observation that nicotine significantly reduces the ibotenate-induced cortical plate lesion without affecting the white matter damage (Laudenbach et al., 2002b), further supports the hypothesis that white matter and cortical plate lesions are largely independent from each other in this model.

Role of Brain Macrophages in Excitotoxic Brain Lesions

Massive activation of brain macrophages has been shown to take place during the early stages of ibotenate-induced lesions in newborn mice (Tahraoui et al., 2001) (Figure 3) or of NMDA-induced lesions in newborn rats (Acarin, Gonzalez, Castro, & Castellano, 1999). Further supporting the hypothesis of a pathophysiological role of brain macrophages, inhibitors of macrophage activation such as minocycline or strategies aiming at macrophage depletion are neuroprotective against ibotenate-induced lesions (Dommergues, Plaisant, Verney, & Gressens, 2003). Immunohistochemical analysis of brain macrophages activated on ibotenate insult reveals that within the first 24 hours post-insult, the vast majority of these cells is derived from resident microglia and is not blood-derived monocytes-macrophages (Dommergues et al., 2003).

In the developing murine periventricular white matter, there is a transient expression of NMDA on brain macrophages between P2 and P10, which strikingly parallels the window of vulnerability of the mouse white matter to excitotoxic lesions (Tahraoui et al., 2001). Therefore, one could make the hypothesis that in preterm infants, transient expression of NMDA receptors by white matter macrophages could participate to the vulnerability of the white matter to perinatal insults. Although this hypothesis remains to be confirmed, preliminary data obtained in human fetuses suggest the presence of NMDA receptors on white matter microglia during the period of vulnerability to periventricular leukomalacia (Monier, Gressens, Evrard, & Verney, 2002).

Role of Preoligodendrocytes in Excitotoxic White Matter Lesions

Extensive *in vitro* studies from Joe Volpe's group have clearly demonstrated the vulnerability of oligodendrocytes to glutamate

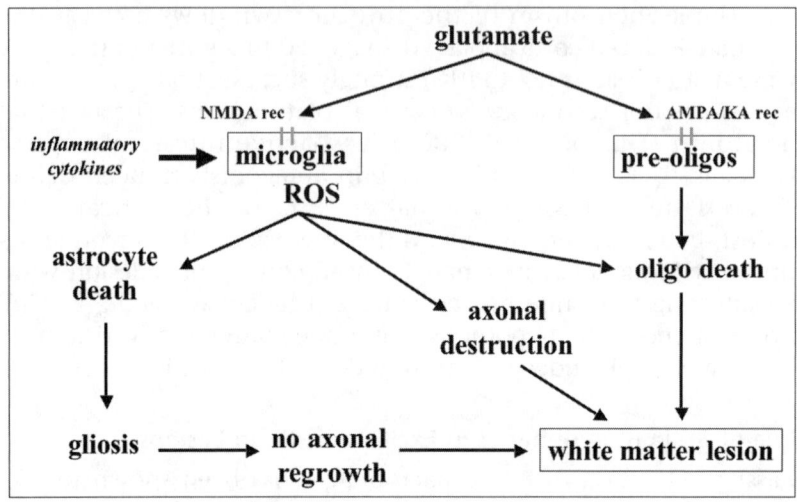

Figure 3. Schematic representation of the potential cellular and molecular pathways of perinatal excitotoxic white matter lesions. Rec, receptors; ROS, reactive oxygen species; KA, kainate; oligo(s), oligodendrocyte(s).

agonists activating AMPA receptors (2001). More recently, *in vivo* approaches from different labs have shown that AMPA or AMPA-kainate receptor agonists produce, in newborn rodents, periventricular white matter lesions, mimicking human periventricular leukomalacia (Follett, Rosenberg, Volpe, & Jensen, 2000; Tahraoui et al., 2001) (Figure 3). Of particular interest, intracerebral injection of AMPA agonists induces massive death of oligodendrocytes in the periventricular white matter (Follett et al., 2000) as well as suppression of oligodendroglial gene expression (Xu, Barks, Liu, & Silverstein, 2001).

EFFECTS OF INFLAMMATORY CYTOKINES ON EXCITOTOXIC BRAIN LESIONS

Findings from several studies support an association between maternal-fetal infection, circulating cytokines, and PVL (Dammann, Kuban, & Leviton, 2002). Furthermore, a striking association has been reported between increased levels of perinatal circulating cytokines, including IL-1-beta, IL-6, IL-8, IL-9, and tumor necrosis factor-alpha (TNF-alpha), and subsequent occurrence of CP in full-term infants (Nelson, Dambrosia, Grether, & Phillips, 1998). Although the epidemiologic and clinical data are quite compelling, we still lack indisputable evidence of a direct link between excess cytokine production and brain lesions in the full- and preterm infants. Animal models could be very useful in testing this hypothesized association.

Intracerebral NMDA injection to neonatal rat brain stimulates production of IL-1-beta (Hagan, Poole, Bristow, Tilders, & Silverstein, 1996). Pretreatment for five days with intraperitoneal IL-1-beta, IL-6, or TNF-alpha significantly exacerbates ibotenate-induced white mater and cortical plate lesions when compared to pretreatment with saline or IL-4 (Dommergues et al., 2000). Pretreatment with systemic IL-1-beta + IL-6 + TNF-alpha does not produce larger effects on excitotoxic lesions than each cytokine taken separately, suggesting common mechanisms of actions for the three pro-inflammatory cytokines. When compared to the toxic effects of systemic administration of TNF-alpha on excitotoxic brain lesions, astrocytic overexpression of TNF-alpha by gene targeting has no detectable effect on the size of ibotenate-induced lesions (Plaisant, Dommergues, Campbell, & Gressens, 2002). These preliminary findings suggest that the deleterious effect of circulating cytokines on perinatal brain lesions requires a systemic target to exert their toxic effects.

In contrast to NMDA receptor-mediated brain lesions, pretreatment with systemic IL-1-beta has no detectable effect on brain lesions induced by an agonist of AMPA-kainate receptors (Plaisant et al., 2002) (Figure 3). One of the potential mechanisms by which pro-inflammatory cytokines can exacerbate neonatal excitotoxic brain lesions could be the recruitment of new macrophage in the periventricular white matter and cortical plate.

Interestingly, systemic administration of pro-inflammatory cytokines does not induce any detectable brain lesions in the absence of an excitotoxic insult, further supporting the concept of a two-hit mechanism where cytokines would play a role of a pro-damage condition (Gressens et al., 2002).

IL-10 is a Th2 cytokine having marked suppressive effects on the production of pro-inflammatory cytokines by monocytes-macrophages, and down-regulating the expression of activating molecules on these cells and dendritic cells. Recent studies performed *in vitro* or in adult models have shown that IL-10 has neuroprotective properties against glutamate-induced (Bachis et al., 2001) or hypoxic-ischemic (Dietrich, Busto, & Bethea, 1999; Grilli et al., 2000) neuronal death, and lipopolysaccharide- or interferon-induced oligodendrocyte cell death (Molina-Holgado, Vela, Arevalo-Martin, & Guaza, 2001). In our mouse model of neonatal excitotoxic brain lesions, exogenous IL-10 completely blunts the toxic effect of IL-1-beta pretreatment (Mesplès, Plaisant, & Gressens, 2003). However, in contrast to studies performed in the adult, endogenous IL-10 does not seem to play a significant role in limiting the post-insult inflammatory response. This apparently low endogenous production of IL-10 during post-lesional brain inflammation could contribute to the high susceptibility of the newborn brain to inflammatory processes.

Effects of IL-9 on Excitotoxic Brain Lesions

In a retrospective human study, mean levels of perinatal circulating proinflammatory cytokines and IL-9 were higher in cases with subsequent occurrence of CP than in controls (Nelson et al., 1998). In that study, levels of pro-inflammatory cytokines were associated with one another, but no correlation was detected between IL-9 levels and the levels of the other cytokines tested. These data could suggest the existence of a subpopulation of CP patients characterized by increased levels of circulating IL-9 at birth.

IL-9 is produced by activated Th2 lymphocytes and is active on various immune cells including mast cells. Mast cells are present in the brain, including the neocortex, where their numbers increase during early postnatal development in rats. Mast cells can produce a variety of potentially toxic factors including histamine, serotonin, neutral proteases, cytokines, chemokines, and free radicals. Mast cells have been implicated in the pathophysiology of brain lesions associated with multiple sclerosis, Guillain-Barré syndrome, or Gayet-Wernicke encephalopathy.

Pretreatment with systemic IL-9 prior to ibotenate injection to newborn mouse pups significantly exacerbate cortical plate and white matter excitotoxic lesions (Dommergues et al., 2000). This toxic effect of IL-9 is largely mediated by brain mast cells (Patkai et al., 2001) and involves transforming growth factor beta-1 (TGF-beta-1) (Mesplès, Fontaine, Lelièvre, Launay, & Gressens, 2005) (Figure 4). Therapeutic targeting mast cells (inhibitors of mast cell degranulation and antihistamine drugs) were neuroprotective in mouse pups exposed to IL-9 prior to ibotenate insult.

In aggregate, these data suggest the existence of two different pathophysiological mechanisms of perinatal brain lesions associated with different circulating cytokine profiles, namely, elevated pro-inflammatory cytokines with potential effects on brain microglia and elevated IL-9 levels with effects on brain mast cells.

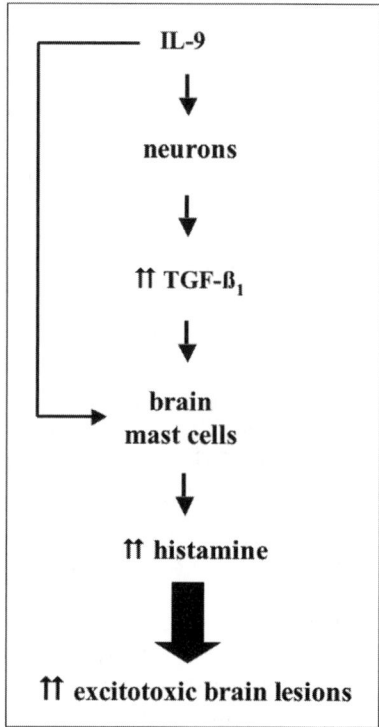

Figure 4. Schematic representation of the potential mechanism by which treatment with IL-9 leads to an exacerbation of excitotoxic lesions the newborn mice. In this model, neurons represent the major source of TGF-β_1 on exposure to IL-9. The main target of this additional TGF-β_1 is the mast cell, which in turn will increase the extracellular histamine concentration primarily by degranulation in the context of an excitotoxic insult. Increased histamine will exacerbate excitotoxic brain lesions. In addition, IL-9 will act directly on mast cells, upregulating the expression of mast cell enzymes, which also could contribute to excitotoxic brain damage, although this remains to be demonstrated.

EFFECTS OF TROPHIC FACTORS AND NEUROPROTECTIVE MOLECULES ON EXCITOTOXIC BRAIN LESIONS

Availability in trophic factors controls neuronal survival and most likely postlesional brain plasticity, two key events in terms of long-term functional consequences following damage to the developing brain. The above-described excitotoxic model allowed us to test the effects of trophic factors such as brain-derived neurotrophic factor (BDNF) as well as of other potential neuroprotective molecules.

Vasoactive intestinal peptide (VIP) is a neuropeptide with trophic properties (Brenneman, Hill, Gressens, & Gozes, 1997). Previous studies have shown that VIP-treated astrocytic cultures produce and/or release trophic factors including BDNF. We have demonstrated that co-injection of VIP or BDNF and ibotenate in P5 mice protected the white matter against the evolution of ibotenate-induced lesions (Gressens et al., 1997; Husson et al., 2005). VIP and BDNF did not prevent the initial appearance of white matter lesions, but rather promoted a secondary decrease of the white matter lesion size, suggesting a role in mediating axonal regrowth or sprouting (Gressens et al., 1998; Husson et al., 2005). We additionally showed that VIP induced BDNF synthesis *in vivo* and *in vitro* and that VIP neuroprotective effects were largely abolished by BDNF blockade. Furthermore, our data showed that protein kinase C (PKC) and MAPK pathways were critical for VIP neuroprotection (Gressens et al., 1998), and MAPK pathway for BDNF neuroprotection (Husson et al., 2005). The combination of these data permit us to propose the following formulation regarding the neuroprotective actions of VIP and BDNF in our mouse model of white matter injury (Figure 5): (1) VIP binds to a specific receptor on white matter astrocytes and activates a PKC pathway; (2) PKC activation promotes astrocytic survival and astrocytic production and/or release of soluble factors including BDNF; and (3) BDNF activates a MAPK cascade in neurons leading to white matter neuroprotection possibly involving axonal sprouting. The functional consequences of this neuroprotective effect remain to be determined.

Similarly, melatonin did not prevent white matter lesion formation but induced a secondary repair, probably involving axonal sprouting (Husson et al., 2002). However, the underlying molecular mechanisms were different as they involved specific melatoninergic receptors and cAMP production.

Other neurotransmitter systems also seem to be involved in the modulation of excitotoxic brain lesions in P5 mice. Indeed, nicotine and alpha4-beta2 nicotinic receptor agonists significantly reduced ibotenate-induced neuronal cell death while alpha7 nicotinic receptor agonists were deleterious (Laudenbach et al., 2002b). Alpha2 adrenergic agonists significantly reduced both white and gray matter lesions induced by ibotenate (Laudenbach et al., 2002a). Activation of the opioid ORL-1 receptor exacerbated ibotenate-induced white matter lesion while activation of classical opioid receptors did not induce detectable effects on excitotoxic brain lesions (Laudenbach et al., 2001). Finally, activation of D1 dopamine receptors induced a moderate but significant reduction of

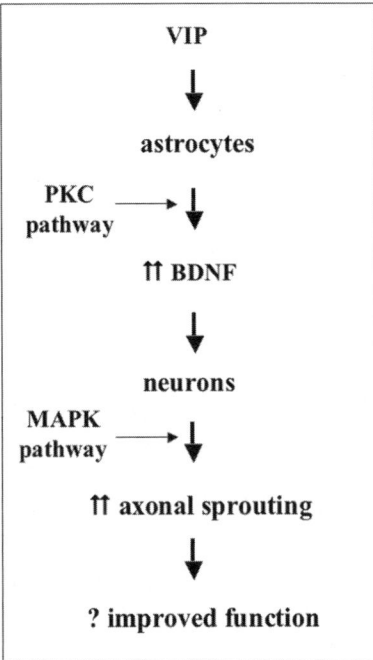

Figure 5. Schematic representation of the potential mechanism by which treatment with VIP and BDNF leads to neuroprotection of the white matter. See text for details.

ibotenate-induced neuronal loss. Altogether, these data underline the complex and selective modulation by numerous neurotransmitters of excitotoxic brain lesions in the developing brain.

In conclusion, experimental administration of excitotoxins at different stages of development has allowed producing a spectrum of brain damage mimicking brain lesions observed in the human fetuses and neonates such as neuronal migration disorders, polymicrogyria, cystic periventricular leukomalacia, and hypoxic-ischemic or ischemic-like cortical and striatal lesions. These models have identified brain macrophages and oligodendrocytes as key cells in white matter lesions mediated by, respectively, NMDA and AMPA receptors. Furthermore, these models have demonstrated a toxic effect of inflammatory cytokines and of IL-9, providing experimental support for epidemiological studies. These studies have also identified potential targets for neuroprotection and the key role of trophic factors in postlesional plasticity.

Address correspondence to: Pierre Gressens, INSERM U 676, Hôpital Robert Debré, 48 boulevard Sérurier, F-75019 Paris, France; E-mail: gressens@rdebre.inserm.fr

REFERENCES

Acarin, L., Gonzalez, B., Castro, A .J., & Castellano, B. (1999). Primary cortical glial reaction versus secondary thalamic glial response in the excitotoxically injured young brain: Microglial/macrophage response and major histocompatibility complex class I and II expression. *Neuroscience, 89,* 549–565.

Bachis, A., Colangelo, A. M., Vicini, S., Doe, P. P., De Bernardi, M. A., Brooker, G., & Mocchetti, I. (2001). Interleukin-10 prevents glutamate-mediated cerebellar granule cell death by blocking caspase-3-like activity. *The Journal of Neuroscience, 21,* 3104–3112.

Brenneman, D. E., Hill, J. M., Gressens, P., & Gozes, I. (1997). Neurotrophic action of VIP: From CNS ontogeny to therapeutic strategy. In S. S. Said (Ed.), *Pro-inflammatory and anti-inflammatory peptides* (pp. 383–408). New York: M. Dekker, Inc.

Dammann, O., Kuban, K. C., & Leviton, A. (2002). Perinatal infection, fetal inflammatory response, white matter damage, and cognitive limitations in children born preterm. *Mental Retardation and Developmental Disabilities Research Reviews, 8,* 46–50.

Dammann, O., & Leviton, A. (1997). Maternal intrauterine infection, cytokines, and brain damage in the preterm newborn. *Pediatric Research, 7*(42), 1–8.

Dietrich, W. D., Busto, R., & Bethea, J. R. (1999). Postischemic hypothermia and IL-10 treatment provide long-lasting neuroprotection of CA1 hippocampus following transient global ischemia in rats. *Experimental Neurology, 158,* 444–450.

Dommergues, M. A., Patkai, J., Renauld, J. C., Evrard, P., & Gressens, P. (2000). Pro-inflammatory cytokines and IL-9 exacerbate excitotoxic lesions of the newborn murine neopallium. *Annals of Neurology, 47,* 54–63.

Dommergues, M. A., Plaisant, F., Verney, C., & Gressens, P. (2003). Early microglial activation following neonatal excitotoxic brain damage in mice, a target for neuroprotection. *Neuroscience, 121,* 619–628.

Eklind, S., Mallard, C., Leverin, A. L., Gilland, E., Blomgren, K., Mattsby-Baltzer, I., & Hagberg, H. (2001). Bacterial endotoxin sensitizes the immature brain to hypoxic-ischaemic injury. *European Journal of Neuroscience, 13,* 1101–1106.

Evrard, P., Miladi, N., Bonnier, C., & Gressens, P. (1992). Normal and abnormal development of the brain. In I. Rapin, & S. J. Segalowitz (Eds.), *Child neuropsychology. Handbook of neuropsychology* (pp. 11–44). Amsterdam: Elsevier Science.

Follett, P. L., Rosenberg, P. A., Volpe, J. J., & Jensen, F. E. (2000). NBQX attenuates excitotoxic injury in developing white matter. *The Journal of Neuroscience, 20,* 9235–9241.

Gressens, P., Marret, S., & Evrard, P. (1996). Developmental spectrum of the excitotoxic cascade induced by ibotenate: A model of hypoxic insults in fetuses and neonates. *Neuropathology and Applied Neurology, 22,* 498–502.

Gressens, P., Marret, S., Hill, J. M., Brenneman, D. E., Gozes, I., Fridkin, I., & Evrard, P. (1997). Vasoactive intestinal peptide prevents excitotoxic hypoxic-like cell death in the murine developing brain. *Journal of Clinical Investigation, 100,* 390–397.

Gressens, P., Marret, S., Martin, J. L., Laquerrière, A., Lombet, A., & Evrard, P. (1998). Regulation of neuroprotective action of vasoactive intestinal peptide in the murine developing brain by protein kinase C and mitogen-activated protein kinase cascades: In vivo and in vitro studies. *Journal of Neurochemistry, 70,* 2574–2584.

Gressens, P., Rogido, M., Paindaveine, B., & Sola, A. (2002). The impact of frequent neonatal intensive care practices on the developing brain. *Journal of Pediatrics, 140,* 646–653.

Grilli, M., Barbieri, I., Basudev, H., Brusa, R., Casati, C., Lozza, G., & Ongini, E. (2000). Interleukin-10 modulates neuronal threshold of vulnerability to ischaemic damage. *European Journal of Neuroscience, 12,* 2265–2272.

Hagan, P., Poole, S., Bristow, A. F., Tilders, F., & Silverstein, F. S. (1996). Intracerebral NMDA injection stimulates production of interleukin-1 beta in perinatal rat brain. *Journal of Neurochemistry, 67,* 2215–2218.

Husson, I., Mesplès, B., Bac, P., Vamecq, J., Evrard, P., & Gressens, P. (2002). Melatoninergic neuroprotection of the murine periventricular white matter against neonatal excitotoxic challenge. *Annals of Neurology, 51,* 82–92.

Husson, I., Rangon, C. M., Lelievre, V., Bemelmans, P. A., Sachs, P., Mallet, J., Kosofsky, B. E., & Gressens, P. (2005). BDNF-induced white matter neuroprotection and stage-dependant neuronal survival following a neonatal excitotoxic challenge. *Cerebral Cortex, 15,* 250–261

Laudenbach, V., Calo, G., Guerrini, R., Lamboley, G., Benoist, J. F., Evrard, P., & Gressens, P. (2001). Nociceptin/orphanin FQ exacerbates excitotoxic white matter lesions in the murine neonatal brain. *Journal of Clinical Investigation, 107,* 457–466.

Laudenbach, V., Mantz, J., Lagercrantz, H., Desmonts, J. M., Evrard, P., & Gressens, P. (2002a). Effects of alpha-2 adrenoceptor agonists on perinatal excitotoxic brain injury: Comparison of clonidine and dexmedetomidine. *Anesthesiology, 96,* 134–141.

Laudenbach, V., Medja, F., Zoli, M., Rossi, F. M., Evrard, P., Changeux, J. P., & Gressens P. (2002b). Selective activation of central subtypes of the nicotinic acetylcholine receptor has opposite effects on neonatal excitotoxic brain injuries. *FASEB Journal, 16,* 423–425.

Marret, S., Gressens, P., & Evrard, P. (1996). Neuronal migration disorders induced by ibotenate in the neocortex. *Proceedings of the National Academy of Sciences USA, 17,* 543–551.

Marret, S., Mukendi, R., Gadisseux, J. F., Gressens, P., & Evrard, P. (1995). Effect of ibotenate on brain development: An excitotoxic mouse model of microgyria and posthypoxic like lesions. *Journal of Neuropathology and Experimental Neurology, 54,* 358–370.

Mesplès, B., Fontaine, R. H., Lelièvre, V., Launay, J. M., & Gressens, P. (2005). Neuronal TGF-b1 mediates IL-9/mast cell interaction and exacerbate excitotoxicity in newborn mouse. *Neurobiology of Disease, 18,* 193–205.

Mesplès, B., Plaisant, F., & Gressens, P. (2003). Effects of interleukin-10 on neonatal excitotoxic brain lesions. *Developmental Brain Research, 141,* 25–32.

Molina-Holgado, E., Vela, J. M., Arevalo-Martin, A., & Guaza, C. (2001). LPS/IFN-gamma cytotoxicity in oligodendroglial cells: Role of nitric oxide and protection by the anti-inflammatory cytokine IL-10. *European Journal of Neuroscience, 13,* 493–502.

Monier, A., Gressens, P., Evrard, P., & Verney, C. (2002). Immunocytochemical study of microglia in white matter injury of the human premature brain. *Pediatric Research, 51,* 448A.

Nelson, K. B., Dambrosia, J. M., Grether, J. K., & Phillips, T. M. (1998). Neonatal cytokines and coagulation factors in children with cerebral palsy. *Annals of Neurology, 44,* 665–675.

Nelson, K. B., & Ellenberg, J. H. (1996). Antecedents of cerebral palsy. Multivariate analysis of risk. *New England Journal of Medicine, 315,* 81–86.

Nelson, K. B., & Grether, J. K. (1998). Potentially asphyxiating conditions and spastic cerebral palsy in infants of normal birth weight. *American Journal of Obstetrics and Gynecology, 179,* 507–513.

Patkai, J., Mesplès, B., Dommergues, M. A., Fromont, G., Thornton, E. M., Renauld, J. C., Evrard, P., & Gressens, P. (2001). Deleterious effects of IL-9-activated mast cells and neuroprotection by antihistamine drugs. *Pediatric Research, 50,* 222–230.

Plaisant, F., Dommergues, M. A., Campbell, I. L., & Gressens, P. (2002). Effects of systemic and CNS pro-inflammatory cytokines on NMDA and AMPA receptors-mediated brain lesions in newborn mice. *Pediatric Research, 51,* 442A.

Redecker, C., Lutzenburg, M., Gressens, P., Evrard, P., Witte, O. W., & Hagemann, G. (1998). Patterns of excitability changes and glucose metabolism in experimentally induced cortical dysplasias. *Cerebral Cortex, 8,* 623–634.

Tahraoui, S. L., Marret, S., Bodénant, C., Leroux, P., Dommergues, M. A., Evrard, P., & Gressens P. (2001). Central role of microglia in neonatal excitotoxic lesions of the murine periventricular white matter. *Brain Pathology, 11,* 56–71.

Volpe, J. J. (2001). Neurobiology of periventricular leukomalacia in the premature infant. *Pediatric Research, 50,* 553–562.

Xu, H., Barks, J. D., Liu, Y. Q., & Silverstein, F. S. (2001). AMPA-induced suppression of oligodendroglial gene expression in neonatal rat brain. *Developmental Brain Research, 132,* 175–178.

Four-color illustrations from Chapter 6, Neuronal Migration and Dyslexia Susceptibility, Joseph J. LoTurco et al.

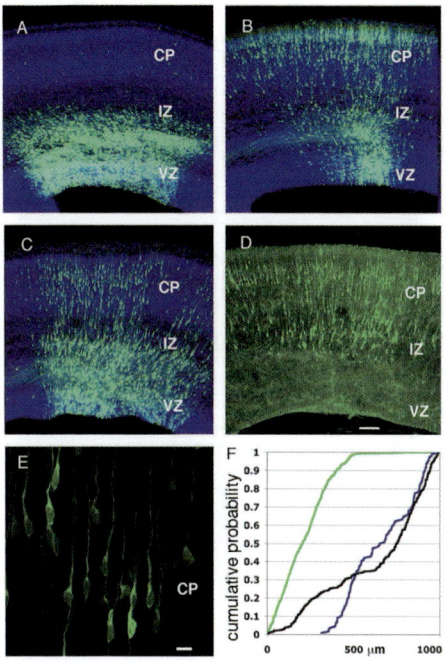

Figure 1: Dyx1c1 RNAi disrupts migration in developing neocortex. A) *In utero* electroporation of Dyx1c1 RNAi causes a block in normal migration to the cortical plate (CP). B) Normal migration of eGFP+ cells when transfected with a control RNAi (RNAi/TUB3) and eGFP. C) Rescue of many migrating neurons from the effects of Dyx1c1/RNAi by cotransfection with a Dyx1c1 expression plasmid. D) Complete rescue of neurons from Dyx1c1 RNAi when cotransfected with Dyx1c1-GFP expression plasmid. All fluorescent cells are cells expressing Dyx1c1 fusion and these migrate normally. E) Rescue of normal radial morphology by Dyx1c1-GFP. F) Cumulative probability migration plot comparing migration after transfection of Dyx1c1/RNAi (green), Dyx1c1/RNAi +Dyx1c1-GFP (rescue; blue), and eGFP control (black). For cumulative probability plots the distance of each labeled cell from the VZ surface was determined. The abscissa is the distance from the VZ surface in μm and the ordinate is the probability of cells occurring at that distance or less. (scale bar same for A-D, 100 μm, 15 μm for E).

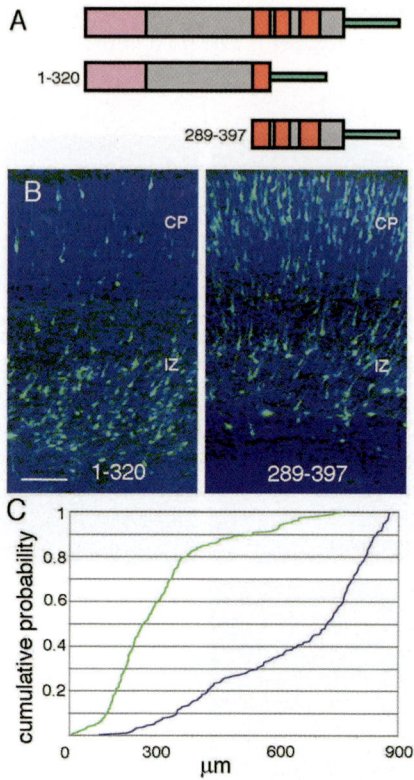

Figure 2: The C-terminus of Dyx1c1 is necessary and sufficient for rescuing migration arrest. A) Diagrams of the three Dyx1c1 constructs used in rescue experiments: full Dyx1c1 fused to GFP(top), a truncation containing code for aa 1-320 fused to GFP, and a C-terminus fragment containing code for aa 289-397 fused to GFP (green bar). Pink bar indicates location of p23 homology domains at the N-terminus and red bars indicate location of 3 TPR domains in Dyx1c1. B) The N-terminus missing the 2 terminal TPR domains fails to rescue (left) migration disruption by Dyx1c1/RNAi; however, the C-terminal alone containing the three TPR domains rescues the effects of Dyx1c1 RNAi (right). C) Cumulative probability plot of the position of cells in the two rescue conditions four days after transfection with Dyx1c1/RNAi and the corresponding Dyx1c1 fragment: green; aa 1-320 construct, and blue; rescue by the aa 289-397 fragment. (scale bar for B, 100 ?m)

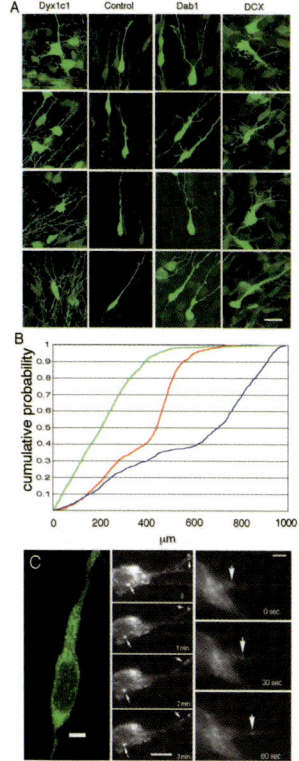

Figure 3: Dyx1c1 functions differently from that of the other migration control genes, Dab1 and DCX. A) Comparison of morphologies induced by RNAi of three different migration control genes: Dyx1c1, Dab1 and DCX. Different RNAi treatment causes development of distinct neuronal morphologies in the IZ. B) Comparison of migration disruption by Dyx1c1 RNAi and DCX RNAi. Cumulative migration distance plots indicate that Dyx1c1 RNAi causes an earlier migration arrest (green) than does DCX RNAi (red). Two components of migration arrest in DCX/RNAi (red) are shown by the bimodal shape of the plot. Migration of control transfected cells (blue) also shows multiple components perhaps reflecting the multiple phases of radial migration in neocortex (Noctor, Martinez-Cerdeno, Ivic, & Kriegstein, 2004). C) Dyx1c1 protein is compartmentalized to the cytoplasm and is dynamic throughout processes and surrounding the nucleus. Middle and right panel sequences (top to bottom) show live cell images of Dyx1c1-GFP in migrating neurons in the IZ. Arrows indicate Dyx1c1 particles: one traffics around the nucleus (middle) and another in the dendrite moves towards the soma (middle). In the right most sequence Dyx1c1 moves along a dendrite away from the soma.

Four-color illustration from Chapter 12, What a Difference a Day Makes: Linking Timing to Mechanisms in Epileptogenic Microgyri, Andrea Zsombok et al.

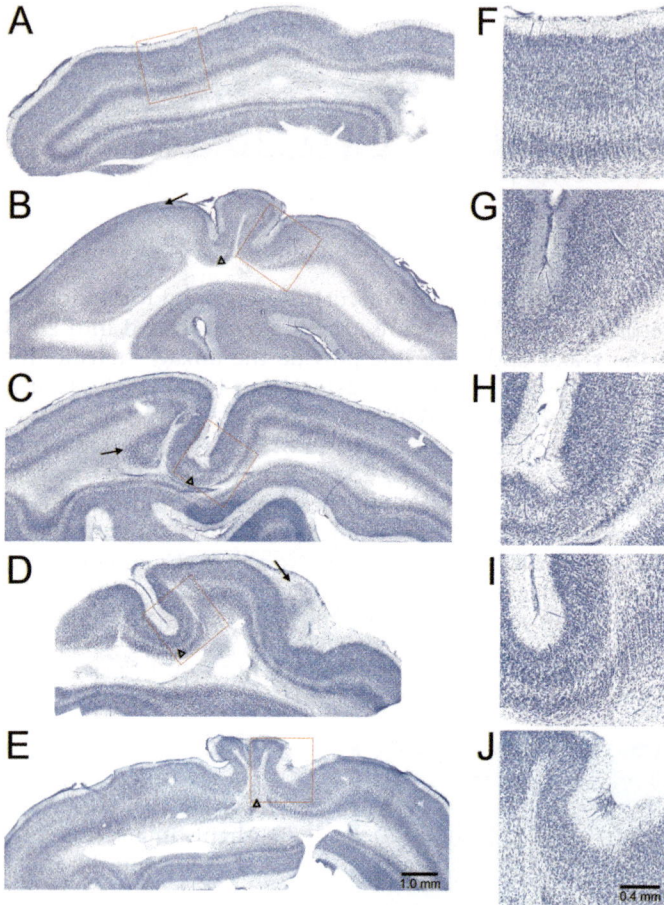

Figure 1. Nissl-stained coronal sections from control (A, F), and experimental ferrets given transcranial freeze-lesions at day 3 (B, C, G, H) or day 6 (D, E, I, J). Box outline in pictures of left column indicates region of high-power picture shown in right column. In P3 lesions, section from a slice in which epileptiform activity was not found (B, G) shows similar laminar abnormality to slice in which epileptiform activity was evoked (C, H). Abnormal lamination, including a microgyral cell-sparse layer (open arrowheads) is present in both P3 and P6 lesions. Ectopic and heterotopic collections of cells were also commonly seen adjacent to the microgyrus (filled arrows).

Four-color illustration from Chapter 13, Structural and Functional Deficits in a Rat Model of Cortical Heterotopia, Kevin S. Lee et al.

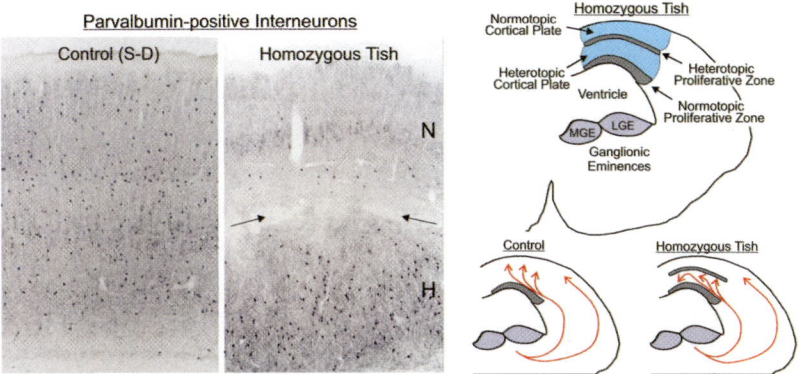

Figure 3. Interneuron distribution is disturbed in the homozygous tish neocortex. The two photomicrographs shown on the left side of the figure are coronal sections stained immunohistochemically for parvalbumin. The control (Sprague-Dawley: S-D) brain shows parvalbumin-positive interneurons distributed throughout the neocortex. In contrast, parvalbumin-positive interneurons are more concentrated in the heterotopic cortex (H) than in the normotopic cortex (N) of the homozygous tish cortex. The right side of the figure shows schematized drawings of the developing neocortex. The upper drawing illustrates the two proliferative zones and two cortical plates in the developing tish neocortex. Two sites of interneuron proliferation, the medial ganglionic eminence (MGE) and lateral ganglionic eminence (LGE), are depicted. In the lower left drawing, routes of tangential interneuron migration are depicted for normal brain. In the lower right drawing, a hypothetical route of disturbed migration is illustrated for the homozygous tish brain. In this model, some migrating interneurons fail to migrate past the heterotopic proliferative zone in the neocortex.

Four-color illustrations from Chapter 15, MRI-based Morphometry in Human Developmental Disorders: Looking Back in Time, David N. Kennedy.

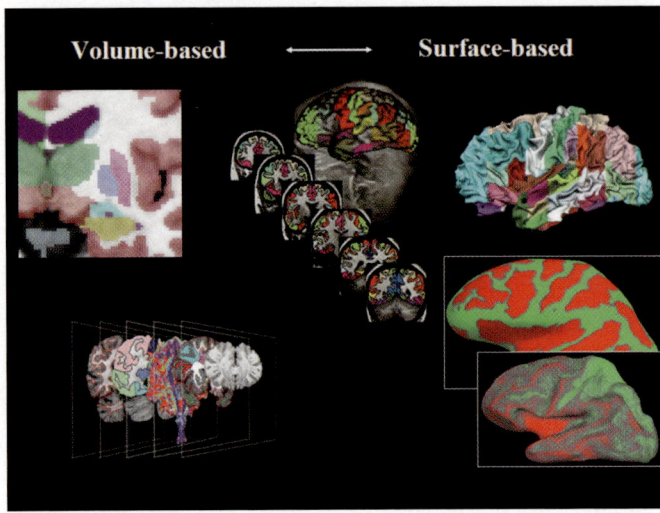

Figure 2. Examples of volume and surface classes of morphometric measures.

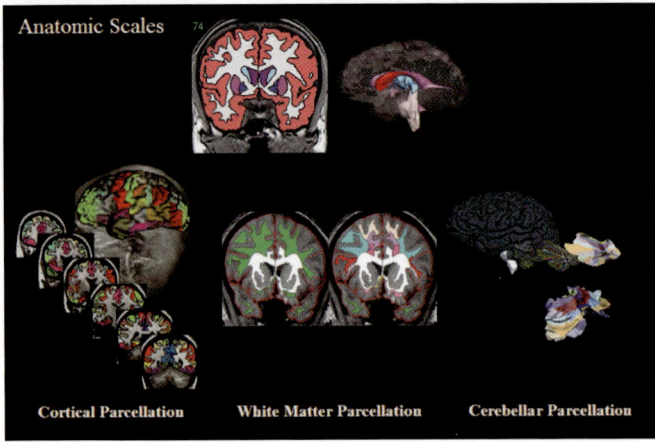

Figure 3. Example scales of neuromorphometric analysis ranging from "general" segmentation of cerebral structures (top) to "parcellation" of cerebral cortex, cerebral white matter, and cerebellum cortex (bottom row).

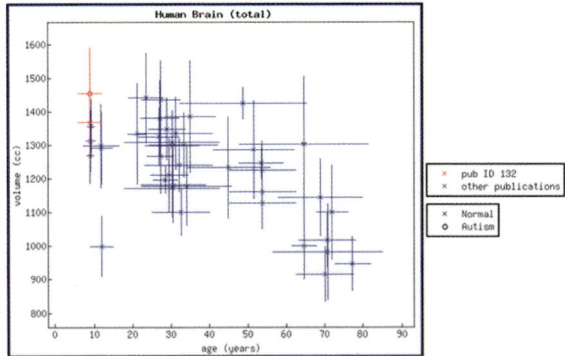

Figure 4. An example report of large total brain volume in autism. Pub ID 132 is (Herbert et al., 2003).

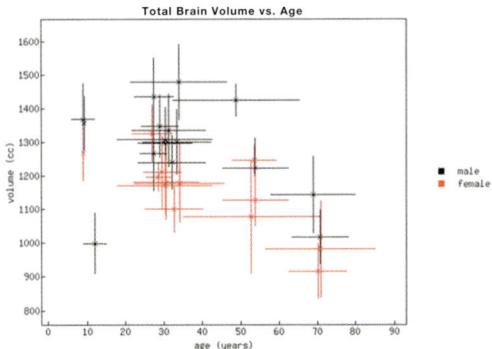

Figure 5. IBVD display of volumetric literature of gender (males in black, females in red) differences in total brain volume.

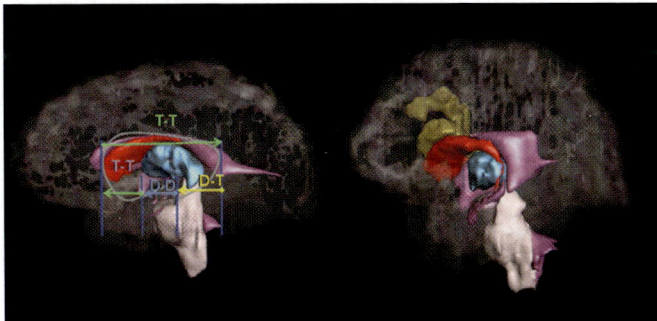

Figure 6. (Left) Normal midline topology showing axis of developmental trajectory. (Right) Altered midline topology in subject with HPE.

Four-color illustrations from Chapter 16, Cortical Plasticity: The Effects of Sensory Deprivation, Hugo Théoret et al.

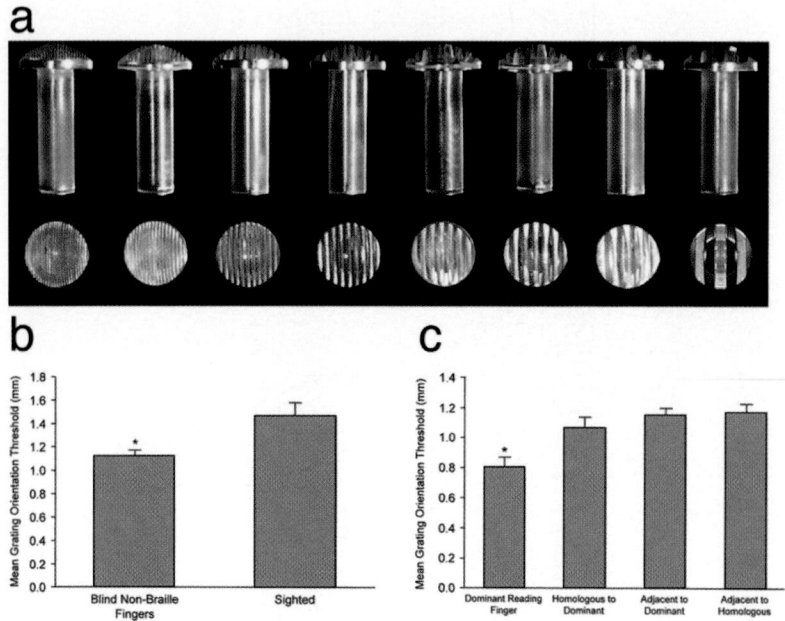

Figure 1. Increased tactile spatial resolution in the blind. (a) Johnson-Van Boven-Phillips domes that were used to assess tactile spatial resolution. (b) The threshold for grating orientation is significantly lower in blind subjects compared to sighted controls. (c) In blind subjects, the sensory threshold in the Braille reading finger is lower than that of other fingers. (Adapted from Van Boven et al., 2000).

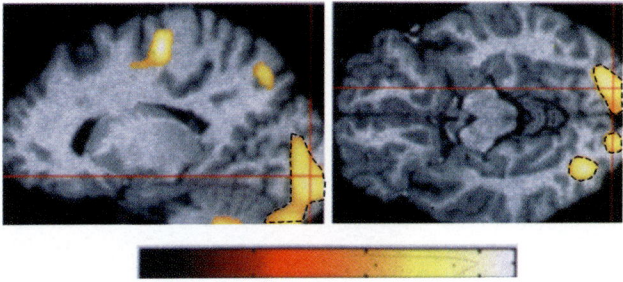

Figure 3. PET activation sites in reponse to tactile stimulation. Evidence for visual involvement in tactile discrimination is apparent (dashed circles). (Adapted from Sadato et al., 1996).

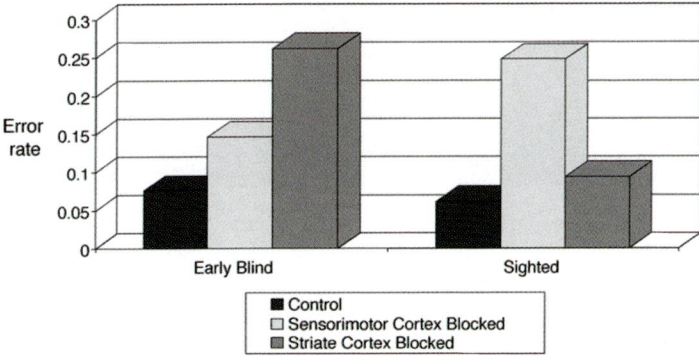

Figure 4. Functional relevance of occipital recruitment. In early blind subjects, rTMS over the occipital pole results in increased errors in a tactile discrimination task. Occipital stimulation in sighted subjects does not increase the error rate. (Adapted from Cohen et al., 1997).

Four-color illustration from Chapter 17, Dyslexia: Advances in Cross-level Research, Albert M. Galaburda.

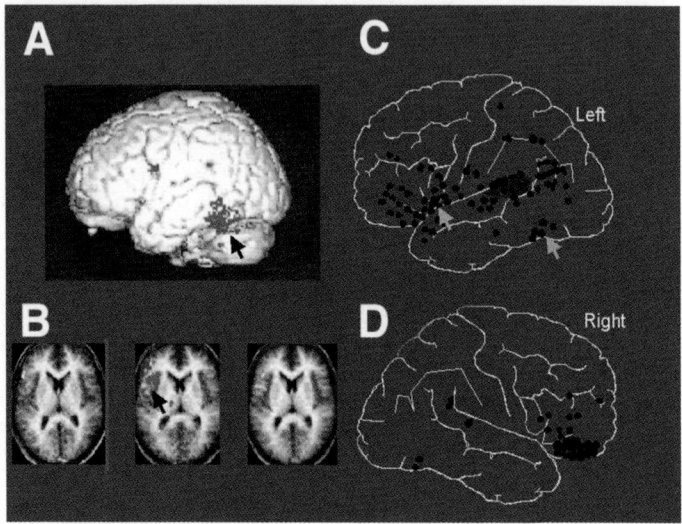

Figure 1: Examples of anomalous activation (arrows) of the letter string/word form area (Brunswick, McCrory, Price, Frith, & Frith, 1999) and left perisylvian cortex (Georgiewa et al., 2002) (A and B, respectively) in dyslexics. A composite map of the location of ectopias over eight brains studied is shown in C and D. The distribution of the anomalies is comparable to that of the activation studies; note arrow.

Chapter • 12

What a Difference a Day Makes: Linking Timing to Mechanisms in Epileptogenic Microgyri

A. Zsombok and K.M. Jacobs

Dyslexia and seizures are just part of the neurological sequelae that result from early damage to the developing cortical plate. To understand mechanisms underlying such neurological deficits associated with cortical malformations, the timing of both the precipitating incident and onset of symptoms are critical issues. The structure of the cortical malformation varies in form and severity with the timing and type of the insult (Ruddick & Khera, 1975; Ferrer, 1993; Cohen & Roessmann, 1994). In addition, there is often a delay between the insult and seizure onset (Raymond et al., 1995; Bartolomei et al., 1999). Although epilepsy is commonly associated with developmental cortical malformations, not every malformation results in seizures, suggesting that in some cases, an additional abnormality or reinforcing activation is necessary to induce epileptogenesis. The rat freeze lesion model of microgyria mimics these clinical characteristics, including association with hyperexcitability in most but not all cases, a structural pathology that varies with insult timing and delayed onset of epileptiform activity (Luhmann & Raabe, 1996; Jacobs, Gutnick, & Prince, 1996; Jacobs, Hwang, & Prince 1999). In this model, a transcranial freeze lesion

---

We greatly appreciate the skills of Jennifer Cooke in slice preparation, histological processing, and animal care. These studies were supported by NIH grant NINDS 1 R21 NS045901-01.

given within the first 48 hours of birth produces a focal abnormal four-layered cortical region that is histopathologically similar to human four-layered polymicrogyria. Lesions given on postnatal day (P) 6 in the rat do not produce microgyria (Dvorak & Feit, 1977). After P0 or P1 lesions, the onset of hyperexcitability is dramatically sudden. It is entirely absent when brain slices are examined from animals aged P9–10, but present in nearly every slice from nearly every animal by P12 (Jacobs, Hwang, & Prince, 1999).

A difference of a single day in lesion timing affects the incidence of epileptiform activity evoked in rats older than P40. When the lesion is made on P0, the cortex shows a severe reduction in epileptiform incidence when examined at P40 relative to younger survival ages, suggesting that there is a "recovery." This does not occur in cortex if the initial lesion is made one day later (Jacobs, Hwang, & Prince, 1999). The microgyrus is produced by lesion of the neurons present in the cortical plate at the time of the lesion. In the rat, migration of neurons into the cortical plate continues until ~P4 (Bayer & Altman, 1991). We have suggested that the greater epileptogenicity of P1 versus P0 lesioned cortex at long survival times may be due to elimination of a particular subgroup of cells or to simply a lesion of a greater number of cells. The neurons that will make up layer IV are migrating into the cortical plate on P0, with most present in the plate by P1. This layer is particularly important in controlling the ultimate pattern of synaptic connection between thalamic afferents and neocortical neurons. Thalamocortical afferent patterns of projection are altered in and around rat microgyri (Jacobs, Kharazia, & Prince, 1999; Rosen, Burstein, & Galaburda, 2000). Our previous work has suggested that hyperinnervation by excitatory afferents occurs in the region adjacent to the malformation (Jacobs, Kharazia, & Prince, 1999). We hypothesize that later lesions that eliminate a greater portion of layer IV will result in more extensive redirection of thalamocortical afferents away from the malformed region toward the surrounding paramicrogyral zone where layer IV neurons are available as synaptic targets. To explore this issue and determine its effect on epileptogenicity, we have created a model of microgyria in the more altricial ferret. Neurons destined for layer IV enter the cortical plate after birth in the ferret (Jackson, Peduzzi, & Hickey, 1989). Thus, lesions that do not eliminate layer IV neurons may be created within a few days of birth and compared to later lesions. Here, we have compared the effects of P3 and P6 lesions in the ferret.

We have also examined the effect of lesion timing on postsynaptic currents in the rat microgyrus model. The neuronal mechanisms underlying recovery from hyperexcitability are not well understood. The rat microgyrus model provides an excellent opportunity to characterize these mechanisms with the clear separation between epileptiform incidence in P0 versus P1 lesioned cortex. We have previously demonstrated that just after hyperexcitability onset, postsynaptic currents are altered within layer V neurons of the paramicrogyral zone relative to those recorded in control cortex (Jacobs, Kharazia, & Prince, 1999). The increases in the frequency of excitatory postsynaptic currents (EPSCs) in PMG cells would obviously be likely to increase overall cortical excitability adjacent to the malformation. However, our results suggested that hyperinnervation of inhibitory interneurons also occurred in the paramicrogyral zone, indicating that compensatory mechanisms may occur simultaneously with cellular changes that promote epileptogenicity. Our current results suggest that the hyperinnervation of inhibitory interneurons occurs only in cortex from P0 lesioned rats, suggesting that these compensatory mechanisms may contribute to recovery.

A standard practice in investigation of epilepsy models is to identify cellular and circuit abnormalities that occur after hyperexcitability onset. This is a helpful first step. Previous studies, however, have suggested that seizures themselves may alter neurological function (Sutula, 2002; Dudek, Hellier, Williams, Ferraro, & Staley, 2002). In addition, animal models exploring cellular mechanisms of hyperexcitability suggest that there is a progression of modifications in receptor components and function (Gibbs, Shumate, & Coulter, 1997; Coulter, 2001). Also, it is well known that the expression of neurochemicals and neurotransmitter receptors varies with the level of activity in the cortex (Huntsman, Isackson, & Jones, 1994; Micheva & Beaulieu, 1997). For these reasons, it is necessary to distinguish cellular changes that are caused by hyperexcitability from those that precede it and may, therefore, play a role in initiation of epileptogenesis. Here, we have examined postsynaptic currents in layer V neurons of the paramicrogyral zone and homologous control cortex during the five days prior to epileptogenic onset. Together, these aspects of lesion timing and survival timing help to identify the causes of neurological dysfunction resulting from malformed cortex.

METHODS

Our goal was to characterize the electrophysiological changes occurring after damage to the developing cortical plate. Malformations were induced in rats and ferrets by transcranial freeze lesion at different stages of cortical development. After variable survival times, we examined the electrophysiological properties of these brains using field potentials and whole cell patch clamp techniques to identify the excitability of populations of neurons and synaptic connections between neurons, respectively.

All experimental procedures were performed under protocols approved by the Virginia Commonwealth University Administrative Panel on Laboratory Animal Care. Transcranial freeze lesions were made under hypothermia anesthesia, as previously described (Jacobs et al., 1996). The freeze probe consisted of a copper bar with a rectangular tip (2 X 5 mm), cooled to −50 to −70°C, and placed with the long axis in an anterior-posterior direction for 5–10 sec. In ferrets three or six days after birth, the probe was placed over Occipital cortex (2–4 mm lateral, with the caudal edge at Lambda). In P0 or P1 rats, the probe was placed over the whisker and face somatosensory representation (centered over 2.5 mm caudal to Bregma, 3.0 mm lateral to the midline) within Parietal cortex. Coronal cortical slices (300–400 μm thick) were prepared using standard procedures. Animals were anesthetized with pentobarbital (55 mg/kg, i.p.), decapitated, and brains removed and placed in a high sucrose slicing solution. Slices were placed in a normal artificial cerebrospinal fluid (aCSF) containing the following (in mM): 126 NaCl; 3.0 KCl; 2.0 $MgCl_2$; 2.0 $CaCl_2$; 1.25 NaH_2PO_4; 10 glucose; and 26 $NaHCO_3$, pH 7.4 when saturated with 95% O_2, 5% CO_2, and warmed to 34°C for 30 minutes and room temperature thereafter.

Glass micropipettes (3–6 MΩ) filled with 1 M NaCl were used to record field potentials (DC, low pass filtered at 1 KHz) from layer II/III of ferret occipital cortex. Recordings were digitized on-line (10 KHz) using Axon Instruments Software. A concentric bipolar electrode (FHC) was placed within deep layers directly beneath the recording site to deliver electrical stimuli. To search for epileptiform activity, single 20 μs square current pulses were applied at a rate ≤ 0.2 Hz with increasing current intensities, beginning with 5 μA. The threshold level of current for short latency events was considered to be the current that evoked a 0.2 mV peak negative field potential. A series of stimulus intensities was then applied (0.1 Hz) at threshold current by increasing the duration of the pulse (20, 40, 80, 160, 320 μsec).

Whole cell patch clamp recordings were made from layer V pyramidal neurons identified with infrared differential interference contrast microscopy, with some subsequently verified with biocytin labeling. The intracellular patch solution consisted of (in mM): 117 CsGluconate; 11 CsCl; 10 Hepes; 11 EGTA; 1 $MgCl_2$;

1 CaCl$_2$; 4 Na-ATP; 0.2 Na-GTP; and 0.5 QX-314, pH adjusted to 7.3 with CsOH and osmolarity to 280–290 mOsmol. EPSCs were recorded at a holding potential of -60 mV, and IPSCs were recorded at a holding potential of 0 or +10 mV (E$_{Cl-}$ = -51 mV) with either an AxoClamp 2B or a Multiclamp 700B amplifier (Axon Instruments). Only recordings with an access resistance less than 20 MΩ that varied <20% were accepted for analysis. Data were digitized online (2–20 KHz) using software from Axon Instruments. For experiments involving blockade of ionotropic glutamate receptors, 20 μM 6,7-Dinitroquinoxaline-2,3(1H,4H)-dione (DNQX) and 50 μM DL-2-Amino-5-phosphonopentanoic acid (APV) were included in the normal aCSF. Miniature synaptic currents were recorded in aCSF containing 1 μM Tetrodotoxin (TTX).

Following electrophysiological recordings, slices were immediately fixed in 4% paraformaldehyde in 0.1 M phosphate buffer, pH 7.4, and maintained at 4°C until resectioning. Slices were cryoprotected by immersion in 30% sucrose in phosphate-buffered saline until they sank and resectioned on a freezing microtome at 60 mm. Ferret sections were stained with cresyl violet in order to relate the histology of the malformation to the electrophysiological results. Rat sections were processed for biocytin using standard procedures.

RESULTS

Ferret Model of Microgyria

Transcranial freeze lesions created within three to six days of birth in ferret kits altered the gross structure of the cortex, such that at least one additional fold (microsulcus) was created (see Figure 1 in the four-color section on page 222-F). These abnormalities were similar to, although more extensive than, those created with freeze lesions made within 48 hours of birth in rats. In ferrets, the abnormally folded region extended from 2 to 4 mm medially-laterally. Laminar abnormalities present in lesioned ferret cortex were also similar to the histopathology of previously described rat microgyri. Cresyl-violet staining showed that the area underneath and surrounding the microsulcus contained: (1) a layer similar to, and contiguous with, layer I; (2) a cell-dense layer, contiguous with the adjacent layer II/III; (3) a thin, cell-sparse layer (arrowheads in Figure 1B-D); and (4) a final cell-dense layer above the white matter. In some cases, a vertical column of cell-sparse tissue separated the microgyrus from adjacent cortex. Heterotopia occurred adjacent to the microgyrus in both P3 and P6 lesions (see arrows, Figure 1B, 1C, and 1D).

Field potentials recorded from control ferret cortex were more complex than those recorded from rat cortex (Figure 2A), typically containing a short latency negativity followed by a second smaller amplitude, long lasting negativity. All cortex from lesioned animals also contained both of these short latency events that were graded with stimulus intensity (see Figure 2). The amplitude of the second negativity appeared larger in P3-lesioned animals than in controls. We expected that transcranial freeze lesions performed on day 3 in the ferret would produce similar results to lesions made on day 0 in rats. On P0 in rats, and P3 in ferrets, layer V and VI neurons are present in the cortical plate, while layer IV is incomplete. Because of our previous results in rats (Jacobs, Gutnick, & Prince, 1996; Jacobs, Hwang, & Prince, 1999), we expected that field potential recordings made from ferrets with P3 freeze lesions would show long latency, variable form, all-or-none events that are typical of interictal-like epileptiform activity.

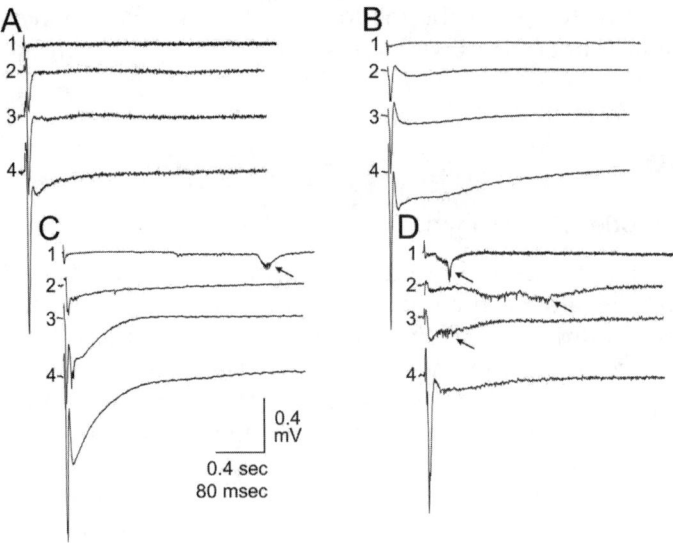

Figure 2. Examples of evoked field potentials recorded from control (A) and experimental ferrets given transcranial freeze lesions at day 3 (B, C) or day 6 (D). Responses to increasing levels of stimulus intensity shown in 1-4 of A-D. Note traces shown in 1 at shorter timebase (0.4 sec), to include longer latency events. Arrows indicate epileptiform activity. Spontaneous epileptiform activity was observed only after P6 lesions (not shown).

However, in only 8 of 24 slices was this type of activity observed (Figure 2C1 and Figure 3). For neuroblasts generated on E36, which will ultimately be found within layer IV, migration into the cortical plate begins by P1 and continues beyond P8 in ferret visual cortex (Jackson, Peduzzi, & Hickey, 1989). We expected that P6 lesions would eliminate a larger proportion of layer IV neurons compared to P3 lesions. In cortical slices from P6-lesioned ferrets, every slice tested (n = 12) showed epileptiform activity (c.f., Figure 2D1 and Figure 3). A z-test showed that this proportion of epileptiform slices was significantly larger than that for slices from P3-lesioned ferrets (Figure 3, $p < 0.001$). Spontaneous interictal-like epileptiform activity was also observed in slices from P6 lesioned ferrets, but not in those from P3 lesions. The evoked epileptiform activity was eliminated with high intensity stimulation (Figure 2D4). Increases in the rate of stimulation from 0.1 to 0.3 Hz also eliminated the epileptiform activity (not shown).

Effect of Lesion Age on Postsynaptic Currents Recorded after Epileptiform Onset in Microgyral Rats

We examined whether our previous results showing an increase in peak conductance of sIPSCs in layer V pyramidal neurons of P13–16 rat PMG were related to the timing of the lesion. In cells recorded from rats lesioned on the day of birth (P0), the sIPSC

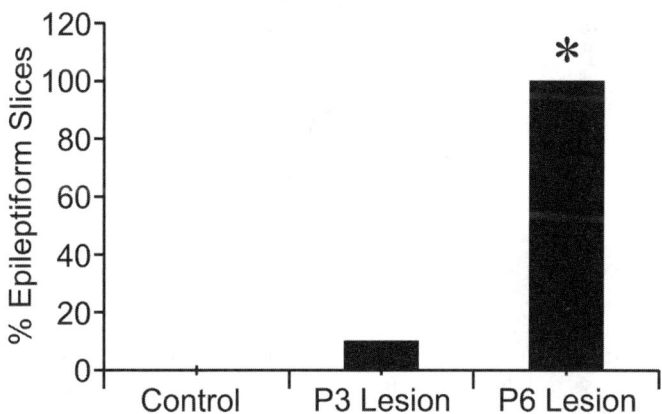

Figure 3. Percent of slices showing epileptiform activity for controls, and ferrets given freeze lesions at P3 and P6. Number of slices tested = 28, 24, and 12, respectively. * = significant difference, z-test, $p < 0.001$. At least four sites within each slice were tested.

peak conductance was significantly larger than that in control cells, and PMG cells from animals lesioned on P1 (Figure 4A, 1-way ANOVA, $p < 0.05$). This difference in peak conductance was no longer present after the application of APV and DNQX in the bathing medium (0.28 ± 0.12, 0.31 ± 0.09, and 0.30 ± 0.07 nS for 15 control, 16 P0 lesion and 13 P1 lesion cells, respectively). In addition, there was no difference after application of TTX in mIPSCs

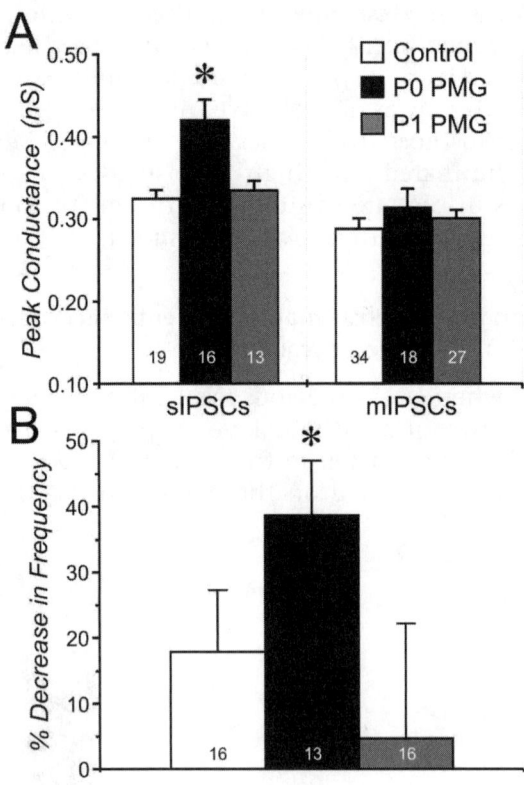

Figure 4. Effect of lesion timing on IPSCs recorded in slices from animals aged 13 to 16 days. A. Mean peak conductance for inhibitory events recorded in layer V pyramidal neurons of the paramicrogyral zone in slices from rats lesioned on P0, P1, or in homotopic control cortex. B. Percent decrease in IPSC frequency after the application of glutamate antagonists to the bathing medium. Larger decrease in cells from P0 lesioned animals shows that a larger portion of these IPSCs are dependent on the activity of excitatory afferents to inhibitory neurons. A greater number of large events may account for the peak conductance differences seen in A. Digits within bars indicate the number of cells for each group. * = significant difference, t-tests, $p < 0.05$.

conductance (Figure 4A). There was also no significant difference in sIPSC rise time or frequency (1.3 ± 0.04, 1.3 ± 0.05, 1.3 ± 0.05 msec, and 4.3 ± 0.4, 4.7 ± 0.7, and 4.8 ± 0.6 Hz for 72 control, 42 P0 lesion, and 38 P1 lesion cells, respectively). In order to test the idea that the increase in peak conductance was due to an increase in excitatory afferents onto inhibitory neurons, we evaluated the percent decrease in IPSC frequency within individual neurons after application of APV and DNQX. The percent decrease in IPSC frequency was significantly greater for cells from P0 lesioned cortex than for controls or P1 lesioned cortex (Figure 4B).

We have also previously described two types of IPSC responses to nearby extracellular electrical stimulation. In one group of PMG layer V pyramidal neurons, stimulation produced long latency all or none multiphasic events having characteristics similar to the field potential epileptiform activity (PMG_E cells). The second group of PMG neurons had only short latency events that decayed smoothly (PMG_S cells) similar to control cells. There was no significant difference in the proportion of PMG_E cells for P0 versus P1 lesions (57%, $n = 60$ versus 63%, $n = 67$, respectively, z-test, NS). A two-way ANOVA on response type (PMG_E, PMG_S) versus lesion date for sIPSC conductance in PMG neurons showed that there was a significant effect of lesion date ($p < 0.01$), but no significant interaction between response type and lesion date, and no significant effect of response type (Table I). We have also previously demonstrated an increase in the frequency of sEPSCs and mEPSCs in PMG cells relative to controls. A two-way ANOVA on sEPSC frequency in PMG neurons showed no significant effects of

Table I. Measures of synaptic currents recorded in layer V pyramidal neurons adjacent to the microgyrus and in homotopic control cortex from animals aged P13–16. PMG_E cells responded to nearby stimulation with long latency all-or-none multiphasic activity in addition to the short latency response that was graded with stimulus intensity. PMG_S cells responded with only the short latency, smoothly decaying IPSC.

	PMG_E	PMG_S	ALL PMG	Control
sIPSC Conductance (nS) mean ±stderr (n)				
P0 lesions	0.44 ± 0.04 (24)	0.40 ± 0.04 (15)	0.43 ± 0.03 (39)	0.32 ± 0.03
P1 lesions	0.34 ± 0.02 (21)	0.32 ± 0.02 (13)	0.33 ± 0.01 (34)	(18)
sEPSC Frequency (Hz)				
P0 lesions	6.4 ± 0.3 (2)	5.3 ± 2.5 (3)	5.2 ± 1.2 (6)	6.0 ± 1.1
P1 lesions	8.1 ± 1.2 (10)	6.5 ± 1.2 (6)	7.7 ± 0.9 (17)	(29)
mEPSC Frequency (Hz)				
P0 lesions	3.3 ± 0.8 (2)	5.1 ± 0.4 (3)	4.4 ± 0.6 (5)	3.1 ± 0.4
P1 lesions	3.5 ± 0.4 (11)	6.4 ± 1.1 (7)	4.6 ± 0.6 (18)	(16)

response type or lesion date, and no interaction (Table I). For mEPSCs in PMG neurons, there was a significant effect of response type ($p < 0.05$), but not of lesion day or the interaction.

POSTSYNAPTIC CURRENTS PRIOR TO EPILEPTIFORM ONSET IN MICROGYRAL RATS

Hyperexcitability onset occurs at P12 (Jacobs, Hwang, and Prince, 1999). Here, we recorded postsynaptic currents from layer V pyramidal neurons in slices from rats aged 7 to 11 days. For this data, lesions were made only at P1. Mean frequency of sEPSCs was significantly higher in cells of PMG cortex relative to control cells (Figure 5A). Frequency of sEPSCs varied from 0.3 to 5.7 Hz in control cells and from 0.1 to 15.3 Hz in PMG cells. Event bursts (two or more overlapping events) were more frequent in PMG than in control cells (5.7 ± 1.3 versus 21.1 ± 6.1 bursts/min for 38 control and 40 PMG cells, respectively, t-test, $p < 0.02$). In control cells, sEPSC frequency did not vary with age from P7 to P11 (Figure 5B, one-way ANOVA, NS). In contrast, within PMG cells, sEPSC frequency increased significantly with age from a mean of 0.8 ± 0.2 at P7 to 5.2 ± 1.3 Hz at P11 (Figure 5B). There was no significant difference between control and PMG cells in mean amplitude, area, rise time, or decay time for sEPSCs (Table II).

Miniature EPSCS (mEPSCs) were recorded after application of TTX. Findings for mEPSCs were similar to those for sEPSCs, with a higher frequency and greater burst frequency in PMG cells relative to controls (Figure 5A, 2.3 ± 0.8 and 19.2 ± 10.0 burst/min for 26 control and 16 PMG cells, respectively). There was no significant difference between control and PMG neurons in mean amplitude, area, rise time, or decay time for mEPSCs (Table II). There was a nonsignificant trend toward an increasing mEPSC frequency with age in PMG cells (Figure 5C).

Table II. Measures of excitatory synaptic currents recorded in layer V pyramidal neurons in slices from animals aged P7–11. For PMG neurons, freeze lesions were made at P1. For sEPSCs, measures from 38 control and 40 PMG neurons. For mEPSCs, measures from 26 control and 16 PMG cells. Values reported as mean ±stderr. No significant differences were found between control and PMG neurons on these measures.

	sEPSCs		mEPSCs	
	Control	PMG	Control	PMG
Amplitude (pA)	23.7 ± 1.5	20.5 ± 0.9	17.1 ± 1.0	16.9 ± 1.0
Area (pA)	185.1 ± 22.7	139.5 ± 7.4	109.3 ± 6.4	116.0 ± 10.8
Rise Time (msec)	1.5 ± 0.1	1.6 ± 0.1	1.6 ± 0.1	1.7 ± 0.2
Decay Time (msec)	11.2 ± 0.5	10.4 ± 0.4	9.9 ± 0.5	10.1 ± 0.7

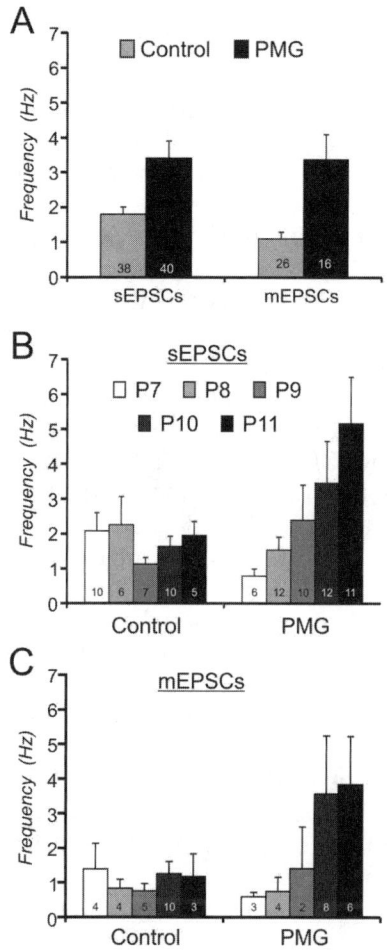

Figure 5. Frequency of excitatory synaptic currents in layer V pyramidal neurons from animals aged 7 to 11 days (prior to epileptogenic onset). PMG cells recorded from rats given freeze lesions on P1. Mean frequency calculated for >50 events per cell. A. Events shown are those recorded under normal bathing medium (sIPSCs) and after addition of TTX (mIPSCs). B. Mean sEPSC frequency for cells recorded at various postnatal ages. A 1-way ANOVA shows a significant difference in the mean frequency among different survival ages for PMG neurons ($p < 0.05$). There is no significant difference among cells recorded at different survival ages within the control group. C. Mean mEPSC frequency for cells recorded at different survival ages. For mEPSCs, there is a similar, but nonsignificant trend of increasing frequency with age within the PMG group and no difference with age among the control group. Digits within bars indicate the number of cells for each group. * = significant difference, t-tests, $p < 0.05$.

DISCUSSION

These results provide evidence that the excitability of cortex as well as the underlying abnormalities in synaptic connectivity vary when the same injury occurs at different developmental ages.

The difference in epileptiform incidence from 33% to 100% in slices from P3 versus P6 freeze-lesioned ferrets is dramatic and will allow for more direct study of the mechanisms underlying epileptogenesis associated with microgyria. Using this ferret model, we may be able to differentiate between cellular alterations that induce epileptogenesis and benign changes more directly due to the lesion. We have previously suggested that there are at least two major contributors to the cortical hyperexcitability of the paramicrogyral zone: (1) hyperinnervation of the PMG by thalamocortical and other afferents; and (2) alterations in postsynaptic receptor subunit composition. The idea of hyperinnervation has been supported by both anatomical and physiological findings from the rat model (Prince & Jacobs, 1998; Jacobs, Kharazia, & Prince, 1999; Rosen, Burstein, & Galaburda, 2000). This newly demonstrated ferret model will allow us to determine whether the degree of thalamocortical afferent rearrangement correlates with incidence of epileptiform activity. Despite the difference in epileptogenicity, the laminar structure of the malformation at P3 versus P6 was relatively similar. This model has further confirmed the idea that the structure of the malformation cannot predict the presence of epileptiform activity (Jacobs, Hwang, and Prince, 1999). This would suggest that simple cell rearrangement is not enough to induce hyperexcitability. The fact that the reeler mutant, with an "upside down" cortex (Caviness, 1976) is also not hyperexcitable further confirms this idea (Ross, 2002). Another model of aberrant cell positioning is the use of teratogenic agents such as methylazoxymethanol acetate (MAM) given to rats at selective stages of pregnancy (Spatz, Dougherty, & Smith, 1967; Chevassus-Au-Louis, Baraban, Gaïarsa, & Ben-Ari, 1999). This produces heterotopic islands of cells subventricularly, within the hippocampus as well as within neocortex. Layer I and white matter ectopias are also common. Despite malpositioned neurons, affected cortex is not hyperexcitable under normal in vitro conditions (Baraban & Schwartzkroin, 1995).

Focal removal of deep layers has significantly different consequences than continuous absence of a single layer. In the MAM model, when layer IV is eliminated throughout neocortex, thalamocortical afferents will synapse on neurons of an inappropriate layer (Jones, Valentino, & Fleshman, 1981), and produce relatively normal receptive fields within somatosensory cortex (Noctor,

Palmer, McLaughlin, & Juliano, 2001). In contrast, the focal freeze lesion dramatically disrupts the structural organization of layer IV neurons (Jacobs, Morgensen, Warren, & Prince, 1999; Rosen, Windzio, & Galaburda, 2001). Hyperexcitable zones associated with microgyria may specifically require the juxtaposition of malformed cortex to a region that contains all six layers. It is also possible that neurons that are damaged but not removed contribute to abnormal activity in the paramicrogyral cortex. Morphological abnormalities that included a simplified dendritic branching pattern have been reported for neurons located adjacent to the malformation (Giannetti, Gaglini, Di Rocco, Di Rocco, & Granato, 2000; Di Rocco, Giannetti, Gaglini, Di Rocco, & Granato, 2001).

Cellular Mechanisms that Vary with Age of Insult

Lesions at either P0 or P1 in rat both result in sudden onset of field epileptiform activity at P12 (Jacobs, Morgensen, Warren, & Prince, 1999), and both produce an increased frequency of sEPSCs and mEPSCs in layer V pyramidal neurons of the PMG. Effects on IPSCs as well as on ultimate recovery from epileptiform activity differ for P0 versus P1 lesions of rat cortex. The increased amplitude of sIPSCs, combined with the greater decrease in frequency after application of glutamate antagonists, suggests that inhibitory interneurons are hyperinnervated specifically in P0 lesioned rats. These changes in inhibitory currents were found at young ages (P13–16), so it is unclear why this might have a delayed effect of promoting reduction in epileptiform activity only after 40 days of age. GABAergic inhibitory receptors are immature at the ages used for recording IPSCs, thus maturation may have strengthened their effectiveness and made the hyperinnervation of inhibitory interneurons more evident.

The fact that the mEPSC frequency is not different for neurons of P0 versus P1 lesions suggests that there is not a simple correlation between hyperinnervation of pyramidal and inhibitory interneurons. This is not surprising in light of a previous study that suggests development of inhibitory synaptic transmission is mediated by mechanisms different from those controlling maturation of excitatory synaptic connections (Groc, Gustafsson, & Hanse, 2003). It is possible that the hyperinnervation of inhibitory neurons is a compensatory action that is due to previously occurring hyperexcitability; however, it is then hard to explain why a similar compensation would not occur in P1 lesioned cortex. A recent finding suggests that during normal development, inhibitory neurons accumulate within layer I at P0 before migrating vertically and tangentially to deeper layers (Hevner, Daza, Englund, Kohtz, & Fink, 2004). It is possible that a P0 lesion kills a greater number of inhibitory neurons than does the P1 lesion due to this accumulation. Afferents that exclusively select inhibitory neurons as targets then would have to find appropriate synapse space on interneurons in the adjacent cortex.

Cellular Mechanisms Prior to Hyperexcitability Onset

Synaptic connectivity between afferents and cortical neurons is well underway by P7. Our results showing that in control cortex mEPSC frequency does not change from P7 to P11, suggests that release probabilities of excitatory afferents and the numbers of these synapses on layer V pyramidal neurons are relatively stable by P7. This suggests that the increase in mEPSC frequency that occurs within PMG neurons might not be a result of normal developmental processes where afferents simply fill available (appropriate) target space. It is possible that this hyperinnervation is an active anomalous process that increases with age. Another possibility is that there is a delay of normal maturation processes that control excitatory synaptic development. Findings that the microgyral area remains immature include the survival of radial glial (Rosen, Sherman, & Galaburda, 1994), and Cajal-Retzius cells (Super, Perez, & Soriano, 1997; Kharazia, Jacobs, Hwang, Parada, & Prince, 2000; Eriksson et al., 2001) in mature cortex and maintenance of normally transient synaptic connections (Innocenti & Berbel, 1991). Growth factors or other soluble compounds may diffuse from the region of the microgyrus to affect synaptic connections in the adjacent region.

The increase in EPSC bursts may be an additional factor that results in onset of epileptiform activity, since "buildup" of excitatory activity appears to occur prior to seizure onset (Cisse, Crochet, Timofeev, & Steriade, 2004). A change in release probability may contribute to the greater frequency of EPSC bursts in PMG cells. If true, this would be expected to cause a greater synchronization of connected pyramidal neurons.

Dyslexia and Epilepsy

Many studies have demonstrated a comorbidity between poor academic performance and epilepsy (Pazzaglia & Frank-Pazzaglia, 1976; Stores, 1978; Seidenberg et al., 1986; Jovic & Vranjesevic, 1989; Aldenkamp, Overweg-Plandsoen, & Arends, 1999). These deficits are apparently due to a combination of psychosocial factors (Williams, 2003), attention and memory problems (Carlsson, Igelbrink-Schulze Neubauer, & Stephani, 2000; Williams et al., 2001; Nolan et al. 2004), disruptions in information processing (Haverkamp, Hanisch, Mayer, & Noeker, 2001) and anomia (Mayeux, Brandt, Rosen, & Benson, 1980; Hermann, Wyler, Steenman, & Richey, 1992). A direct link between hyperexcitability and dyslexia is suggested by the fact that patients with left temporal lobe epileptic foci perform more poorly than those with right hemisphere foci (Hermann et al., 1992; Breier et al., 1997; Butterbaugh et al., 2004). In addition, in studies where intelligence measures are controlled, reading disabilities are still apparent (Bailet & Turk, 2000), suggesting an underlying biological cause rather than psychological (low self-esteem) or economic factors (low socioeconomic status) (Williams et al., 2001).

It is important to differentiate between cognitive decline caused by seizures or damage from seizures, and that initiated by preexisting conditions. Examinations of epilepsy severity variables such as seizure frequency or age at seizure onset have failed to find a strong correlation between these measures and cognitive disability (Mitchell, Chavez, Lee, & Guzman, 1991; Bailet & Turk, 2000; Williams et al., 2001). Language impairment appears to be lifelong in these patients, even when seizures are well controlled (Mayeux et al., 1980; Hermann et al., 1988). Follow-up studies also demonstrate that these deficits do not improve with time, but also do not worsen (Austin, Huberty, Huster, & Dunn, 1999). These findings suggest that neuronal mechanisms producing dyslexia exist independent of abnormalities induced by hyperexcitability. It is possible, however, that both neuropathologies are instigated by the same initial anomalous processes. Findings that patients with less severe or well-controlled epilepsy do not show significant differences from control populations in reading or memory abilities (Austin, Huberty, Huster, & Dunn, 1999; Williams et al., 2001) may reflect a more subtle underlying cause of this type of epilepsy. In contrast, epilepsy associated with developmental malformations is often difficult to treat with currently available medications (Farrell et al., 1992; Dowd, Dillon, Barbaro, & Laxer, 1992; Wolf et al., 1993). It is not surprising that aberrant synaptic connectivity, believed to occur in malformed cortex (Rosen & Galaburda, 1998; Jacobs, Kharazia, & Prince, 1999), would not be ameliorated through pharmacological means. Studies of reading ability in epilepsy patients with developmental malformations have not been done. A challenge for the future will be to prevent the initial miswiring or its reinforcement, and to determine if that lessens both hyperexcitability and cognitive dysfunction.

CONCLUSIONS

Manipulating the time of injury to the cortical plate has demonstrated that the mechanisms that create laminar irregularities and structural malformation are separate from those that produce hyperexcitability. These results have also shown that multiple abnormal cellular processes with distinct temporal characteristics are simultaneously active. Hyperinnervation of pyramidal neurons by excitatory afferents occurs prior to onset of epileptiform activity and may, therefore, initiate buildup of synchronizing events leading to epileptiform activity. Epileptogenesis is one symptom of neurological dysfunction in a malformed, abnormally wired brain. Future experiments should address whether the same mechanisms that induce hyperexcitability are also responsible for cognitive deficits associated with dyslexia.

Address correspondence to: Kimberle M. Jacobs, Ph.D., Department of Anatomy & Neurobiology, Virginia Commonwealth University, P.O. Box 980709, Richmond, VA 23298; E-mail: kmjacobs@vcu.edu

REFERENCES

Aldenkamp, A. P., Overweg-Plandsoen, W. C., & Arends, J. (1999). An open, nonrandomized clinical comparative study evaluating the effect of epilepsy on learning. *Journal of Child Neurology 14*, 795–800.

Austin, J. K., Huberty, T. J., Huster, G. A., & Dunn, D. W. (1999). Does academic achievement in children with epilepsy change over time? *Developmental Medicine and Child Neurology, 41*, 473–479.

Bailet, L. L., & Turk, W. R. (2000). The impact of childhood epilepsy on neurocognitive and behavioral performance: A prospective longitudinal study. *Epilepsia, 41*, 426–431.

Baraban, S. C., & Schwartzkroin, P. A. (1995). Electrophysiology of CA1 pyramidal neurons in an animal model of neuronal migration disorders: Prenatal methylazoxymethanol treatment. *Epilepsy Research, 22*, 145–156.

Bartolomei, F., Gavaret, M., Dravet, C., Guye, M., Bally-Berard, J. Y., Genton, P., Raybaud, C., Régis, J., & Gastaut, J. L. (1999). Late-onset epilepsy associated with regional brain cortical dysplasia. *European Neurology, 42*, 11–16.

Bayer, S. A., & Altman, J. (1991). *Neocortical development.* New York: Raven Press.

Breier, J. I., Brookshire, B. L., Fletcher, J. M., Thomas, A. B., Plenger, P. M., Wheless, J. W., Willmore, L. J., & Papanicolaou, A. (1997). Identification of side of seizure onset in temporal lobe epilepsy using memory tests in the context of reading deficits. *Journal of Clinical and Experimental Neuropsychology, 19*, 161–171.

Butterbaugh, G., Olejniczak, P., Roques, B., Costa, R., Rose, M., Fisch, B., Carey, M., Thomson, J., & Skinner, J. (2004). Lateralization of temporal lobe epilepsy and learning disabilities, as defined by disability-related civil rights law. *Epilepsia, 45,* 963–970.

Carlsson, G., Igelbrink-Schulze, N., Neubauer, B. A., & Stephani, U. (2000). Neuropsychological long-term outcome of rolandic EEG traits. *Epileptic Disorders, 2*(Suppl. 1), S63–S66.

Caviness, V. S., Jr. (1976). Patterns of cell and fiber distribution in the neocortex of the reeler mutant mouse. *The Journal of Comparative Neurology, 170,* 435–447.

Chevassus-Au-Louis, N., Baraban, S. C., Gaïarsa, J. L., & Ben-Ari, Y. (1999). Cortical malformations and epilepsy: New insights from animal models. *Epilepsia, 40,* 811–821.

Cisse, Y., Crochet, S., Timofeev, I., & Steriade, M. (2004). Synaptic responsiveness of neocortical neurons to callosal volleys during paroxysmal depolarizing shifts. *Neuroscience, 124,* 231–239.

Cohen, M., & Roessmann, U. (1994). In utero brain damage: Relationship of gestational age to pathological consequences. *Developmental Medicine and Child Neurology, 36,* 263–268.

Coulter, D. A. (2001). Epilepsy-associated plasticity in gamma-aminobutyric acid receptor expression, function, and inhibitory synaptic properties. *International Review of Neurobiology, 45,* 237–252.

Di Rocco, F., Giannetti, S., Gaglini, P., Di Rocco, C., & Granato, A. (2001). Dendritic anomalies in a freezing model of microgyria: A parametric study. *Pediatric Neurosurgery, 34,* 57–62.

Dowd, C. F., Dillon, W. P., Barbaro, N. M., & Laxer, K. D. (1992). Intractable complex partial seizure: Correlation of magnetic resonance imaging with pathology and electroencephalography. *Epilepsy Research Supplement, 5,* 101–110.

Dudek, F. E., Hellier, J. L., Williams, P. A., Ferraro, D. J., & Staley, K. J. (2002). The course of cellular alterations associated with the development of spontaneous seizures after status epilepticus. In T. Sutula (Ed.), *Do seizures damage the brain?* (pp. 53–65). Boston: Elsevier.

Dvorak, K., & Feit, J. (1977). Migration of neuroblasts through partial necrosis of the cerebral cortex in newborn rats. Contribution to the problems of morphological development and developmental period of cerebral microgyria. *Acta Neuropathologica (Berlin), 38,* 203–212.

Eriksson, S. H., Thom, M., Heffernan, J., Lin, W. R., Harding, B. N., Squier, M. V., & Sisodiya, S. M. (2001). Persistent reelin-expressing Cajal-Retzius cells in polymicrogyria. *Brain, 124,* 1350–1361.

Farrell, M. A., DeRosa, M. J., Curran, J. G., Lenard Secor, D., Cornford, M. E., Comair, Y. G., Peacock, W. J., Shields, W. D., & Vinters, H. V. (1992). Neuropathologic findings in cortical resections (including hemispherectomies) performed for the treatment of intractable childhood epilepsy. *Acta Neuropathologica, 83,* 246–259.

Ferrer, I. (1993). Experimentally induced cortical malformations in rats. *Child's Nervous System, 9,* 403–407.

Giannetti, S., Gaglini, P., Di Rocco, F., Di Rocco, C., & Granato, A. (2000). Organization of cortico-cortical associative projections in a rat model of microgyria. *Neuroreport, 11,* 2185–2189.

Gibbs, J. W., III, Shumate, M. D., & Coulter, D. A. (1997). Differential epilepsy-associated alterations in postsynaptic GABA(A) receptor function in dentate granule and CA1 neurons. *Journal of Neurophysiology, 77,* 1924–1938.

Groc, L., Gustafsson, B., & Hanse, E. (2003). Early establishment of multiple release site connectivity between interneurons and pyramidal neurons in the developing hippocampus. *European Journal of Neuroscience, 17*, 1873–1880.

Haverkamp, F., Hanisch, C., Mayer, H., & Noeker, M. (2001). Evidence of a specific vulnerability for deficient sequential cognitive information processing in epilepsy. *Journal of Child Neurology, 16*, 901–905.

Hermann, B. P., Seidenberg, M., Haltiner, A., & Wyler, A. R. (1992). Adequacy of language function and verbal memory performance in unilateral temporal lobe epilepsy. *Cortex, 28*, 423–433.

Hermann, B. P., Wyler, A. R., & Richey, E. T. (1988). Wisconsin card sorting test performance in patients with complex partial seizures of temporal-lobe origin. *Journal of Clinical and Experimental Neuropsychology, 10*, 467–476.

Hevner, R. F., Daza, R. A., Englund, C., Kohtz, J., & Fink, A. (2004). Postnatal shifts of interneuron position in the neocortex of normal and reeler mice: Evidence for inward radial migration. *Neuroscience, 124*, 605–618.

Huntsman, M. M., Isackson, P. J., & Jones, E. G. (1994). Lamina-specific expression and activity-dependent regulation of seven GABAA receptor subunit mRNAs in monkey visual cortex. *The Journal of Neuroscience, 14*, 2236–2259.

Innocenti, G. M., & Berbel, P. (1991). Analysis of an experimental cortical network: II. Connections of visual areas 17 and 18 after neonatal injections of ibotenic acid. *Journal of Neural Transplantation & Plasticity, 2*, 29–54.

Jackson, C. A., Peduzzi, J. D., & Hickey, T. L. (1989). Visual cortex development in the ferret. I. Genesis and migration of visual cortical neurons. *The Journal of Neuroscience, 9*, 1242–1253.

Jacobs, K. M., Gutnick, M. J., & Prince, D. A. (1996). Hyperexcitability in a model of cortical maldevelopment. *Cerebral Cortex, 6*, 514–523.

Jacobs, K. M., Hwang, B. J., & Prince, D. A. (1999). Focal epileptogenesis in a rat model of polymicrogyria. *Journal of Neurophysiology, 81*, 159–173.

Jacobs, K. M., Kharazia, V. N., & Prince, D. A. (1999). Mechanisms underlying epileptogenesis in cortical malformations. *Epilepsy Research, 36*, 165–188.

Jacobs, K. M., Mogensen, M., Warren, L., & Prince, D. A. (1999). Experimental microgyri disrupt the barrel field pattern in rat somatosensory cortex. *Cerebral Cortex, 9*, 733–744.

Jones, E. G., Valentino, K. L., & Fleshman, J. W. J. (1982). Adjustment of connectivity in rat neocortex after prenatal destruction of precursor cells of layers II-IV. *Brain Research, 254*, 425–431.

Jovic, N., & Vranjesevic, D. (1989). Reading disorders in children with partial epilepsy. *Neurologija, 38*, 191–200.

Kharazia, V. N., Jacobs, K. M., Hwang, J., Parada, I., & Prince, D. A. (2000). Persistent reelin-like immunoreactive neurons may contribute to an epileptogenic neocortical malformation. *Society for Neuroscience Abstracts, 26*, 661.10

Luhmann, H. J., & Raabe, K. (1996). Characterization of neuronal migration disorders in neocortical structures: I. Expression of epileptiform activity in an animal model. *Epilepsy Research, 26*, 67–74.

Mayeux, R., Brandt, J., Rosen, J., & Benson, D. F. (1980). Interictal memory and language impairment in temporal lobe epilepsy. *Neurology, 30,* 120–125.

Micheva, K. D., & Beaulieu, C. (1997). Development and plasticity of the inhibitory neocortical circuitry with an emphasis on the rodent barrel field cortex: A review. *Canadian Journal of Physiology and Pharmacology, 75,* 470–478.

Mitchell, W. G., Chavez, J. M., Lee, H., & Guzman, B. L. (1991). Academic underachievement in children with epilepsy. *Journal of Child Neurology, 6,* 65–72.

Noctor, S. C., Palmer, S. L., McLaughlin, D. F., & Juliano, S. L. (2001). Disruption of layers 3 and 4 during development results in altered thalamocortical projections in ferret somatosensory cortex. *The Journal of Neuroscience, 21,* 3184–3195.

Nolan, M. A., Redoblado, M. A., Lah, S., Sabaz, M., Lawson, J. A., Cunningham, A. M., Bleasel, A. F., & Bye, A. M. (2004). Memory function in childhood epilepsy syndromes. *Journal of Paediatrics and Child Health 40,* 20–27.

Pazzaglia, P., & Frank-Pazzaglia, L. (1976). Record in grade school of pupils with epilepsy: An epidemiological study. *Epilepsia, 17,* 361–366.

Prince, D. A., & Jacobs, K. (1998). Inhibitory function in two models of chronic epileptogenesis. *Epilepsy Research, 32,* 83–92.

Raymond, A. A., Fish, D. R., Sisodiya, S. M., Alsanjari, N., Stevens, J. M., & Shorvon, S. D. (1995). Abnormalities of gyration, heterotopias, tuberous sclerosis, focal cortical dysplasia, microdysgenesis, dysembryoplastic neuroepithelial tumour and dysgenesis of the archicortex in epilepsy. Clinical, EEG and neuroimaging features in 100 adult patients. *Brain, 118*(pt. 3), 629–660.

Rosen, G. D., Burstein, D., & Galaburda, A. M. (2000). Changes in efferent and afferent connectivity in rats with induced cerebrocortical microgyria. *The Journal of Comparative Neurology, 418,* 423–440.

Rosen, G. D., & Galaburda, A. M. (1998). Efferent and afferent connectivity of induced neocortical microgyria. *Society for Neuroscience Abstracts, 24,* 561.

Rosen, G. D., Sherman, G. F., & Galaburda, A. M. (1994). Radial glia in the neocortex of adult rats: Effects of neonatal brain injury. *Developmental Brain Research, 82,* 127–135.

Rosen, G. D., Windzio, H., & Galaburda, A. M. (2001). Unilateral induced neocortical malformation and the formation of ipsilateral and contralateral barrel fields. *Neuroscience, 103,* 931–939.

Ross, M. E. (2002). Brain malformations, epilepsy, and infantile spasms. *International Review of Neurobiology, 49,* 333–352.

Ruddick, J. A., & Khera, K. S. (1975). Pattern of anomalies following single oral doses of ethylenethiourea to pregnant rats. *Teratology, 12,* 277–281.

Seidenberg, M., Beck, N., Geisser, M., Giordani, B., Sackellares, J. C., Berent, S., Dreifuss, F. E., & Boll, T. J. (1986). Academic achievement of children with epilepsy. *Epilepsia, 27,* 753–759.

Spatz, M., Dougherty, W. J., & Smith, D. W. (1967). Teratogenic effects of methylazoxymethanol. *Proceecings of the Society for Experimental Biology and Medicine, 124,* 476–478.

Stores, G. (1978). School-children with epilepsy at risk for learning and behaviour problems. *Developmental Medicine and Child Neurology, 20,* 502–508.

Super, H., Perez, S. P., & Soriano, E. (1997). Survival of Cajal-Retzius cells after cortical lesions in newborn mice: A possible role for Cajal-Retzius cells in brain repair. *Developmental Brain Research, 98,* 9–14.

Sutula, T. (2002). Seizure-induced axonal sprouting: Assessing connections between injury, local circuits, and epileptogenesis. *Epilepsy Currents, 2,* 86–91.

Williams, J. (2003). Learning and behavior in children with epilepsy. *Epilepsy and Behavior, 4,* 107–111.

Williams, J., Phillips, T., Griebel, M. L., Sharp, G. B., Lange, B., Edgar, T., & Simpson, P. (2001). Factors associated with academic achievement in children with controlled epilepsy. *Epilepsy and Behavior, 2,* 217–223.

Wolf, H. K., Zentner, J., Hufnagel, A., Campos, M. G., Schramm, J., Elger, C. E., & Wiestler, O. D. (1993). Surgical pathology of chronic epileptic seizure disorders: Experience with 63 specimens from extratemporal corticectomies, lobectomies and functional hemispherectomies. *Acta Neuropathologica, 86,* 466–472.

Chapter • 13

Structural and Functional Deficits in a Rat Model of Cortical Heterotopia

*Kevin S. Lee, Matthew J. Anzivino,
Maro G. Machizawa, Fayong Zhang,
Cedric Williams, Frank Schottler,
Sara Tsuchitani, Jessica Drummond,
Cindy L. Kinard, Edward Bertram,
Stacey Trotter, Jaideep Kapur, and
Zong-Fu Chen*

SUMMARY

Cortical malformations are commonly associated with developmental delays, dyslexia, and certain forms of mental retardation. It is generally assumed that the functional disorders observed in individuals with brain malformations are the result of disturbances in the cells and/or circuits associated with the malformations. However, in most cases, the relation between a structural malformation and its associated functional deficit is not well characterized. This chapter examines structural abnormalities and behavioral deficits that occur in a seizure-prone animal (the tish rat). This animal exhibits large groups of misplaced neurons in the neocortex, termed subcortical band heterotopia. Seizure activity in the tish brain does not appear to emanate from the cortical heterotopia, but rather from the normal-appearing areas of

---

Supported by NIH grants NS34124 (KSL). We thank Meredith Temple and Oswald Steward for important contributions to the initial behavioral studies, and Aaron Dumont for assistance in preparing the manuscript.

cortex neighboring the heterotopia. In addition, the behavioral deficits observed in this animal occur, at least in part, in a manner that is independent of the primary cortical malformation. These latter findings suggest that other, more subtle disturbances in neural cells and/or their circuitries can play a key role in functional disturbances associated with cortical malformations.

BACKGROUND

Malformations of the cerebral cortex are surprisingly common. It is estimated that 1% to 2% of the general population exhibits some type of cellular misplacement or disorganization in the cerebral cortex, and the incidence of cortical malformation increases dramatically in certain neurological disorders (Meencke &Veith, 1992; Meencke & Janz, 1984; Hardiman et al., 1988; Farrell et al., 1992). The relatively high incidence of cortical malformations is a reflection of the complex choreography required for proper cortical development. Minor disturbances in any of a myriad of overlapping events—such as cellular proliferation, migration, and differentiation—can disrupt the strict timing and precise cellular communication needed to produce intricate cortical patterning. Although a surprisingly high percentage of brains harbor a cortical malformation, many of these malformations are not manifested as a functional deficit. Nonetheless, cortical malformations are a very common feature in a range of neurological disorders including dyslexia, epilepsy, and certain forms of mental retardation. It is, therefore, of critical importance to characterize the relation between cortical malformations and specific functional disorders. A clear understanding of the genetic, cellular, and molecular underpinnings of such disorders could provide insights into potential preventative and palliative interventions.

This chapter examines an animal model of cortical malformation that exhibits subcortical band heterotopia and a proclivity for epilepsy. The animal is termed the "tish" rat, which is an acronym for "telencephalic internal structural heterotopia". Studies performed over the last few years have elucidated several key features of the development and adult organization of the tish brain. In addition, electrophysiological investigations have helped clarify the relation between altered cortical structure and seizure activity. Finally, recent studies examining the behavioral impact of cortical malformation in the tish brain have begun to reveal a subtle interaction between cortical organization and behavioral deficits. A general description of cortical organization and development in the tish brain is presented here. In addition, findings will be discussed indicating that functional deficits can occur in a manner that is either dependent on, or independent of, the primary cortical malformation in this animal.

OVERVIEW OF THE TISH RAT

The defining characteristic of the homozygous tish rat is a prominent cortical malformation involving the misplacement of large collections of cells in the white matter below the neocortex (Lee et al., 1997). These bilateral subcortical band heterotopia affect primarily the frontal and parietal areas of the neocortex (Figure 1). The heterotopia sometimes extend into the occipital cortex, while temporal areas are typically unaffected. The neocortical areas located above the heterotopia (termed normotopic cortex; see Figure 1) are thinner than normal, but the primary neurons display characteristic lamination and orientation (Lee et al., 1997; Lee, Collins, Anzivino, Frankel, & Schottler, 1998; Lee et al., 1999). In contrast, the primary neurons in the heterotopia (termed heterotopic cortex) appear to lack proper lamination and orientation. Despite these anomalies, projection neurons in both normotopic and heterotopic areas are capable of establishing efferent connections in a regionally and topographically appropriate manner (Schottler, Couture, Rao, Kahn, & Lee, 1998; Schottler et al., 2001). For instance, the axons of large pyramidal neurons in the heterotopia

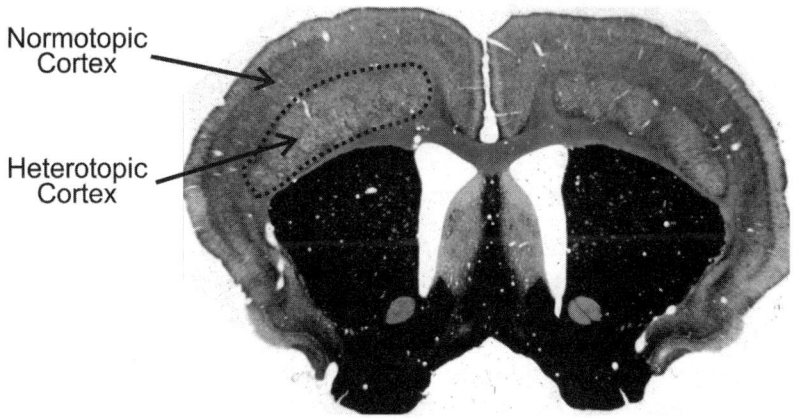

Figure 1. Coronal section of a homozygous tish brain stained using acetylcholinesterase histochemistry. Prominent subcortical band heterotopia (heterotopic cortex) are present bilaterally. The overlying normotopic cortex is thinned somewhat compared to wild-type cortex.

project to their most distant targets in the spinal cord with similar precision to that observed for the axons of large layer 5 pyramidal neurons in the normal cortex. In addition, afferents to the homozygous tish cortex terminate in a regionally and topographically appropriate manner in both normotopic and heterotopic areas (Lee et al., 1997; Schottler et al., 1998). Together, these findings indicate that although heterotopic neurons fail to position and orient themselves properly, they retain the capacity to send and receive connections with appropriate targets.

The phenotype of subcortical band heterotopia observed in the tish brain is similar to the human disorder of double cortex (e.g., Palmini et al., 1991). However, unlike double cortex in humans, which is inherited in a hemizygous X-linked manner, the large neocortical heterotopia observed in tish rats are inherited in an autosomal recessive pattern (Lee et al., 1997). Consequently, cortical heterotopia are present in homozygous tish rats, but are absent in heterozygous animals. The gene affected in human double cortex has been identified (*doublecortin*: Gleeson et al., 1998, this volume; des Portes et al., 1998a, 1998b), and its gene product is a microtubule associated protein that plays a key role in neuronal migration (Gleeson, Lin, Flanagan, & Walsh, 1999; Francis et al., 1999; see also Gleeson, this volume). Recent work using RNA interference techniques to disrupt doublecortin production in rats *in utero* demonstrates that doublecortin is critical for proper radial migration of cortical neurons *in vivo*, and that knocking down the production of this gene product results in the development of subcortical band heterotopia (Bai et al., 2003; see also LoTurco, this volume). The gene or genes responsible for the disturbed development of the tish brain are unknown and are a matter of ongoing investigation.

DEVELOPMENT OF THE TISH NEOCORTEX

Neocortical development requires multiple phases of proliferation, migration, and differentiation, and involves diverse cellular populations. During the early stages of development, a cortical preplate is formed, followed later by the establishment of the cortical plate. The cortical preplate is comprised of superficial Cajal-Retzius cells, and deeper cells that will eventually become the cortical subplate. The majority of cortical neurons, which comprise the later-forming cortical plate, proliferate in the cortical ventricular (and subventricular) zone. The cells forming the cortical plate migrate into the neocortex, and are intercalated between the Cajal-Retzius cells and subplate cells. The cortical plate cells establish an inside-out neurogenetic gradient as later-born cells migrate to progressively more superficial positions in the developing cortical plate. In the homozygous tish rat, normotopic areas of the affected neocortex display a distinct cortical preplate during early development. However, the deeper-situated area that is destined to contain the heterotopic neurons does not contain preplate cells (Lee et al., 1998). As development continues in the tish neocortex, the normotopic cortical plate develops in a typical inside-out manner with neurons migrating into the area between the Cajal-Retzius and subplate cells. In contrast, the neurons in the heterotopic cortical plate exhibit a more complex pattern of migration in which earlier-born cells are positioned around the rim of the heterotopia, while later-born cells are located toward the core of the structure. This unique neurogenetic pattern is thought to result from the presence of a secondary, misplaced region of cellular proliferation in the developing tish cortex (Lee et al., 1998). Cellular proliferation in the developing tish neocortex occurs in both the typical dorsal ventricular zone and in an atypical position in the intermediate zone (Figure 2). Heterotopic cellular proliferation is among the earliest disturbances observed in the tish neocortex, and is established prior to the generation or migration of the vast majority of cortical plate neurons.

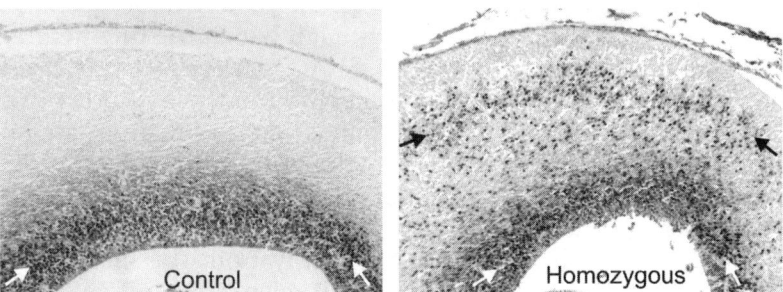

Figure 2. Heterotopic cellular proliferation occurs in the homozygous tish neocortex. Coronal sections of embryonic day 18 brains from control and homozygous tish animals stained immunohistochemically for proliferating cell nuclear antigen (PCNA) are shown. PCNA is expressed in mitotically active cells, and the stain provides an index of regions of active cellular proliferation. In the control brain, PCNA-positive cells are observed primarily in the typical cortical proliferative zone located in the vicinity of the lateral ventricle (white arrows). In the homozygous tish brain, proliferative activity is observed near the ventricle (white arrows), and also in a secondary, heterotopic area of proliferation in the intermediate zone (black arrows).

The proliferation and migration of interneuons in the neocortex entails a rather different process than that for primary cortical neurons. Strong evidence has accrued in recent years indicating that the majority of interneurons in the neocortex are not derived from the dorsal neocortical proliferative zone, but rather are generated in the ventral telencephalon, and migrate tangentially into the neocortex (for a recent review, see Nadarajah & Parnevalas, 2002; Xu, de la Cruz, & Anderson, 2003). Moreover, there are multiple subtypes of interneurons in the adult neocortex, and these may derive from different regions of the ventral telencephalon (Xu, Cobos, de la Cruz, Rubenstein, & Anderson, 2004). Preliminary evidence from our laboratory indicates that interneuron positioning is disturbed in the homozygous tish neocortex. Based on the distribution of GAD67-immunopositive neurons in adult homozygous tish brains, there appear to be more interneurons in heterotopic areas than in the normotopic areas of the neocortex. However, this disturbance in interneuronal distribution is apparently not uniform for all subtypes of interneurons. Preliminary findings suggest that there are increased numbers of parvalbumin-positive interneurons in heterotopic areas (see Figure 3 in the four-color section on page 222-G); however, this distribution pattern does not hold for all interneuronal subtypes. The reason(s) for this alteration in interneuronal positioning is not known. One possibility is that the presence of a heterotopic proliferative zone in a region of cortex through which the interneurons typically migrate disrupts the migratory patterns of these cells (Figure 3). Heterotopic cellular proliferation in the neocortex is already established during the time frame that interneurons are migrating into the neocortex. Another possibility is that the interneuronal proliferative and/or migratory zones are differentially affected in the tish rat. For instance, parvalbumin-positive interneurons appear to originate primarily from the medial ganglionic eminence (MGE) in the ventral telencephalon (Xu et al., 2004). It is conceivable that a selective disturbance of the proliferative and/or migratory characteristics of interneurons derived from restricted portions of the ganglionic eminence could lead to a selective disturbance in the distribution of interneuron subtypes in the tish neocortex. Clarification of the precise mechanism(s) responsible for altered interneuronal distribution awaits further investigation.

In summary, the developmental events necessary to construct a typical neocortex are quite complex. Multiple disturbances involving both proliferative and migratory processes appear to play roles in the malformation of the tish neocortex. One of the earliest events is misplaced cellular proliferation. Heterotopic neurogenesis is postulated to produce the primary malformation in which cortically generated neurons establish normotopic and heterotopic cortical plates. However, this process likely involves a disturbance in migration as well because the typical inside-out neurogenetic gradient seen in neocortex is disturbed in heterotopic areas. Alterations in the positioning of neocortical interneurons may also involve a disruption in cellular migration. It is postulated that the normal process of tangential interneuronal migration into the neocortex is disrupted by the presence of a secondary, heterotopic proliferative zone in the developing neocortex.

TISH RATS ARE SEIZURE-PRONE

Some homozygous tish animals exhibit spontaneous, recurrent seizure activity that begins a month or so after birth and continues throughout their lifespan. These epileptic animals exhibit partial seizures with variable secondary generalization (Lee et al., 1997). The seizures affect neocortical and limbic structures, while subcortical structures are not prominently activated (Chen et al., 2000). Heterozygous animals, which do not exhibit neocortical heterotopia, do not display seizure activity. This suggests that some aspect of the heterotopia, such as intrinsic neuronal properties or circuit-based interactions, plays a key role in epileptogenesis in the tish brain. However, seizure activity in these animals does not appear to originate in the heterotopic areas of the affected cortex. Instead, the normal-appearing (normotopic) areas of cortex in the vicinity of the cortical heterotopia are more excitable. *In vitro* electrophysiological experiments utilizing slices of the tish neocortex have examined neuronal spiking activity in the presence of proconvulsant compounds (Chen et al., 2000). These studies demonstrate that when connections between the normotopic and heterotopic areas are disrupted physically or pharmacologically, the normotopic area continues to exhibit spike bursting activity, while the heterotopic area does not. These results suggest that aberrant discharge activity is initiated in the normotopic cells and that this activity recruits the heterotopic cells (Figure 4). Thus, although both normotopic and heterotopic areas of the tish neocortex display seizure activity when depth recordings are performed during *in vivo* seizures, the normotopic area may be responsible for initiating the seizures.

The reasons for the instability in the normotopic area are still under investigation. However, one possible explanation is the differential distribution of interneurons in the normotopic and

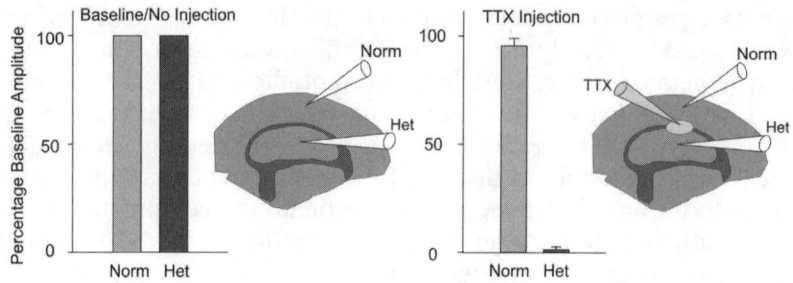

Figure 4. Normotopic areas of the tish neocortex are more susceptible to exhibit aberrant discharge activity. Recordings were performed from normotopic (Norm) and heterotopic (Het) areas of the tish neocortex using *in vitro* slices from homozygous tish brains. Addition of a proconvulsant concentration of penicillin-G to the solution bathing the slices resulted in spontaneous, interictal-like bursts in both the normotopic and heterotopic areas (left bar graph and drawing). The Y axis on the graphs represents the percentage of the baseline amplitude of discharges recorded in the presence of penicillin-G. In the right bar graph and drawing, action potentials were blocked in axons traversing the area between the normotopic and heterotopic areas by focally injecting the sodium channel blocker, tetrodotoxin (TTX). The injection of TTX did not have a significant effect on bursting in the normotopic area, but nearly eliminated bursting in the adjacent heterotopic area. These findings indicate that proconvulsant-induced discharges emanate from the normotopic area, and that the heterotopic area is recruited by synaptic drive from the normotopic area.

heterotopic areas. As described earlier, our preliminary findings indicate that parvalbumin-positive interneurons are present in lower numbers in the normotopic areas as compared to heterotopic areas. These interneurons provide a substantial inhibitory influence in the neocortex, and a paucity of such cells in the normotopic cortex could serve to destabilize neuronal activity. The potential role of altered inhibitory function in the tish neocortex is currently being evaluated by examining the cellular actions of the inhibitory neurotransmitter GABA. Preliminary findings from experiments using whole-cell voltage clamp recordings from slices of homozygous tish neocortex are consistent with the concept that reduced inhibition in the normotopic cortex plays a role in destabilizing neuronal activity (Trotter, Anzivino, Lee, & Kapur, 2004).

BEHAVIORAL DEFICITS IN THE TISH RAT

Morris Water Maze

A broad range of functional deficits have been observed in conjunction with cortical malformations. These include reduced IQ, impaired psychomotor development, generalized developmental delays, dyslexia, and mental retardation (e.g., Palmini et al., 1991; see also Galaburda, this volume). Interestingly, some of the affected individuals exhibit profound deficits, while others are only minimally impaired. The reasons for such disparities are not well understood, but are often ascribed to the extent to which (or site at which) neural circuitry is altered by a cortical malformation, or to the amount of damage induced by secondary events such as seizures. We have begun to evaluate the underlying causes of behavioral impairments linked to subcortical band heterotopia by characterizing functional deficits in the tish rat. The performance of tish rats on two behavioral tasks designed to test learning, memory, and cognitive function will be described.

The first behavioral task examined spatial learning using a Morris Water Maze (MWM). In this task, an animal is placed in a tank containing opaque water, and the animal is required to locate a submerged (hidden) platform. The time required for the animal to find the platform, its swimming speed, and the distance traversed are monitored. The tish rats utilized in the MWM tests did not display clinical seizures, thus reducing the possible role of seizure-induced corruption of behavioral function. Sprague-Dawley rats were used as controls in these and other experiments because they represent the parent strain for the tish rat. The swimming speed and distance traversed did not differ significantly between control and homozygous tish rats, indicating that an impairment of motor function does not complicate the performance of tish rats on this task. This is an important issue because impaired motor function could affect performance on the MWM without implicating a change in learning capacity. The latency to find the hidden platform was progressively reduced over the four days of testing in both the control and homozygous tish rats. This indicates that performance improved in both groups over the daily trials. Notably, the latency to find the hidden platform did not differ statistically between the two groups on any of the four days of testing. Consequently, it was not possible to distinguish between homozygous tish rats and controls based on their performance on this standard visual-spatial learning task.

Eight-arm Radial Maze

It is conceivable that the MWM task utilized in the preceding experiment does not provide an adequate test of the circuitries affected in the tish brain. It is also possible that the task selected in the MWM was not sufficiently challenging to reveal a deficit in the homozygous tish rat. We, therefore, tested the performance of tish rats on a more complex task in which animals must employ a win-shift strategy on an eight-arm radial maze. Rats were placed on a food-restricted diet to reduce their weight to 85% of baseline. The animals were then acclimatized to the eight-arm maze and trained to perform a win-shift task (e.g., Williams, Packard, & McGaugh, 1994). Briefly, this task involves the placement of a rat in the middle of an eight-arm maze with four arms randomly baited with food pellets at the end of the arms. The unbaited arms are blocked with removable plexiglas barriers during this "initial trial" phase of the task. The maze is surrounded by visual cues that are constant throughout the entire task. After retrieving the food pellets in the four baited arms, the animal is removed from the maze and placed in its cage for five minutes. The animal is then returned to the maze for the "retention test" phase of the procedure. During the retention test phase, all of the arms are open (no plexiglas barriers in place) and only the four arms that were previously unbaited are now baited. In this task, the animal learns that the most effective strategy to obtain food is to select the arms that were previously unbaited, and to avoid the previously baited arms. A correct choice occurs when an animal enters a previously unbaited arm for the first time during the retention test phase and obtains a food pellet. An incorrect choice occurs when an animal enters a previously baited arm, or re-enters an arm that it has already visited during the retention test phase. Successful performance of the task is based on a strict criterion of no incorrect choices on two consecutive days of testing. When the animal reaches this criterion for the five-minute interval, the interval between training and the retention testing is increased to 15 minutes. Once an animal achieved criterion performance at the 15 minute interval, the interval between the initial trial phase and the retention test phase is extended to three hours. This task was selected because it is a relatively complex and challenging learning paradigm. The experiments tested three groups of animals: control (Sprague-Dawley), homozygous tish, and heterozygous tish rats.

All control rats were able to master the longest intertrial interval tested (i.e., three hours). In contrast, homozygous tish rats were significantly impaired in terms of the longest interval that could be mastered. An unexpected finding in this study was that the performance of the heterozygous tish rats was also significantly impaired relative to control rats. These findings indicate that the tish rat possesses functional deficits when tested on a complex learning and memory task. The results also suggest that this impairment is due, at least in part, to a functional disturbance that is independent of the subcortical band heterotopia. The heterozygous tish rats do not display subcortical band heterotopia, but are significantly impaired on the win-shift task. The mechanistic basis for this deficit is unknown, but could reside in a more subtle disturbance in the cells and/or circuitries that is present in the tish animals.

IS THERE A HETEROZYGOUS PHENOTYPE FOR THE TISH RAT?

The most striking features of the homozygous tish rat are bilateral subcortical band heterotopia and a proclivity for epilepsy. Consequently, most previous studies of the tish rat have focused on understanding structural and functional features of the subcortical band heterotopia, including how they are organized, how they develop, how they relate to epilepsy, and how they might contribute to behavioral deficits. However, the results presented in the preceding section indicate that heterozygous animals are also behaviorally impaired, even though they do not exhibit subcortical band heterotopia or epilepsy. This suggests that performance deficits observed in tish animals are due, at least in part, to a disturbance that is independent of subcortical band heterotopia or epilepsy. These findings have prompted a more intensive analysis of the heterozygous phenotype in the tish rat with the long-term goal of identifying mechanisms that could contribute to impaired performance on complex learning and memory tasks.

Recent findings indicate that tish animals exhibit a more subtle structural alteration that affects the hippocampus. Hippocampal mossy fibers project to atypical postsynaptic sites in both heterozygous and homozygous tish animals (Anzivino, Kinard, Thompson, Trotter, & Lee, 2004). The hippocampal mossy fiber system is a critical synaptic circuit in the hippocampal formation. Mossy fibers are the axons and terminals of dentate gyrus granule cells, which typically project to the proximal apical dendrites (*stratum lucidum*) of CA3 pyramidal neurons. In tish rats, the mossy fiber system projects not only to the apical dendritic field, but also to the basal dendritic field (*stratum oriens*) of the CA3 pyramidal cells (see Figure 5). This effect is more profound in the homozygous animals than in heterozygous animals. Mossy fiber innervation of the basal dendritic field appears to occur at the cost of innervation of the apical dendritic field in the tish rat. The width of the band of innervation in the apical dendrites is reduced as a function of the added innervation in the basal dendrites.

It is possible that altered circuitry of this type could be the result of developmental errors or seizure-induced reorganization.

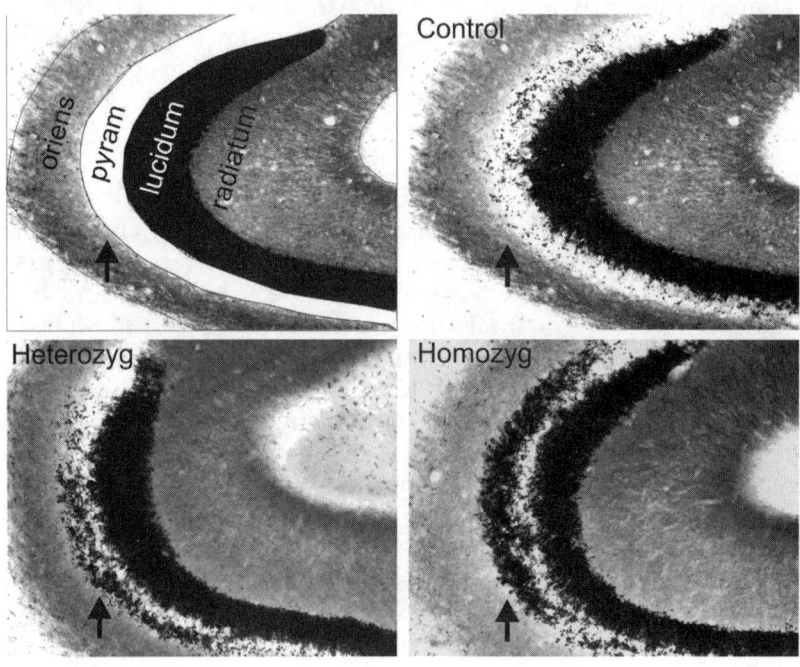

Figure 5. Hippocampal mossy fiber distribution is altered in heterozygous (Heterozyg) and homozygous (Homozyg) tish rats. Coronal sections of the CA3 region of control and tish rats are shown. The sections were stained using Timm's method, which allows the visualization of hippocampal mossy fibers (black in appearance). The upper left image illustrates the layers of the CA3 region of the hippocampus using the control section as a template. *Stratum lucidum* is the primary target for the mossy fibers, and is stained darkly in all three animals. The control animal exhibits sparse staining in *stratum pyramidale* (pyram; the pyramidal cell body layer), and virtually no staining in *stratum oriens*. In contrast, heterozygous and homozygous tish rats exhibit denser staining in *stratum pyramidale*, and distinct bands in *stratum oriens*. Staining of *stratum oriens* is most prominent in the homozygous animals, and intermediate in the heterozygous animal. Arrows in each frame indicate the proximal *stratum oriens* (basal dendritic area) of CA3.

Previous studies have demonstrated that seizures involving the temporal lobe can result in the reorganization of mossy fiber circuitry, including the aberrant innervation of the infrapyramidal (i.e., basal dendritic) area of CA3 (e.g., Liu et al., 1999). However, two lines of evidence argue against seizure-induced reorganization as a cause of mossy fiber alterations in the tish rat. First, the atypical innervation is seen in heterozygous animals, which have not been shown to display seizure activity. Second, the misdirected axons are present in homozygous animals at developmental stages that precede the onset of seizures. These findings indicate that the altered organization of mossy fiber circuitry in the tish rat is a developmental event, and does not occur as a result of seizure-induced reorganization.

It is not known whether this modification in hippocampal mossy fiber circuitry contributes to the behavioral deficits observed in the tish rat. Previous studies have demonstrated that the pattern of mossy fiber termination varies considerably among different strains of mice (reviewed in Schwegler & Crusio, 1995). Moreover, some studies have demonstrated that performance on spatial tasks covaries with the pattern of mossy fiber termination (Crusio, Schwegler, & Lipp, 1987; Prior, Schwegler, & Ducker, 1997). However, in most of these studies, better spatial performance was correlated with a larger infrapyramidal band of mossy fibers. This finding does not correspond with the observations in the tish rat in which poorer spatial learning was associated with a larger infrapyramidal band of mossy fibers. The possible mechanistic relationship between behavioral performance and mossy fiber distribution thus remains unclear. Differences in genetic backgrounds can influence behavioral strategies (Sluyter, Marican, Roubertoux, & Crusio, 1999), and could conceivably influence the behavioral impact of mossy fiber reorganization. It is not known how the genetic background of the tish rat may influence circuitry-associated behavioral deficits. The fact that the heterozygous tish phenotype is intermediate to control and homozygous phenotypes may ultimately provide insights into this issue if an intermediate behavioral deficit can be identified that covaries with the magnitude of the circuitry changes.

CONCLUSIONS

The mechanisms through which cortical malformations produce specific functional disorders are just beginning to be understood. In some cases, the relation between structure and function is relatively straightforward, while in others the influences appear to be more subtle. The tish rat serves as a useful model system for examining interactions of this type. Fundamental disturbances in cortical development, including alterations in proliferation and migration, produce a striking and reproducible structural phenotype in the homozygous animal. The large heterotopia observed in the tish neocortex are reminiscent of a human cortical syndrome, even though the genetic underpinnings appear to differ. The disorganized and misplaced neurons in the heterotopia would seem the logical candidates to destabilize cortical activity and predispose the animal to seizures; however, it is the normal-appearing cortical tissue in the vicinity of the heterotopia that is more susceptible to aberrant discharge activity. Recent findings indicate that the performance of tish rats is impaired on a complex spatial learning task. Perhaps the most surprising observation from these studies is that heterozygous animals, which do not display neocortical heterotopia or seizures, are also impaired behaviorally. This latter finding suggests that more subtle disturbances in brain organization and function contribute to behavioral deficits in these animals. Ongoing investigations into the genetic, molecular, and cellular characteristics of the tish rat seek to further elucidate the mechanisms responsible for failed cortical development, and to clarify the links between structural anomalies and specific functional deficits.

Address correspondence to: Kevin S. Lee, Box 801392, Department of Neuroscience, University of Virginia, Charlottesville, VA 22908; E-mail: ksl3h@virginia.edu

REFERENCES

Anzivino, M. J., Kinard, C. L., Thompson, R. C., Trotter, S. A., & Lee, K. S. (2004). Non-neocortical structural anomalies in the brains of heterozygous and homozygous tish rats. *Society for Neuroscience Annual Meeting Abstracts, 679*, 21.

Bai, J., Ramos, R. L., Ackman, J. B., Thomas, A. M., Lee, R. V., & LoTurco, J. J. (2003). RNAi reveals doublecortin is required for radial migration in rat neocortex. *Nature Neuroscience, 6*, 1277–1283.

Chen, Z. F., Schottler, F., Bertram, E., Gall, C. M., Anzivino, M. J., & Lee, K. S. (2000). Distribution and initiation of seizure activity in a rat brain with subcortical band heterotopia. *Epilepsia, 41*, 493–501.

Crusio, W. E., Schwegler, H., & Lipp H.-P. (1987). Radial-maze performance and structural variation of the hippocampus in mice: A correlation with mossy fibre distribution. *Brain Research, 425*, 182–185.

des Portes, V., Pinard, J.-M., Billuart, P., Vinet, M. C., Koulakoff, A., Carrie, A., Gelot, A., Dupuis, E., Motte, J., Berwald-Netter, Y., Catala, C., Kahn, A., Beldjord, C., & Chelly, J. (1998a). Identification of a novel CNS gene required for neuronal migration and involved in X-linked subcortical laminar heterotopia and lissencephaly syndrome. *Cell, 92,* 51–61.

des Portes, V., Francis, F., Pinard, J.-M., Desguerre, I., Moutard, M.-L., Snoeck, I., Meiners, L. C., Capron, F., Cusmai, R., Ricci, S., Motte, J., Echenne, B., Ponsot, G., Dulac, O., Chelly, J., & Beldjord, C. (1998b). Doublecortin is the major gene causing X-linked subcortical laminar heterotopia (SCLH). *Human Molecular Genetics, 7,* 1063–1070.

Farrell, M. A., DeRosa, M. J., Curran, J. G., Secor, D. L., Cornford, M. E., Comair, Y. G., Peacock, W. J., Shields, W. D., & Vinters, H. V. (1992). Neuropathologic finding in cortical resection (including hemispherectomies) performed for the treatment of intractable childhood epilepsy. *Acta Neuropathologica (Berl), 83,* 246–259.

Francis, F., Koulakoff, A., Boucher, D., Chafey, P., Schaar, B., Vinet, M. C., Friocourt, G., McDonnell, N., Reiner, O., Kahn, A., McConnell, S. K., Berwald-Netter, Y., Denoulet, P., & Chelly, J. (1999). Doublecortin is a developmentally regulated, microtubule-associated protein expressed in migrating and differentiating neurons. *Neuron, 23,* 247–256.

Gleeson, J. G., Allen, K. M., Fox, J. W., Lamperti, E. D., Berkovic, S., Scheffer, I., Cooper, E. C., Dobyns, W. B., Minnerath, S. R., Ross, M. E., & Walsh, C. A. (1998). Doublecortin, a brain-specific gene mutated in human X-linked lissencephaly and double cortex syndrome, encodes a putative signaling protein. *Cell, 92,* 63–72.

Gleeson, J. G., Lin, P. T., Flanagan, L. A., & Walsh, C. A. (1999). Doublecortin is a microtubule-associated protein and is expressed widely by migrating neurons. *Neuron, 23,* 257–271.

Hardiman, O., Burke, T., Phillips, J., Murphy, S., O'Moore, B., Staunton, H., & Farrell, M. A. 1988. Microdysgenesis in resected temporal neocortex: Incidence and clinical significance in focal epilepsy. *Neurology, 38,* 1041–1047.

Lee, K. S., Schottler, F. Collins, J. L., Lanzino, G., Couture, D., Rao, A., Hiramatsu, K. I., Goto, Y., Hong, S. C., Caner, H., Yamamoto, H., Chen, Z. F., Bertram, E., Berr, S., Omary, R., Scrable, H., Jackson, T., Goble, J., & Eisenman, L. (1997). A genetic animal model of human neocortical heterotopia associated with seizures. *The Journal of Neuroscience, 17,* 6236–6242.

Lee, K. S., Collins, J. L., Anzivino, M. J., Frankel, E. A., & Schottler, F. (1998). Heterotopic neurogenesis in a rat with cortical heterotopia. *The Journal of Neuroscience, 18,* 9365–9375.

Lee, K. S., Schottler, F., Anzivino, M. J., Collins, J. L., Frankel, E. A., Chen, Z.-F., & Bertram, E. (1999). Neuronal development in an epileptic rat with cortical heterotopia. In R. Spreafico, G. Avanzini, & F. Andermann (Eds.), *Abnormal cortical development and epilepsy* (pp. 145–157). London: John Libbey and Co.

Liu, Z., Yang, Y., Silveira, D. C., Sarkisian, M. R., Tandon, P., Huang, L.-T., Stafstrom, C. E., & Holmes, G. L. (1999). Consequences of recurrent seizures during early brain development. *Neuroscience, 92,* 1443–1454.

Meencke, H., & Janz, D. (1984). Neuropathological findings in primary generalized epilepsy: A study of eight cases. *Epilepsia, 25,* 8–21.

Meencke, H., & Veith, G. (1992). Migration disturbances in epilepsy. *Epilepsy Research,* (suppl 9), 31–40.

Nadarajah, B., & Parnavelas, J. G. (2002). Modes of neuronal migration in the developing cerebral cortex. *Nature Reviews Neuroscience, 3*, 423–432.

Palmini, A., Andermann, A., Aicardi J., Dulac, O., Chaves, F., Ponsot, G., Pinard, J. M., Goutieres, F., Livingston, J., Tampieri, D., Andermann, E., & Robitaille, Y. (1991). Diffuse cortical dysplasia, or the "double cortex" syndrome: The clinical and epileptic spectrum in 10 patients. *Neurology, 41*, 1656–1662.

Prior, H., Schwegler, H., & Ducker, G. (1997). Dissociation of spatial reference memory, spatial working memory and hippocampal mossy fiber distribution in two rat strains differing in emotionality. *Behavioural Brain Research, 87*, 183–194.

Schottler, F., Couture, D., Rao, A., Kahn, H., & Lee, K. S. (1998). Subcortical connections of normotopic and heterotopic neurons in sensory and motor cortices of the tish mutant rat. *The Journal of Comparative Neurology, 395*, 29–42.

Schottler, F., Fabiato, H., Leland, J. M., Chang, L.-Y., Lotfi, P., Getachew, F., & Lee, K. S. (2001). Normotopic and heterotopic cortical representations of mystacial vibrissae in rats with subcortical band heterotopia. *Neuroscience, 108*, 217–235.

Schwegler, H., & Crusio, W. E. (1995). Correlations between radial-maze learning and structural variations of septum and hippocampus in rodents. *Behavioural Brain Research, 67*, 29–41.

Sluyter, F., Marican, C. C. M., Roubertoux, P. L., & Crusio, W. E. (1999). Radial maze learning in two inbred mouse strains and their reciprocal congenics for the non-pseudoautosomal region of the Y chromosome. *Brain Research, 835*, 68–73.

Trotter, S. A., Anzivino, M. J., Lee, K. S., & Kapur, J. (2004). Altered synaptic inhibition in an animal model for cortical malformation. *Society for Neuroscience Annual Meeting Abstracts, 228.13.*

Williams, C. L., Packard, M. G., & McGaugh, J. L. (1994). Amphetamine facilitation of win-shift radial arm maze retention: The involvement of peripheral adrenergic and central dopaminergic systems. *Psychobiology, 22*, 141–148.

Xu, Q., de la Cruz, E., & Anderson, S. A. (2003). Cortical interneuron fate: Diverse sources for distinct subtypes? *Cerebral Cortex, 13*, 670–676.

Xu, Q., Cobos, I., de la Cruz, E., Rubenstein, J. L., & Anderson, S. A. (2004). Origins of cortical interneuron subtypes. *The Journal of Neuroscience, 24*, 2612–2622.

Chapter • 14

Behavioral Consequences of Focal Anomalies in the Cerebral Cortex

R. Holly Fitch and Ann M. Peiffer

AUDITORY PROCESSING DEFICITS AND LANGUAGE DISABILITY

It has been reported that 7%–8% of preschool children are diagnosed with a language disability or impairment of unknown cause (Beitchman et al., 1986). Such children may be identified based on an abnormal discrepancy between verbal and nonverbal IQ, or a low individual language score as compared to population norms. Even though clinical definitions vary, most clinicians agree that language learning impairment (LLI) is a receptive/expressive language difficulty that is not predicted or expected from general intelligence.

Multiple, convergent behavioral studies of children with LLI have pointed to a common underlying difficulty in processing rapidly occurring sensory events for this population (e.g., nonverbal stimuli—Tallal & Piercy, 1973; Tallal & Stark, 1981; Tomblin, Freese, & Records, 1992; Wright et al., 1997; Duffy, McAnulty, & Waber, 1999; verbal stimuli—Tallal & Piercy, 1974, 1975; Werker & Tees, 1987; Reed, 1989; Kraus et al., 1995, 1996; Leppänen, Pihko, Eklund, & Lyytinen, 1999; visual stimuli—Badcock & Lovegrove, 1981; DiLollo, Hanson, & McIntyre, 1983; Stanley & Hall, 1973; see Farmer & Klein, 1995 for review; tactile—Laasonen, Service, & Virsu 2001, 2002). For example, LLI children have difficulty in discriminating 75 ms tones separated by interstimulus intervals (ISI) of shorter than 300 ms, while normal children can discriminate up to an 8 ms ISI (Tallal & Piercy, 1973). Of 160 ". . . sensory, perceptual, motor, neurodevelopmental, speech and demographic variables . . . ," Tallal, Stark, and Mellits (1985) extracted six rapid temporal processing variables that could accurately differentiate 98% of 59 subjects as LLI or controls. These six composite variables included both verbal and nonverbal indices of tactile, auditory, and visual sensory modalities. Temporal processing variables in the same sensory modalities, but with stimuli of longer duration, were not effective discriminators. For example, LLI children were found to be impaired at discriminating speech syllables characterized by rapid frequency changes of 40 ms in length (e.g., /ba/ from /da/; Tallal & Piercy, 1975; Tallal, Stark, and Mellits, 1985). However, when the defining formant frequency transition was lengthened to 80 ms for /ba/ and /da/, the syllables could be discriminated by LLI children (Tallal, Stark, & Mellitis, 1985).

In addition, temporal resolution in infancy has been linked to language ability later in development. For example, Trehub and Henderson (1996) examined relationships between performance on gap detection tasks—that is, the ability to detect a short silent gap in a background of sound (usually white noise)—and language scores at six or 12 months of age. Subjects with lower gap detection thresholds in infancy were found to have larger vocabularies, more irregular word forms, and more complex sentences in the toddler and preschool years as compared to subjects with poorer temporal resolution. When infants with a positive family history (FH+) of language impairments were assessed on detecting a gap between two complex tone pairs, they had higher (i.e., worse) auditory processing thresholds than infants with a negative family history (FH-) (Benasich & Tallal, 1996). Subsequently, when these same infants were assessed for language ability at 16, 24, and 36 months of age, FH+ infants had poorer language scores than FH- infants (Benasich & Tallal, 1996, 2002; Benasich, Thomas, Choudhury, & Lappänen, 2002).

Preschoolers with LLI move on to elementary school where they experience more reading problems than unimpaired peers (up to 80% meeting criteria for dyslexia) (Stark et al., 1984; Tallal, 1988; Beitchman & Inglis, 1991). For example, in a longitudinal study, kindergarten children with LLI were at high risk for reading disabilities in second and fourth grades; however, if LLI children received assistance and showed an improvement in their spoken language abilities, their subsequent reading outcomes were better than for those children with persistent language impairments (Catts, Fey, Tomblin, & Zhang, 2002). Children labeled as reading disordered and/or learning disabled have also been found to perform worse than controls on tasks of auditory gap detection (McCroskey & Kidder, 1980). Similarly, in a study of children with dyslexia compared to age matched controls (10–12 years of age), a rapid auditory processing deficit was confirmed on a task using complex tones (Heiervang, Stevenson, & Hugdahl, 2002).

In the auditory modality, same/different identification tasks of paired speech syllables (e.g., ba/da, pa/ta) and tones have shown that reading disabled children have difficulty discriminating among specific syllable pairs (Reed, 1989; De Weirdt, 1988; Tallal, 1980). Interestingly, Reed (1989) presented vowels in the same/different task, and found that reading disabled children were not impaired at discriminating these items. Vowels require the least temporal auditory differentiation, while stop consonants require the most (e.g., /b/, /d/, /p/, and /t/) (Phillips & Farmer, 1990). Interestingly, preverbal infants (six months old) with a FH+ of dyslexia also respond differently to the temporal structure of speech sounds, both in initial responsiveness and change-detection response when compared to FH- infants using electrical brain activation measures (Leppänen et al., 2002). Therefore, just as for children with LLI, reading disabled children appear to show difficulty processing rapid auditory temporal variables (e.g., speech stop consonants), but can process similar but more slowly changing variables (e.g., speech vowels). Not surprisingly, tests assessing poor readers for the most difficult aspects of auditory processing indicate that the greatest deficit in poor readers compared to good readers occurs when spectral discriminations are made with brief stimulus forms or with stimuli in rapid succession (Ahissar, Protopapas, Reid, & Merzenich, 2000).

Studies in the visual modality have found that reading disabled children need longer ISIs than controls to detect blanks between two sine waves, blanks between vertical lines, or different parts of the same stimulus (Badcock & Lovegrove, 1981; DiLollo, Hanson, & McIntyre, 1983; Stanley & Hall, 1973; see Farmer & Klein, 1995 for review). Kinsbourne, Rufo, Gamzu, Palmer, and Berliner (1991) also found dyslexic subjects to be impaired at temporal order judgments in both auditory (clicks) and visual (light flashes) modalities, suggesting that a general cross modal temporal processing difficulty also exists in dyslexics. Laasonen and colleagues (Laassonen, Service, & Virsu, 2001, 2002) extended the cross modal investigation to include tactile perception (in addition to visual and auditory), and found that a temporal input processing impairment is generally correlated to dyslexia in both children and adults while nontemporal experimental aspects are not.

Based on temporal processing research in children with developmental LLI and/or dyslexia, Tallal (1984) asserted that a rapid processing deficit may underlie some cases of LLI. Tallal, Miller, and Fitch (1993) further propose a developmental cascade of impairments, which stem from a basic deficit in auditory temporal processing (or an even more general cross-modal temporal processing deficit). Specifically, auditory processing deficits may lead to poor acquisition of phonological elements, which then manifests in phonological processing deficits (Leonard, 1998; Tallal, Merzenich, Miller, & Jenkins, 1998; Wright, Bowen, & Zecker, 2000; Montgomery, 2003). This cascade is supported by experiments indicating the presence of a phonological processing deficit (a well-defined dyslexic symptom; e.g., see Liberman & Shankweiler, 1985) in populations with LLI (Edwards & Lahey, 1996; Tallal et al., 1998). Together, these deficits may contribute not only to the impairment of speech perception and language development, but also to impairments in later reading ability. In fact, some have proposed that temporal information embedded in speech sounds (rather than phonetic information per se) causes dyslexics to perform poorly on certain behavioral measures (Schulte-Korne, Deimel, Bartling, & Remschmidt, 1999). Despite compelling data, there is ongoing controversy as to whether or not a rapid auditory processing deficit underlies the phonemic processing deficits seen in dyslexia. Evidence of a specific neurobiological cause has not been found for any part of this proposed cascade, and greater knowledge about the etiology underlying rapid auditory and phonological processing deficits may shed light on the debate regarding a putative relationship between such deficits and language and reading disability.

SEX DIFFERENCES IN THE OCCURRENCE OF LANGUAGE DISABILITY

In general, males are found to be at a disadvantage (increased risk) for neurodevelopmental disorders including epilepsy, autism, hyperactivity, mental retardation, cerebral palsy, and dyslexia. These disorders are diagnosed significantly more often in males than females (Gualtieri & Hicks, 1985). Recently, male sex was also identified as one of three risk factors (the others being low maternal education and a positive family history) that indicated a child was 7.7 times as likely to have a speech delay of unknown origin than a child without these three factors (Campbell et al., 2003). With respect to dyslexia, a number of researchers have reported a higher predominance in males (Finucci, Isaacs, Whitehouse, & Childs,

1983; Gualtieri & Hicks, 1985; Neils & Aram, 1986; Tallal, 1991; Liederman & Flannery, 1993), though controversy exists (Shaywitz, Shaywitz, Fletcher, & Escobar, 1990).

This controversy stems, in part, from the assertion that more males than females are referred and evaluated due to the greater tendency for extroverted expression amongst males, leading, in turn, to an artificially biased result that males are more often diagnosed. Numerous studies have been performed to address this potential referral bias. For example, in a large prospective cohort of children (N = 32,223), boys were twice as likely as girls to have a reading disability irrespective of race, severity of disability, or exclusion of children with high activity levels or attentional disturbances (Flannery, Liederman, Daly, & Schultz, 2000). Similarly, using a population-based retrospective birth cohort study (N = 5,718) and four different research criteria for establishing a reading disability (two regression-based discrepancy, one nonregression-based discrepancy, and one low achievement), boys were still found to be two to three times more likely to be affected than girls, regardless of the assessment method applied (Katusic, Colligan, Barbaresi, Schaid, & Jacobson, 2001).

In view of the lack of knowledge about the underlying etiology of dyslexia and the reliance on imposed behavioral criteria for diagnosis, this debate is likely to continue for some time. The suggested sex difference is intriguing, given observational evidence that the focal anomalies in the brains of male and female dyslexics differ (i.e., males tend to develop microgyria and ectopia while females tend to develop glial scarring and few ectopias) (see Beaton, 1997). Moreover, the evidence of putative sex differences in language disability, and the development of an animal model linking focal cortical malformations and auditory processing deficits, specifically in male rats, allows for the question of sex differences in dyslexia and language impairment to be empirically addressed.

POSTMORTEM ANALYSIS OF DYSLEXIC BRAINS

Postmortem analysis of the brains of dyslexic individuals, some having suggested developmental language complications, has revealed the presence of neural anomalies. These include cortical anomalies (i.e., microgyria, ectopias, glial scaring) reflecting, in turn, complications in early neural migration presumably occurring around the sixth month of fetal life (Galaburda, Sherman, Rosen, Aboitiz, & Geschwind, 1985; Humphreys, Kaufmann, & Galaburda, 1990). Interestingly, this time period has been identified as the beginning of a critical or sensitive period of phonologic language development that extends through the 12th month of infancy, which is dependant on a model of central auditory nervous system flexibility (Ruben, 1997).

As stated above, observational evidence suggests that the nature of these cortical anomalies appear to show a sex difference with males having the tendency to develop microgyria or ectopias, and females to develop glial scarring (Beaton, 1997). The anomalies are, however, seen in similar cortical regions across the sexes (heavily concentrated around the perisylvian regions of the left hemisphere), at least in the small sample to date. This phenomenon has lead some to propose that the sexes differ due to females' faster neuronal maturation rate (Beaton, 1997). Specifically, it has been postulated that the as yet unknown causal factors of focal anomalies occur during a specific time frame, and that because the sexes may differ in rate of maturation, these factors may lead to different types of anomalies in males and females (Fitch, Miller, & Tallal, 1997b; Fitch et al., 1997a). Such an assertion could further contribute to the observation that fewer females than males are affected with dyslexia and language impairments (Gualtieri & Hicks, 1985).

Additional anatomical analyses of these same postmortem dyslexic brains focused on the lateral geniculate nucleus (LGN) and the medial geniculate nucleus (MGN) of the thalamus. Specifically, Livingstone, Rosen, Drislane, and Galaburda (1991) found that the LGN of dyslexics exhibited fewer large magnocellular cells and comparable numbers of small parvocellular cells as compared to controls. Magnocellular LGN cells are known to process quickly changing visual information, and dyslexics have been shown to have aberrant neural activation on tasks that depend on these magnocellular cells (Lovegrove, Garzia, & Nicholson, 1990; Livingstone et al., 1991). Galaburda, Menard, and Rosen (1994) found a similar pattern of morphological change in the MGN, with dyslexics showing a shift toward fewer large and more small cells when compared to control brains. These findings further establish a link between abnormal thalamic development and abnormal cortical development in dyslexics.

The abnormal thalamic development may be related to rapid temporal processing deficits seen in dyslexics and children with LLI. Since the postmortem studies of Galaburda and colleagues lack a large enough sample size, however, they could not empirically address any sex difference in morphology in either the LGN or MGN, nor the relation between these thalamic nuclei affects and the types of cortical anomalies seen. This remains an area for future research. Perhaps as precision and depth of neuroimaging techniques increase, the subsequently greater number of dyslexic individuals assessed for morphological differences and for functional differences in thalamic response will be able to shed more light on this sex difference debate and whether the magnocellular changes impact the behavior deficits seen in dyslexics.

ANIMAL MODELS LINKING BEHAVIORAL AND ANATOMICAL FEATURES OF LANGUAGE DISABILITY

Microgyria, Auditory Processing, and Thalamic Morphology in Rats

Following the discovery of cellular developmental anomalies in the brains of dyslexics, rodent models were developed to simulate these anomalies through perinatal intervention. For example, Humphreys, Rosen, Press, Sherman, and Galaburda (1991) found that focal freezing lesions on the skull of postnatal day 1 (P1) rats produced neocortical microgyria with striking histological similarity to those seen in dyslexic humans (see also Dvorák & Feit, 1977; Dvor·k, Feit, & Jurankova, 1978; Rosen, Press, Sherman, & Galaburda, 1992; see Galaburda, this volume). The next step in studying a potential neurobehavioral framework linking focal developmental anomalies with behavioral deficits was to assess the behavioral profile of subjects with these induced microgyria. Accordingly, Fitch, Tallal, Brown, Galaburda, and Rosen (1994) adapted an operant conditioning paradigm to test auditory processing in rats, training subjects to perform a target-identification of a two-tone sequence. The temporal parameters of the two-tone stimuli (i.e., total stimulus duration) were shortened across days of testing so that subjects were tested at long as well as short stimulus duration conditions. Results showed that microgyric male rats exhibited auditory processing deficits only at short stimulus durations (see Figure 1). This deficit was strikingly similar to that seen in children with LLI using a similar two-tone sequence discrimination task (Tallal & Piercy, 1973, 1974).

These results provided evidence of a link between a known neuropathological correlate of dyslexia and a known behavioral deficit associated with language disability. Moreover, the results contradict the notion that the effects occurred via direct (local) disruption of cortex (e.g., through local hyperexcitability associated with increased seizure activity as seen in slice studies of microgyric cortex; see Jacobs, Gutnick, & Prince, 1996; Jacobs, Hwang, & Prince, 1999; Zsombok & Jacobs, this volume). Indeed, many colleagues and reviewers have expressed surprise over the fact that

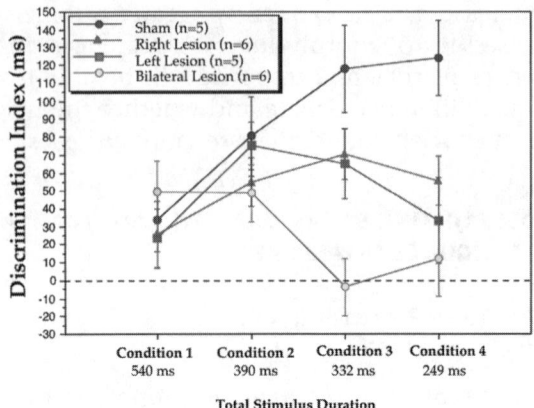

Figure 1. Discrimination indices for sham and microgyric rats tested in a two-tone sequence target identification task as a function of treatment group and total stimulus duration. For Discrimination Indices, zero represents chance while positive values reflect discrimination of the target. From Fitch et al. (1994).

focal freezing lesions were induced in primary sensory-motor cortex (SM-I)—not temporal cortex—and that these SM-I lesions somehow led to rate-specific auditory processing deficits. Interestingly, it has been shown in multiple studies that bilateral P1 freezing lesions placed in the sensory-motor, occipital, and frontal cortices of male rats all lead to significant auditory processing deficits in adulthood (Herman, Galaburda, Fitch, Carter, and Rosen, 1997; see also Clark, Rosen, Tallal, & Fitch, 2000b). Moreover, in these same studies, male rats with neonatally induced microgyria also exhibited morphological changes in the medial geniculate nucleus (MGN)—specifically, a significant shift toward more smaller and fewer large cells (Herman et al., 1997)—much like that seen in the MGN of human dyslexic brains (Galaburda, Menard, & Rosen, 1994). Again, this effect was seen regardless of focal lesion location in cortex.

In sum, these collective results support the view that developmental focal damage of the male rat cortex exerts pervasive reorganizational effects, which ultimately may be associated with anomalies in auditory thalamic (MGN) morphology. The mechanisms underlying this effect may involve developmental propagation from disrupted cortex to the thalamus, potentially via descending projections that develop postnatally in rodents (e.g., Miller, Chou, & Finlay, 1993; see also Goldman-Rakic & Rakic,

1978; Schneider, 1981; Rosen, Burstein, & Galaburda, 2000). These MGN anomalies, in turn, appear to be associated with severely deleterious effects on auditory processing of stimuli that incorporate rapid sequential change. In language-disabled humans, similar anatomical and behavioral effects are seen. We can hypothesize that anatomically based defects in auditory processing may exert cascading effects on phonological perception and, potentially, the development of language and reading skills (see Fitch et al., 1997; Fitch, Read, & Benasich, 2000, for further discussion).

More recently, the above rodent model has been adapted to an acoustic startle reduction (reflex modification) paradigm. The startle reduction paradigm does not require motivation or attention, and data can be collected from the first day of testing (e.g., Wecker, Ison, & Foss, 1985). This paradigm utilizes a loud (105–110 dB) 50 ms burst of white noise, presented at random intervals and unpredictable to the subject (see Hoffman & Ison, 1980; Ison & Hoffman, 1983, for reviews). When the noise bursts are presented, large amplitude motor responses (startle responses) occur. These movements are measured by placing subjects on load-sensing platforms, which transduce and transmit movement information that can be recorded, quantified, and analyzed. In a simple version of the acoustic startle paradigm, some trials include a 75 dB pre-pulse cue (such as a tone) that immediately precedes the noise burst. If the pre-pulse stimulus (or cue) is detected, this cue produces a significant attenuation of the startle response on that trial (i.e., startle reduction or reflex modification). More complex versions of this paradigm include the presentation of a silent gap embedded in low-level background white noise as the pre-pulse cue (e.g., Ison, 1982; Ison & Pinckney, 1983; Ison, O'Connor, Bowen, & Bocirnea, 1991; Leitner et al., 1993). Response attenuation data can then be analyzed to provide an index of pre-pulse stimulus detectability. The startle reduction paradigm has also been adapted to incorporate a repeating background of two-tone sequences, paired with the presentation of a reverse sequence (oddball) immediately before the noise burst on cued trials. Such a format derives from the oddball stimulus presentation design used in electrophysiological research (e.g., Kraus et al., 1994; Clark, Rosen, Tallal, & Fitch, 2000a). Assessment of sham and microgyric males rats using this paradigm showed: (1) a highly significant reduction in subjects' startle response on cued (oddball) trials for both groups using a two-tone sequence separated by 350 ms (indicating that all subjects were able to detect the oddball [deviant] two-tone sequence as different from the background two-tone sequence); and (2) significant sham/microgyric differences for stimuli of total duration less than 89 ms (with microgyric males showing significantly less response attenuation for "short" duration stimuli) (see Figure 2; Clark et al., 2000a).

Since identical acoustic stimuli were used in both the operant target ID auditory discrimination task and the startle reduction paradigm, a comparison could be made between the stimulus properties that elicited processing deficits in microgyric animals as a function of these different test paradigms. This provides an important comparison because the operant task is a fairly demanding task that requires subjects to learn a target, listen to a stimulus, make a comparison, and then determine if that stimulus is the subject's target. The startle reduction paradigm, in contrast, requires only the passive recognition of a stimulus change and is thus considerably less demanding. Interestingly, while two-tone sequences of 249 ms duration have been found to elicit highly significant processing deficits in microgyric animals in the operant paradigm, the startle reduction paradigm (in which the same tone sequences were presented but in a passive oddball detection format) showed that only tone sequences shorter than 89 ms total duration would elicit response differences between control and microgyric animals. This suggests, in turn, that cognitive demand or "load" may interact, in some fashion, with basic auditory processing deficits evidenced in the microgyric group. The notion of parallel (and possibly interactive) deficits in auditory processing and, for example, working memory, is discussed further below.

As an aside, Clark, Tallal, Rosen, Peiffer, and Fitch (2000c) also tested synthetic speech processing in sham and microgyric male rats.

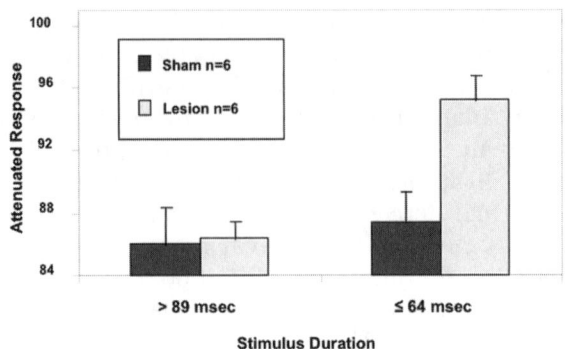

Figure 2. Attenuated startle response as a function of stimulus duration for sham and microgyric male rats (from Clark et al., 2000a). Responses at/near 100% indicate lack of stimulus discrimination.

Preliminary results showed that: 1) neither group exhibited significant discrimination of the synthetic syllables /da/ versus /ga/ on any day; but 2) microgyric subjects were significantly impaired relative to shams in the discrimination of /ba/ from /wa/ on day 1 of testing. The latter stimuli are discriminable based solely on differences in the duration of formant transitions. These preliminary findings have also been replicated in young (P20–35) sham and microgyric male rats (Thomas, Clark, Benasich, & Fitch, 2001). Such findings further support the relationship between malformations of the cerebral cortex and deficits in rapid auditory and speech processing, and validate the continued assessment of the behavioral consequences of cerebrocortical microgyria in the rat as a tool in understanding the etiology of developmental language disabilities.

More recently, we have used the startle reduction auditory discrimination paradigm to explore additional features of the association between focal anomalies and auditory processing deficits in rodents. For example, we have found that deficits are typically more pronounced in juvenile as compared to adult subjects, at least for simpler versions of auditory discrimination tasks such as silent gap detection (Peiffer, Friedman, Rosen, & Fitch, 2004a) (see Figure 3). Moreover, additional cortical damage as induced through increased number of bilateral microgyria is associated with more severe auditory processing deficits in adult male rats as compared to single-pair microgyria (Peiffer, McClure, Threlkeld, Rosen, & Fitch, 2004b) (see Figure 4).

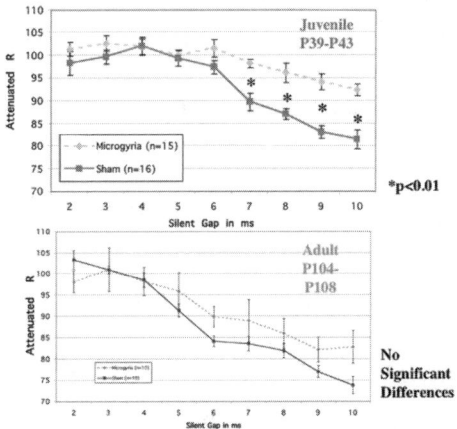

Figure 3. Silent gap detection indices for juvenile and adult sham and microgyric male rats. From Peiffer et al., 2004a.

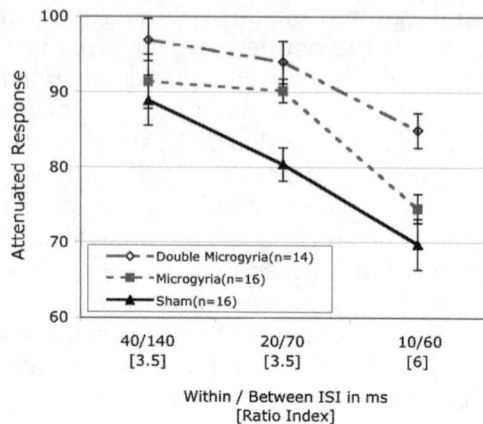

Figure 4. Oddball two-tone sequence results for adult male rats with single-pair or double-pair bilateral microgyria or shams, as a function of within and between stimulus ISI durations. Adapted from Peiffer et al., 2004b.

These results will have critical implications for our understanding of the etiology that underlies the association between early disruption of brain development, auditory processing deficits, and subsequent disruptions of language development in human populations.

Auditory Processing Deficits in Ectopic Mice

Studies have also been performed to examine auditory processing in mice that exhibit spontaneously forming focal malformations of cortex (ectopias). Specifically, in certain strains of mice (including NZB/BlNJ, NXSM-D/Ei, and BXSB/MpJ), neocortical ectopias (mushroom-like clusters of misplaced neurons in layer I of cortex) spontaneously occur (Sherman, Galaburda, & Geschwind, 1985; Sherman, Galaburda, Behan, & Rosen, 1987; Sherman, Morrison, Rosen, Behan, & Galaburda, 1990a). These spontaneous neocortical anomalies are histologically similar to those found in the postmortem analysis of dyslexic human brains (Galaburda et al., 1985). Consequently, these mice have been proposed and studied as animal models of learning disabilities, including developmental dyslexia (Galaburda, Menard, & Rosen, 1994; Galaburda, Schrott, Sherman, Rosen, & Denenberg, 1996; Sherman, Galaburda, & Geschwind, 1985). Although NZB/BlNJ and BXSB/MpJ are autoimmune, embryo transfer studies have indicated that the incidence of ectopias is not a function of the intrauterine autoimmune environment of the dam (Denenberg, Sherman, Schrott, Rosen, & Galaburda, 1991; Denenberg et al., 1992, 1996). Genetic analysis has determined that the predisposition to develop ectopias is a polygenetic trait inherited in an autosomal recessive fashion (Sherman, Stone, Denenberg, & Beier, 1994).

In mice, ectopias are formed between embryonic day 12 and 15, and are thought to be the result of abnormal neuronal migration (Sherman, Rosen, Stone, Press, & Galaburda, 1992a; Sherman, Stone, Press, Rosen, & Galaburda, 1990b). Ectopias are characterized by a ruptured pia-glial limiting membrane, and are associated with densely packed neurofilament axon bundles and radial glial fibers (Sherman et al., 1992a). Frequently, dysplasia—defined as an extensive disruption of the normal lamination of the cortical layers below the ectopia—is also evident (Sherman et al., 1992a, 1990b). The presence of highly localized excitotoxic dendritic damage within the ectopia is suggested by ultra-structural analyses (Boehm et al., 1995). Several types of neurons have been identified within the ectopia, and these neurons receive direct inhibitory and excitatory inputs from the surrounding normatopic cortex (Gabel & LoTurco, 2001). The ectopia shows altered connections with other parts of cortex, as well as the thalamus (Jenner, Galaburda, & Sherman, 2000). Further, ectopic mice show a morphological cell size distribution shift to more small and fewer large cells in the MGN (NZB/BlNJ and NXSM-D/Ei—Jenner, Galaburda, & Sherman, 2000; BXSB/MpJ—Sherman, Hinton, & Galaburda, 1998).

Ectopias spontaneously occur in roughly 40%–60% of these particular mouse strains. BXSB/MpJ mice typically develop ectopias in prefrontal and/or motor regions of cortex, while NZB/BlNJ mice typically develop ectopias in somatosensory cortex (Sherman, Galaburda, & Geschwind, 1985; Sherman et al., 1987; Sherman et al., 1990a). Since ectopias form during development and alter structures in the brain where they are found, they might be expected to affect adult behavior. In fact, results show clear evidence of auditory processing deficits similar to those seen in the microgyric rat model and in ectopic subjects of both the BXSB/MpJ and NZB/B1NJ mouse strains.

In the case of BXSBs, ectopic male mice were found to be significantly worse than nonectopics in detecting the shortest detectable silent gap presented in a background of white noise (Clark, Sherman, Bimonte, & Fitch, 2000d) (see Figure 5). These behavioral data were paralleled by auditory evoked response potential (AERP) data from adult male BXSB mice. AERP results showed that ectopic male BXSB had a smaller negative deflection

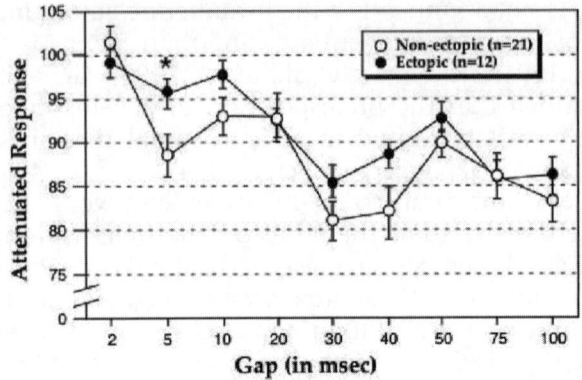

Figure 5. Attenuated startle response (vertical axis) as a function of gap duration (horizontal axis) for ectopic and nonectopic BXSB mice. Responses at or near 100% indicate lack of discrimination of the stimulus. The * indicates a significant difference between ectopics and controls for the 5 ms gap (from Clark et al., 2000d).

for the onset of a second acoustic stimulus following a short, but not long, inserted tone (Frenkel, Sherman, Bashan, Galalburda, & LoTurco, 2000). Interestingly, a similar result was found for dyslexic as compared to control adults using MEG (Nagarajan et al., 1999). Moreover, ectopic NZB/BlNJ male mice demonstrated evidence of impaired auditory processing as compared to nonectopics for short duration stimuli, and again, AERP recordings from a subset of these same animals confirmed that ectopic subjects displayed a reduced negative deflection to the onset of a second acoustic stimulus following a short, but not long, inserted tone (Peiffer et al., 2001) (Figure 6).

Cognitive and Memory Effects in Ectopic Mice

Data obtained by Denenberg and colleagues have also shown differential patterns of learning and memory for ectopic as compared to nonectopic mice of the BXSB/MpJ and NZB/BlNJ strains (Balogh, Sherman, Hyde, & Denenberg, 1998; Boehm, Sherman, Rosen, Galaburda, & Denenberg, 1996a; Boehm et al., 1996b; Denenberg et al., 1991, 1996; Hyde, Sherman, & Denenberg, 2000; Hyde, Sherman, Hoplight, & Denenberg, 2000; Schrott et al., 1992). In this important series of studies, Denenberg & colleagues showed that the presence of cortical ectopias has a significant impact on learning and memory measures in both strains of mice that were studied. These effects include (1) a significant working

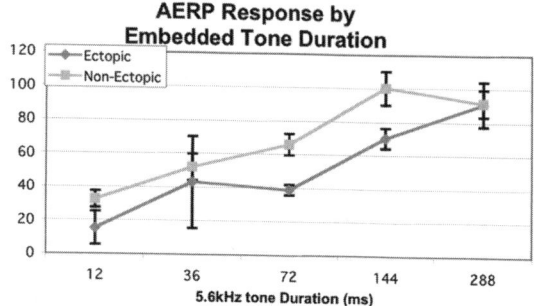

Figure 6. Ratio of peak AERP to first and second onsets of 10.5 KHz tone (A2/A1 X 100, vertical axis), with an inserted 5 KHz tone of variable duration (horizontal axis). Data from ectopic and nonectopic NZB mice. Results show that groups were the same at long durations (288 ms), whereas at shorter durations (144 and 72 ms), NZB ectopics respond significantly less to the second onset than NZB nonectopics. A2=AERP amplitude to second onset; A1=AERP amplitude to first onset (from Peiffer et al., 2001).

memory deficit associated with the presence of ectopias in frontal cortex, and (2) a reference memory deficit associated with ectopias in SM-I. Interestingly, evidence of potential enhancements in reference memory are also seen to be associated with frontal cortical ectopias (e.g., Hyde, Sherman, & Denenberg, 2000; Hyde, Sherman, Hoplight, & Denenberg, 2000).

Thus, ectopia effects on learning and memory processes appear to be more sensitive to cortical ectopia location, (i.e., effects differ for the two strains studied, with effects of frontal versus SM-I ectopias on learning/memory being quite different). This location sensitivity contrasts directly with the location-insensitive effects of cortical malformations on auditory processing deficits, and suggests that different neurodevelopmental pathways may underlie these effects. It has been suggested, for example, that working memory deficits associated with frontal ectopias might be mediated through local alterations in cortical circuitry (e.g., see Gabel & LoTurco, 2001). Auditory deficits associated with these malformations, on the other hand, are more likely the result of reorganizational changes at the thalamic level initiated by cortical malformations, and appear to be insensitive to cortical lesion location (e.g., Herman et al., 1997). In addition, ectopic effects on auditory processing appear to be sensitive to the effects of sex, with deficits seen in males but not females (e.g., Peiffer, Rosen, & Fitch, 2002; see further discussion below), while learning and memory effects of ectopias on mice are apparently insensitive to the effects of sex (Balogh et al., 1998; Boehm et al., 1996a, 1996b; Denenberg et al., 1991, 1996; Hyde, Sherman, Hoplight, & Denenberg, 2000; Hyde et al., 2000; Schrott et al., 1992).

Sex Differences in the Behavioral and Morphological Consequences of Focal Cortical Anomalies in Animal Models

As noted above, Humphreys, Kaufmann, and Galaburda (1990) assessed the postmortem brains of three dyslexic women, and suggested that the anomalies characterizing dyslexic female brains may differ from those seen in dyslexic males. Although the sample size was too small to empirically assess the sex difference, considerable related data supports the existence of fundamental sex differences in brain organization and development (Bachevalier, Brickson, Hagger, & Mishkin, 1990; Bachevalier & Hagger, 1991; Beatty, 1992; Breedlove, 1992; Clark & Goldman-Rakic, 1989; Fitch, Brown, & Tallal, 1993; Kimura & Harshman, 1984; Kulynych, Vladar, Jones, & Weinberger, 1994; McGlone, 1980; Raz, Lauterbach, Hopkins, Glogowski, & Porter, 1995; Shaywitz et al., 1995). In order to address potential sex differences in response to early brain injury, the Fitch et al. (1994) operant study was repeated using both male and female rats with P1 bilateral freezing lesions of SM-I, or sham surgery. A substantial sex difference was found. Behavioral deficits at rapid rates of stimulus presentation were replicated in males but were not seen in females. Female rats with induced microgyria showed no deficits in auditory discrimination performance at any condition (Fitch et al., 1997a). Subsequent anatomical analyses found that lesioned females also had no aberrant morphology of the medial geniculate nucleus (MGN), although male littermates with identical cortical lesions did show significant changes in the distribution of cell size within the MGN (Herman et al., 1997). Subsequent analyses of the MGN in microgyric male, female, and testosterone-treated female rats revealed that these sex effects appear to be mediated by interactions between response to early injury and exposure to testosterone (Rosen, Herman, & Galaburda, 1999). These behavioral results have subsequently been replicated for adult male and female microgyric rats using the startle reduction paradigm described above (Peiffer, Rosen, & Fitch, 2004c) (see Figure 7).

In addition, analyses of BXSB/MpJ mice have revealed sex differences in the behavioral consequence of spontaneously occurring ectopias. Specifically, when BXSB/MpJ mice were tested with

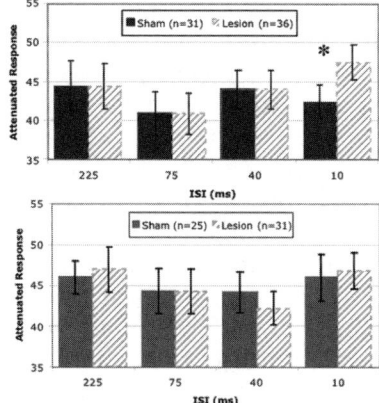

Figure 7. Auditory discrimination indices for male and female sham and microgyric rats as a function of interstimulus interval duration. From Peiffer et al., 2004c.

the oddball reflex modification procedure used in the Clark et al. study (2000a), male but not female ectopic mice were impaired at detecting the two-tone oddball sequence with short (40 and 10 ms) but not long (225 and 75 ms) duration ISI when compared to nonectopic littermates (Peiffer et al., 2002) (Figure 8). Therefore, in addition to the cross-species temporal consistency of the impairment (i.e., being seen at short but not long durations), there appears to be a consistent impairment for male but not female rodents with cortical anomalies, even though the amount of damage is consistent between the sexes.

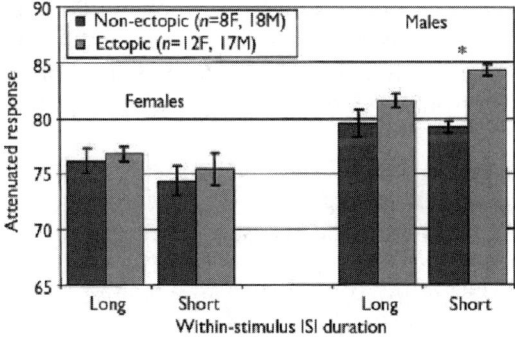

Figure 8. Auditory discrimination indices for long and short duration stimuli, for ectopic and nonectopic male and female mice. From Peiffer et al., 2002.

The factors underlying a female advantage in response to focal developmental cortical damage remain unclear. However, we have previously reported a sex difference in functional organization of the rat brain, with males exhibiting greater asymmetry than females for rapid auditory processing (Fitch et al., 1993). In humans, sex differences in language recovery following left-hemisphere damage have been consistently observed, with females showing significantly better recovery (McGlone, 1980). Sex differences in the magnitude of the right ear advantage (REA) for the discrimination of verbal material have also been reported, with males showing a larger and more consistent REA (Kimura & Harshman, 1984). Sex differences have been reported in the pattern of cerebral blood flow during the performance of verbal tasks (Wood, Flowers, & Naylor, 1991), in asymmetry as measured by fMRI during verbal tasks (Shaywitz et al., 1995), and in structural asymmetry of the right and left plenum temporale as measured by MRI (Kulynych et al., 1994). These results all support the notion of sex differences in the pattern of cerebral organization, particularly for language related functions. Such findings speak in turn to a possible hormonal role in establishing cerebral organization of language functions, and possibly in mediating behavioral response to focal injury (see Lambe, 1999, for discussion). Animal studies support this assertion by demonstrating hormonally mediated differences in the maturation rate of specific cortical regions, which in turn, critically influence the behavioral effects of lesioning these regions (e.g., Bachevalier et al., 1990; Bachevalier & Hagger, 1991; Clark & Goldman-Rakic, 1989; Kolb & Cioe, 1996). Geschwind and Galaburda (1985) postulated that differential androgen exposure *in utero* may influence the development of cerebral organization, particularly for language, and further suggested that exposure to androgens may render the male brain more susceptible to adverse effects following developmental injury. Other studies suggest that female hormones may protect the brain from the deleterious consequences of cortical damage (e.g., see Roof, Duvdevani, & Stein, 1993).

It is possible that sex differences in early hormonal exposure, neural maturation, brain organization, and response to focal brain injury may relate to our reported sex difference in behavioral and morphological defects in response to P1 cortical injury (Fitch, Brown, Tallal, & Rosen, 1997a). These collective data may further relate to reports of a higher incidence of language and reading impairments among males as compared to females (Finucci & Childs, 1983; Flannery & Liederman, 1996; Flannery, Liederman, Daly, & Schultz, 2000; Gualtieri & Hicks, 1985; Liederman & Flannery, 1995; Niels & Aram, 1986).

MECHANISMS OF CORTICAL EFFECTS ON AUDITORY PROCESSING

As can be seen in both postmortem analysis of human brains and rodent models, focal cortical anomalies co-occur with structural changes in thalamic nuclei as well as associated auditory processing deficits. An auditory processing impairment could be related to the change in MGN cell size distribution (i.e., decrease in the number of large cells). However, how does a P1 freezing lesion to cortex affect MGN morphology? It has been proposed that a top-down propagation of reorganization, which affects the thalamus along with other brain areas, is somehow triggered by the insult that produces the focal cortical anomaly itself (i.e., cerebrocortical microgyria) (Galaburda, Menard, & Rosen, 1994). In support of this hypothesis, Herman et al. (1997; Rosen, Herman, & Galaburda, 1999) argue that the relationship between microgyria and MGN cell size could not be explained by direct damage to the thalamus, or to cortical structures directly overlaying the thalamus. Herman et al. (1997) further suggest that connectional changes resulting from early focal injury to developing cortex may link cortical anomalies and changes in thalamic nuclei's cell size distribution. These early freezing lesions may disrupt the formation of afferent and efferent connections associated with damaged cortex (Goldman & Galkin, 1978), and lead to the maintenance of otherwise transient developmental connections (Innocenti & Berbel, 1991).

Moreover, evidence of abnormal cortico-cortical connections formed in association with microgyria exists, along with evidence of a disruption in thalamic connections directly to the cortical anomaly (Rosen, Burstein, & Galaburda, 2000). Based on the timing of the injury and the state of the developing cortical plate, the specific connectivity changes associated with the presence of a microgyria include the following: (1) increased heterotopic contralateral connections to frontal and secondary sensorimotor cortex as compared to controls; (2) homologous contralateral projections, when present, are less dense than those in control animals; (3) efferent projections from the homotopic region of the opposite hemisphere that terminate in the medial portion of the malformation (if it enters it at all); (4) almost no thalamocortical or corticothalamic projections between the cortical region with the malformation (Primary Parietal cortex, or Par1) and the ventrobasal complex; and (5) a dense plexus of thalamocortical fibers often seen at the border of the malformation and normal cortex (Rosen, Burstein, & Galaburda, 2000). Giannetti, Gaglini, Granato, and DiRocco (1999) also showed that following induction of microgyria in frontal cortex, the laminar distribution of callosal neurons in normal cortex near the lesion moves so that the greatest majority of projections originate in layer VI instead of II/III and V, as seen in control animals. When the ipsilateral corticocortical connections traveling across the frontal cortex were studied, Giannetti, Gaglini, Di Rocco, Di Rocco, and Granato (2000) observed that origination of projections was limited to infragranular layers when running through a microgyric zone, but arose in supragranular and infragranular layers in controls. These cortical changes may impact the flexibility of the central auditory nervous system and subsequent processing of both verbal and nonverbal auditory information.

DISCUSSION AND CONCLUSIONS

Human clinical data strongly support a relationship between basic processing defects for the discrimination of rapidly changing acoustic stimuli, and subsequent emergence of disruptions in language acquisition and development. Parallel research suggests that disabilities of reading may be related to focal cortical anomalies that arise at the time of neuronal migration to the cortex. Our research has made use of rodent models to link these behavioral and anatomical correlates of language disability, and our studies have demonstrated a clear relationship between the presence of a focal cortical malformation and disruptions in rapid auditory processing. Evidence also shows that these behavioral effects are more pronounced in juvenile as compared to adult subjects, and are seen primarily for males not females. Finally, despite evidence that an increase in the number of focal anomalies of cortex is associated with more severe behavioral deficits, data also suggest that focal cortical disruption per se is probably not the sole causal candidate for behavioral effects since the location of the anomaly does not appear to affect the emergence of auditory processing deficits (either in rats or mice), even though such location-based effects are evidently seen in behavioral consequences for learning and memory deficits (thus suggesting two separate mechanisms mediating auditory versus learning and memory deficits associated with focal malformations) (see Figure 9).

Convergent findings suggest that behavioral effects are at least, in part, the consequence of pervasive organizational changes triggered by the initial focal injury, an interpretation consistent with evidence of thalamic disruptions in both dyslexic human brains and male microgyric rats. Combined evidence supports a view that despite limitations in the study of language deficits in a

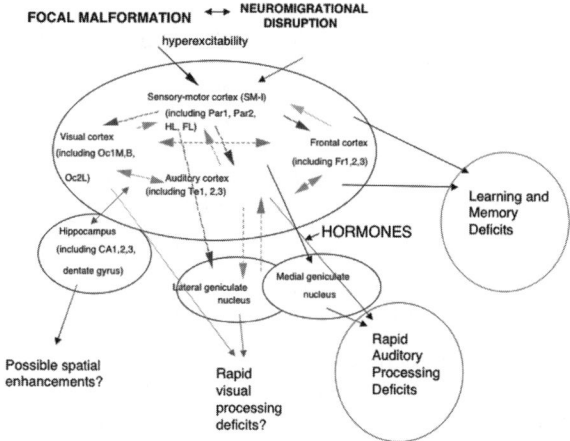

Figure 9. Schematic diagram illustrating possible pathways relating focal neurodevelopmental disruptions to behavioral deficits, which may in turn relate (in humans) to disruption of language. Figure 9 summarizes, in schematic form, data discussed throughout the current chapter and book. 1) Alterations in MGN morphology and rapid auditory processing, as well as 2) alterations in learning and memory, have been established in rodent models of focal cortical anomalies. These deficits may, in humans, disrupt the ability to aquire fundamental components of language, and thus exert secondary (or primary) effects on the acquisition of reading. 3) Evidence of spatial enhancements in rodents with focal malformation is reviewed here, but the physiological basis (and possible human expression) of such enhancements is not established. 4) Alterations in LGN morphology and rapid visual processing have been shown in human dyslexic populations, and will be studied in animal models in future research.

nonhuman model, a rodent model can provide useful insights into the etiology that may underlie at least some disruptions of language in humans.

Address correspondence to: R. Holly Fitch, Ph.D., Department of Psychology, Division of Behavioral Neuroscience, University of Connecticut, Unit 4154, Storrs, CT 06269; Phone: 860/486-2554, Fax: 860/486-3827

REFERENCES

Ahissar, M., Protopapas, A., Reid, M., & Merzenich, M. M. (2000). Auditory processing parallels reading abilities in adults. *PNAS, 97*, 6832–6837.

Bachevalier, J., Brickson, M., Hagger, C., & Mishkin, M. (1990). Age and sex differences in the effects of selective temporal lobe lesions on the formation of visual discrimination habits in rhesus monkeys (Macaca mulatta). *Behavioural Neuroscience, 6,* 885–889.

Bachevalier, J., & Hagger, C. (1991). Sex differences in the development of learning abilities in primates. *Psychoneuroendocrinology, 16,* 177–188.

Badcock, D., & Lovegrove, W. (1981). The effects of contrast, stimulus duration, and spatial frequency on visible persistence in normal and specifically disabled readers. *Journal of Experimental Psychology: Human Perception & Performance, 7,* 495–505.

Balogh, S. A., Sherman, G. F., Hyde, L. A., & Denenberg, V. H. (1998). Effects of neocortical ectopias upon the acquisition and retention of a non-spatial reference memory task in BXSB mice. *Brain Development and Developmental Brain Research, 111,* 291–293.

Beaton, A. A. (1997). The relation of planum temporale asymmetry and morphology of the corpus callosum to handedness, gender, and dyslexia: A review of the evidence. *Brain and Langage, 60,* 255–322.

Beatty, W. (1992). Gonadal hormones and sex differences in nonreproductive behaviors. In A. A. Gerall, H. Moltz, & I. L. Ward (Eds.), *Handbook of behavioral neurobiology* (pp. 85–128) New York: Plenum.

Beitchman, J. H., & Inglis, A. (1991). The continuum of linguistic dysfunction from pervasive developmental disorders to dyslexia. *Psychiatric Clinics of North America, 14,* 95–111.

Beitchman, J. H., Nair, R., Clegg, M., Patel, P. G., Ferguson, B., Pressman, E., & Smith, A. (1986). Prevalence of speech and language disorders in 5-year-old kindergarten children in the Ottawa-Carleton region. *Journal of Speech and Hearing Disorders, 51,* 98–110.

Benasich, A. A., & Tallal, P. (1996). Auditory temporal processing thresholds, habituation, and recognition memory over the first year. *Infant Behavior and Development, 19,* 339–357.

Benasich, A. A., Thomas, J. J., Choudhury, N., & Leppänen, P. H. (2002). The importance of rapid auditory processing abilities to early language development: Evidence from converging methodologies. *Developmental Psychobiology, 40,* 278–292.

Boehm, G. W., Goss, M. W., Seaman, A. J., Galaburda, A. M., Denenberg, V. H., & Sherman, G. F. (1995). Ultrastructural analysis of neocortical ectopias in NXSM-D recombinant inbred mice. *Society for Neuroscience Abstracts, 21,* 1712.

Boehm, G. W., Sherman, G. F., Hoplight, B. J., 2nd, Hyde, L. A., Waters, N. S., Bradway, D. M., Galaburda, A. M., & Denenberg, V. H. (1996b). Learning and memory in the autoimmune BXSB mouse: Effects of neocortical ectopias and environmental enrichment. *Brain Research, 726,* 11–22.

Boehm, G. W., Sherman, G. F., Rosen, G. D., Galaburda, A. M., & Denenberg, V. H. (1996a). Neocortical ectopias in BXSB mice: Effects upon reference and working memory systems. *Cerebral Cortex, 6,* 696–700.

Breedlove, S. M. (1992). Sexual differentiation of the brain and behavior. In J. B. Becker, S. M. Breedlove, & D. Crews (Eds.), *Behavioral endocrinology* (pp. 39–68). Cambridge, MA: MIT Press.

Campbell, T. F., Dollaghan, C. A., Rockette, H. E., Paradise, J. L., Feldman, H. M., Shriberg, L. D., Sabo, D. L., & Kurs-Lasky, M. (2003). Risk factors

for speech delay of unknown origin in 3-year-old children. *Child Development, 74*, 346–357.
Catts, H. W., Fey, M. E., Tomblin, J. B., & Zhang, X. (2002). A longitudinal investigation of reading outcomes in children with language impairments. *Journal of Speech and Language Hearing Research, 45*, 1142.
Clark, A. S., & Goldman-Rakic, P. S. (1989). Gonadal hormones influence the emergence of cortical function in nonhuman primates. *Behavioral Neuroscience, 103*, 1287–1295.
Clark, M. G., Rosen, G. D., Tallal, P., & Fitch, R. H. (2000a). Impaired processing of complex auditory stimuli in rats with induced cerebro-cortical microgyria: An animal model of developmental language disabilities. *Journal of Cognitive Neuroscience, 12*, 828–839.
Clark, M. G., Rosen, G. D., Tallal, P., & Fitch, R. H. (2000b). Impaired two-tone processing at rapid rates in male rats with induced microgyria. *Brain Research, 871*, 94–97.
Clark, M. G., Tallal, P., Rosen, G. D., Peiffer, A. M., & Fitch, R. H. (2000c). Impaired perception of speech stimuli in rats with induced microgyria. *Society for Neuroscience Abstracts, 26*, 30.12.
Clark, M. G., Sherman, G. F., Bimonte, H. A., & Fitch, R. H. (2000d). Perceptual auditory gap detection deficits in ectopic male BXSB mice. *NeuroReport, 11*, 693–696.
De Weirdt, W. (1988). Speech perception and frequency discrimination in good and poor readers. *Applied Psycholinguistics, 9*, 163–183.
Denenberg, V. H., Sherman, G. F., Morrison, L., Schrott, L. M., Waters, N. S., Rosen, G. D., Behan, P. O., & Galaburda, A. M. (1992). Behavior, ectopias and immunity in BD/DB reciprocal crosses. *Brain Research, 571*, 323–329.
Denenberg, V. H., Sherman, G. F., Schrott, L. M., Rosen, G. D., & Galaburda, A. M. (1991). Spatial learning, discrimination learning, paw preference and neocortical ectopias in two autoimmune strains of mice. *Brain Research, 562*, 98–104.
Denenberg, V. H., Sherman, G., Schrott, L. M., Waters, N. S., Boehm, G. W., Galaburda, A. M., & Mobraaten, L. E. (1996). Effects of embryo transfer and cortical ectopias upon the behavior of BXSB-Yaa and BXSB-Yaa plus mice. *Developmental Brain Research, 93*, 100–108.
DiLollo, V., Hanson, D., & McIntyre, J. S. (1983). Initial stages of visual information processing in dyslexics. *Journal of Experimental Psychology: Human Perception & Performance, 9*, 923–935.
Duffy, F. H., McAnulty, G. B., & Waber, D. P. (1999). Auditory evoked responses to single tones and closely spaced tone pairs in children grouped by reading or matrices abilities. *Clinical Electroencephalography, 30*(3), 84–93.
Dvorák, K., & Feit, J. (1977). Migration of neuroblasts through partial necrosis of the cerebral cortex in newborn rats-contribution to the problems of morphological development and developmental period of cerebral microgyria. Histological and autoradiographical study. *Acta Neuropathology (Berlin), 38*(3), 203–212.
Dvorák, K., Feit, J., & Jurankova, Z. (1978). Experimentally induced focal microgyria and status verrucosus deformis in rats—pathogenesis and interrelation. Histological and autoradiographical study. *Acta Neuropathology (Berlin), 44*(2), 121–129.

Edwards, J., & Lahey, M. (1996). Auditory lexical decisions of children with specific language impairment. *Journal of Speech and Hearing Research, 39*(6), 1263–1273.

Farmer, M. E., & Klein, R. M. (1995). The evidence for a temporal processing deficit linked to dyslexia: A review. *Psychonomic Bulletin and Review, 2*(4), 460–493.

Finucci, J. M., & Childs, B. (1983). Dyslexia: Family studies. In C. Ludlow and J. A. Cooper (Eds.), *Genetic aspects of speech and language disorders.* New York: Academic Press.

Finucci, J. M., Isaacs, S. D., Whitehouse, C. C., & Childs, B. (1983). Classification of spelling errors and their relationship to reading ability, sex, grade placement, and intelligence. *Brain and Language, 20*(2), 340–355.

Fitch, R. H., Brown, C., & Tallal, P. (1993). Functional lateralization for auditory temporal processing in male and female rats. *Behavioral Neuroscience, 107,* 844–850.

Fitch, R. H., Brown, C. P., Tallal, P., & Rosen, G. D. (1997a). Effects of sex and MK-801 on auditory-processing deficits associated with developmental microgyric lesions in rats. *Behavioral Neuroscience, 111*(2), 404–412.

Fitch, R. H., Miller, S., & Tallal, P. (1997b). Neurobiology of speech perception. *Annual Review of Neuroscience 20,* 331–353.

Fitch, R. H., Read, H. L., & Benasich, A. A. (2000). Neurophysiology of speech perception in normal and impaired systems. In A. F. Jahn & J. Santos-Sachi (Eds.), *Physiology of the ear.* San Diego, CA: Singular Publishing.

Fitch, R. H., Tallal, P., Brown, C. P., Galaburda, A. M., & Rosen, G. D. (1994). Induced microgyria and auditory temporal processing in rats: A model for language impairment? *Cerebral Cortex, 4,* 260–270.

Flannery, K. A., & Liederman, J. (1996). A re-examination of the sex ratios of families with neurodevelopmentally disordered child. *Journal of Child Psychology and Psychiatry, 37,* 621–623.

Flannery, K. A., Liederman, J., Daly, L., & Schultz, J. (2000). Male prevalence for reading disability is found in a large sample of black and white children free from ascertainment bias. *Journal of International Neuropsychology, 6*(4), 433–442.

Frenkel, M., Sherman, G. F., Bashan, K. A., Galaburda, A. M., & LoTurco, J. J. (2000). Neocortical ectopias are associated with attenuated neurophysiological responses to rapidly changing auditory stimuli. *NeuroReport, 11*(3), 575–579.

Gabel, L. A., & LoTurco, J. J. (2001). Electrophysiological and morphological characterization of neurons within neocortical ectopias. *Journal of Neurophysiology, 85*(2), 495–505.

Galaburda, A. M., Menard, M. T., & Rosen, G. D. (1994). Evidence for aberrant auditory anatomy in developmental dyslexia. *Proceedings of the National Academy of Science USA, 91*(17), 8010–8013.

Galaburda, A. M., Schrott, L. M., Sherman, G. F., Rosen, G. D., & Denenberg, V. H. (1996). Animal models of developmental dyslexia. In C. H. Chase, G. D. Rosen, & G. F. Sherman (Eds.), *Developmental dyslexia: Neural, cognitive, and genetic mechanisms* (pp. 3–14). Baltimore: York Press.

Galaburda, A. M., Sherman, G. F., Rosen, G. D., Aboitiz, F., & Geschwind, N. (1985). Developmental dyslexia: Four consecutive patients with cortical anomalies. *Annals of Neurology, 18*(2), 222–233.

Geschwind, N., & Galaburda, A. M. (1985). Cerebral lateralization. Biological mechanisms, associations, and pathology: I. A hypothesis and a program for research. *Archives of Neurology, 42*(5), 428–459.

Giannetti, S., Gaglini, P., Di Rocco, F., Di Rocco, C., & Granato, A. (2000). Organization of cortico-cortical associative projections in a rat model of microgyria. *NeuroReport, 11*, 2185–2189.

Giannetti, S., Gaglini, P., Granato, A., & Di Rocco, C. (1999). Organization of callosal connections in rats with experimentally induced microgyria. *Childs Nervous System, 15*, 444–448; discussion 449–450.

Goldman, P. S., & Galkin, T. W. (1978). Prenatal removal of frontal association cortex in the fetal rhesus monkey: Anatomical and functional consequences in postnatal life. *Brain Research, 152*, 451–485.

Gualtieri, T., & Hicks, R. E. (1985). An immunoreactive theory of selective male affliction. *Behavioral Brain Science, 8*, 427–441.

Heiervang, E., Stevenson, J., & Hugdahl, K. (2002). Auditory processing in children with dyslexia. *Journal of Child Psychology and Psychiatry, 43*(7), 931–938.

Herman, A. E., Galaburda, A. M., Fitch, R. H., Carter, A. R., & Rosen, G. D. (1997). Cerebral microgyria, thalamic cell size and auditory temporal processing in male and female rats. *Cerebral Cortex, 7*(5), 453–464.

Hoffman, H. S., & Ison, J. R. (1980). Reflex modification in the domain of startle: I. Some empirical findings and their implications for how the nervous system processes sensory input. *Psychological Review, 87*(2), 175–189.

Humphreys, P., Kaufmann, W. E., & Galaburda, A. M. (1990). Developmental dyslexia in women: Neuropathological findings in three patients. *Annals of Neurology, 28*(6), 727–738.

Humphreys, P., Rosen, G. D., Press, D. M., Sherman, G. F., & Galaburda, A. M. (1991). Freezing lesions of the developing rat brain: A model for cerebrocortical microgyria. *Journal of Neuropathology and Experimental Neurology, 50*(2), 145–160.

Hyde, L. A., Sherman, G. F., & Denenberg, V. H. (2000). Non-spatial water radial-arm maze learning in mice. *Brain Research, 863*(1–2), 151–159.

Hyde, L. A., Sherman, G. F., Hoplight, B. J., & Denenberg, V. H. (2000). Working memory deficits in BXSB mice with neocortical ectopias. *Physiology and Behavior, 70*(1–2), 1–5.

Innocenti, G. M., & Berbel, P. (1991). Analysis of an experimental cortical network II: Connections of visual areas 17 and 18 after neonatal injections of ibotenic acid. *Journal of Neural Transplant, 2*(1), 29–54.

Ison, J. R. (1982). Temporal acuity in auditory function in the rat: Reflex inhibition by brief gaps in noise. *Journal of Comparative Physiological Psychology, 96*(6), 945–954.

Ison, J. R., & Hoffman, H. S. (1983). Reflex modification in the domain of startle: II. The anomalous history of a robust and ubiquitous phenomenon. *Psychology Bulletin, 94*(1), 3–17.

Ison, J. R., & Pinckney, L. A. (1983). Reflex inhibition in humans: Sensitivity to brief silent periods in white noise. *Perception and Psychophysics, 34*(1), 84–88.

Ison, J. R., O'Connor, K., Bowen, G. P., & Bocirnea, A. (1991). Temporal resolution of gaps in noise by the rat is lost with functional decortication. *Behavioral Neuroscience, 105*(1), 33–40.

Jacobs, K. M., Gutnick, M. J., & Prince, D. A. (1996). Hyperexcitability in a model of cortical maldevelopment. *Cerebral Cortex, 6*, 514–523.

Jacobs, K. M., Hwang, B. J., & Prince, D. A. (1999). Focal epileptogenesis in a rat model of polymicrogyria. *Journal of Neurophysiology, 81*, 159–173.

Jenner, A. R., Galaburda, A. M., & Sherman, G. F. (2000). Connectivity of ectopic neurons in the molecular layer of the somatosensory cortex in autoimmune mice. *Cerebral Cortex, 10*, 1005–1013.

Katusic, S. K., Colligan, R. C., Barbaresi, W. J., Schaid, D. J., & Jacobsen, S. J. (2001). Incidence of reading disability in a population-based birth cohort, 1976–1982, Rochester, Minn. *Mayo Clinical Proceedings, 76*, 1081–1092.

Kimura, D., & Harshman, R. (1984). Sex diffferences in brain organization for verbal and nonverbal functions. In G. J. DeVries, et al. (Eds.), *Progress in brain research* (vol. 61). Amsterdam: Elsevier.

Kinsbourne, M., Rufo, D. T., Gamzu, E., Palmer, R. L., & Berliner, A. K. (1991). Neuropsychological deficits in adults with dyslexia. *Developmental Medicine & Child Neurology, 33*, 763–775.

Kolb, B., & Cioe, J. (1996). Sex related differences in corrtical function after medial frontal lesions in rats. *Behavioral Neuroscience, 110*, 1271–1281.

Kraus, N., McGee, T., Carrell, T., King, C., Littman, T., & Nicol, T. (1994). Discrimination of speech-like contrasts in the auditory thalamus and cortex. *Journal of the Acoustic Society of America, 96*(5), 2758–2768.

Kraus, N., McGee, T., Carrell, T. D., King, C., Tremblay, K., & Nicol, T. (1995). Central auditory system plasticity associated with speech discrimination training. *Journal of Cognitive Neuroscience, 7*(1), 25–32.

Kraus, N., McGee, T. J., Carrell, T. D., Zecker, S. G., Nicol, T. G., & Koch, D. B. (1996). Auditory neurophysiologic responses and discrimination deficits in children with learning problems. *Science, 273*(5277), 971–973.

Kulynych, J. J., Vladar, K., Jones, D. W., & Weinberger, D. R. (1994). Gender differences in the normal lateralization of the supratemporal cortex: MRI surface-rendering morphometry of Heschls gyrus and the planum temporale. *Cerebral Cortex, 4*, 107–118.

Laasonen, M., Service, E., & Virsu, V. (2001). Temporal order and processing acuity of visual, auditory, and tactile perception in developmentally dyslexic young adults. *Cognitive Affect Behavioral Neuroscience, 1*(4), 394–410.

Laasonen, M., Service, E., & Virsu, V. (2002). Crossmodal temporal order and processing acuity in developmentally dyslexic young adults. *Brain and Language, 80*, 340–354.

Lambe, E. (1999). Dyslexia, gender, and brain imaging. *Neuropsychologia, 37*, 532–536.

Leitner, D. S., Hammond, G. R., Springer, C. P., Ingham, K. M., Mekilo, A. M., Bodison, P. R., Aranda, M. T., & Shawaryn, M. A. (1993). Parameters affecting gap detection in the rat. *Perception and Psychophysics, 54*(3), 395–405.

Leonard, C. (1998). *Children with specific language impairment.* Cambridge, MA: MIT Press.

Leppänen, P. H., Pihko, E., Eklund, K. M., & Lyytinen, H. (1999). Cortical responses of infants with and without a genetic risk for dyslexia: II. Group effects. *NeuroReport, 10*(5), 969–973.

Leppänen, P. H., Richardson U., Pihko E., Eklund K. M., Guttorm T. K., Aro M., & Lyytinen, H. (2002). Brain responses to changes in speech sound durations differ between infants with and without familial risk for dyslexia. *Developmental Neuropsychology, 22*(1), 407–422.

Liederman, J., & Flannery, K. A. (1993). Male prevalence for reading disability is found in a large sample free from ascertainment bias. *Society for Neuroscience Abstracts 19.*

Liederman, J., & Flannery, K. A. (1995). The sex ratios of families with a neurodevelopmentally disordered child. *Journal of Child Psychology and Psychiatry, 36,* 511–517.

Liberman, I. Y., & Shankweiler, D. (1985). Phonology and the problems of learning to read and write. *Remedial and Special Education, 6*(6), 8–17.

Livingstone, M. S., Rosen, G. D., Drislane, F. W., & Galaburda, A. M. (1991). Physiological and anatomical evidence for a magnocellular defect in developmental dyslexia [published erratum appears in Proc Natl Acad Sci USA (1993) Mar 15; 90(6), 2556]. *Proceedings of the National Academy of Science USA, 88*(18), 7943–7947.

Lovegrove, W. J., Garzia, R. P., & Nicholson, S. B. (1990). Experimental evidence for a transient system deficit in specific reading disability. *Journal of the American Optomology Association, 61*(2), 137–146.

McCroskey, R. L., & Kidder, H. C. (1980). Auditory fusion among learning disabled, reading disabled, and normal children. *Journal of Learning Disabilities, 13*(2), 69–76.

McGlone, J. (1980). Sex differences in human brain asymmetry: A critical review. *Behavioral and Brain Sciences, 3,* 215–263.

Miller, B., Chou, L., & Finlay, B. L. (1993). The early development of thalamocortical and corticothalamic projections. *The Journal of Comparative Neurology, 335,* 16–41.

Montgomery, J. W. (2003). Working memory and comprehension in children with specific language impairment: What we know so far. *Journal of Communication Disorders, 36,* 221–231.

Nagarajan, S., Mahncke, H., Salz, T., Tallal, P., Roberts, T., & Merzenich, M. M. (1999). Cortical auditory signal processing in poor-reading adults. *Proceeding of the National Academy of Sciences USA, 96,* 6483–6488.

Neils, J. R., & Aram, D. M. (1986). Handedness and sex of children with developmental language disorders. *Brain and Language, 28*(1), 53–65.

Peiffer, A. M., Dunleavy, C. K., Frenkel, M., Gabel, L. A., LoTurco, J. J., Rosen, G. D., & Fitch, R. H. (2001). Impaired detection of variable duration embedded tones in ectopic NZB/BLNJ mice. *NeuroReport, 12*(13), 2875–2879.

Peiffer, A. M., Friedman, J. T., Rosen, G. D., & Fitch, R. H. (2004a). Impaired gap detection in juvenile microgyric rats. *Developmental Brain Research, 152,* 93–98.

Peiffer, A. M., McClure, M. M., Threlkeld, S. W., Rosen, G. D., & Fitch, R. H. (2004b). Severity of focal microgyria and associated rapid auditory processing deficits. *NeuroReport, 15*(12), 1923–1926.

Peiffer, A. M., Rosen, G. D., & Fitch, R. H. (2002). Sex differences in rapid auditory processing deficits in ectopic BXSB/MpJ mice. *NeuroReport, 13,* 277–280.

Peiffer, A. M., Rosen, G. D., & Fitch, R. H. (2004c). Sex differences in rapid auditory impairments in microgyric rats. *Developmental Brain Research, 148*(1), 53–57.

Phillips, D. P., & Farmer, M. E. (1990). Acquired word deafness, & the time frame of processing in the primary auditory cortex. *Behavioural Brain Research, 40*, 85–94.

Raz, S., Lauterbach, M. D., Hopkins, T. L., Glogowski, B. K., & Porter, C. L. (1995). A female advantage in cognitive recovery from early cerebral insult. *Developmental Psychology, 31*, 958–966.

Reed, M. A. (1989). Speech perception and the discrimination of brief auditory cues in reading disabled children. *Journal of Experimental Child Psychology, 48*, 270–292.

Roof, R., Duvdevani, R., & Stein, D. (1993). Gender influenceoutcome of brain injury. Progesterone plays a protective role. *Brain Research, 607*, 333–336.

Rosen, G. D., Burstein, D., & Galaburda, A. M. (2000). Changes in efferent and afferent connectivity in rats with induced cerebrocortical microgyria. *The Journal of Comparative Neurology, 418*, 423–440.

Rosen, G. D., Herman, A. E., & Galaburda, A. M. (1999). Sex differences in the effects of early neocortical injury on neuronal size distribution of the medial geniculate nucleus in the rat are mediated by perinatal gonadal steroids. *Cerebral Cortex, 9*, 27–34.

Rosen, G. D., Press, D. M., Sherman, G. F., & Galaburda, A. M. (1992). The development of induced cerebrocortical microgyria in the rat. *Journal of Neuropathology and Experimental Neurology, 51*(6), 601–611.

Ruben, R. J. (1997). A time frame of critical/sensitive periods of "language development." *Acta Otolaryngology, 117*(2), 202–205.

Schneider, G. E. (1981). Early lesions and abnormal neuronal connections. *Trends in Neuroscience, 4*, 187–192.

Schrott, L. M., Denenberg, V. H., Sherman, G. F., Waters, N. S., Rosen, G. D., & Galaburda, A. M. (1992). Environmental enrichment, neocortical ectopias, and behavior in the autoimmune NZB mouse. *Developmental Brain Research, 67*(1), 85–93.

Schulte-Korne, G., Deimel, W., Bartling, J., & Remschmidt, H. (1999). Preattentive processing of auditory patterns in dyslexic human subjects. *Neuroscience Letters, 276*(1), 41–44.

Shaywitz, S. E., Shaywitz, B. A., Fletcher, J. M. & Escobar, M. D. (1990). Prevalence of reading disability in boys and girls: Results of the Connecticut longitudinal study. *Journal of the American Medical Association, 264*, 998–1002.

Shaywitz, B. A., Shaywitz, S. E., Pugh, K. R., Constable, R. T., Skudlarski, P., Fulbright, R. K. et al. (1995). Sex differences in the functional organization of the brain for language. *Nature, 373*, 307–309.

Sherman, G. F., Galaburda, A. M., Behan, P. O., & Rosen, G. D. (1987). Neuroanatomical anomalies in autoimmune mice. *Acta Neuropathologica, 74*(3), 239–242.

Sherman, G. F., Galaburda, A. M., & Geschwind, N. (1985). Cortical anomalies in brains of New Zealand mice: A neuropathologic model of dyslexia? *Proceedings of the National Academy of Science USA, 82*(23), 8072–8074.

Sherman, G. F., Hinton, W. R., & Galaburda, A. M. (1998). Neuronal size differences in the anterior thalamic nucleus of mice with neocortical ectopias. *Society for Neuroscience Abstracts, 24*.

Sherman, G. F., Morrison, L., Rosen, G. D., Behan, P. O., & Galaburda, A. M. (1990a). Brain abnormalities in immune defective mice. *Brain Research 532*(1–2), 25–33.

Sherman, G. F., Rosen, G. D., Stone, L. V., Press, D. M., & Galaburda, A. M. (1992a). The organization of radial glial fibers in spontaneous neocortical ectopias of newborn New Zealand black mice. *Developmental Brain Research, 67*(2), 279–283.

Sherman, G. F., Stone, L.V., Denenberg, V. H., & Beier, D.R. (1994). A genetic analysis of neocortical ectopias in New Zealand black mice. *NeuroReport, 5*(6), 721–724.

Sherman, G. F., Stone, J. S., Press, D. M., Rosen, G. D., & Galaburda, A. M. (1990b). Abnormal architecture and connections disclosed by neurofilament staining in the cerebral cortex of autoimmune mice. *Brain Research. 529*(1–2), 202–207.

Stanley, G., & Hall, R. (1973). A comparison of dyslexics and normals in recalling letter arrays after brief presentation. *British Journal of Education Psychology, 43*, 34.

Stark, R. E., Bernstein, L. E., Condino, R., Bender, M., Tallal, P., & Catts, H. (1984). Four-year follow-up study of language-impaired children. *Annals of Dyslexia, 34*, 49–68.

Tallal, P. (1980). Auditory temporal perception, phonics, and the reading disabilities in children. *Brain and Language, 9*, 182–198.

Tallal, P. (1984). Temporal or phonetic processing deficit in dyslexia? That is the question. *Applied Psycholinguistics, 5*(2), 167–169.

Tallal, P. (1988). Developmental language disorders: Part 1-Definition. *Human Communication Canada 9*, 7–22.

Tallal, P. (1991). Hormonal influences in developmental learning disabilities. *Psychoneuroendocrinology, 16*, 203–211.

Tallal, P., Merzenich, M., Miller, S., & Jenkins, W. (1998). Language learning impairment: Integrating research and remediation. *Scandinavian Journal of Psychology, 39*(3), 197–199.

Tallal, P., Miller, S., & Fitch, R. H. (1993). Neurobiological basis of speech: A case for the preeminence of temporal processing. *Annals of the New York Academy of Science, 682*, 27–47.

Tallal, P., & Piercy, M. (1973). Defects of nonverbal auditory perception in children with developmental aphasia. *Nature, 241*(5390), 468–469.

Tallal, P., & Piercy, M. (1974). Developmental aphasia: Rate of auditory processing and selective impairment of consonant perception. *Neuropsychologia, 12*, 83–93.

Tallal, P., & Piercy, M. (1975). Developmental aphasia: The perception of brief vowels and extended stop consonants. *Neuropsychologia, 13*(1), 69–74.

Tallal, P., & Stark, R. E. (1981). Speech acoustic-cue discrimination abilities of normally developing and language-impaired children. *Journal of the Acoustical Society of America, 69*(2), 568–574.

Tallal, P., Stark, R. E., & Mellits, E. D. (1985). Identification of language-impaired children on the basis of rapid perception and production skills. *Brain and Language, 25*(2), 314–322.

Thomas, J., Clark, M., Benasich, A. A., & Fitch, R. H. (2001, March). Developmental changes in gap detection thresholds in the rat. Paper presented at The Cognitive Neuroscience Society, San Francisco, CA.

Tomblin, J. B., Freese, P. R., & Records, N. L. (1992). Diagnosing specific language impairment in adults for the purpose of pedigree analysis. *Journal of Speech and Hearing Research, 35*(4), 832–843.

Trehub, S. E., & Henderson, J. L. (1996). Temporal resolution in infancy and subsequent language development. *Journal of Speech and Hearing Research, 39,* 1315–1320.

Wecker, J. R., Ison, J. R., & Foss, J. A. (1985). Reflex modification as a test for sensory function. *Neurobehavioral Toxicology & Teratology, 7*(6), 733–738.

Werker, J. F., & Tees, R. C. (1987). Speech perception in severely disabled and average reading children. *Canadian Journal of Psychology, 41*(1), 48–61.

Wood, F. B., Flowers, D. L., & Naylor, C. E. (1991). Cerebral laterality in functional neuroimaging. In F. L. Kitterle (Ed.), *Cerebral laterality: Theory and research* (pp. 103–116). Hillsdale, NJ: Lawrence Erlbaum.

Wright, B. A., Bowen, R. W., & Zecker, S. G. (2000). Nonlinguistic perceptual deficits associated with reading and language disorders. *Current Opinions in Neurobiology, 10,* 482–486.

Wright, B. A., Lombardino, L. J., King, W. M., Puranik, C. S., Leonard, C. M., & Merzenich, M. M. (1997). Deficits in auditory temporal and spectral resolution in language-impaired children. *Nature, 387*(6629), 176–178.

Section • IV

Brain Plasticity

INTRODUCTION

The chapter by David Kennedy explores the utility of advanced imaging techniques in the study of development of the brain. Kennedy's goal is to link observable changes in the brain in the postnatal period to events that occurred in the prenatal period (when direct observation of the brain is not possible). Using examples from three different groups, Kennedy illustrates exactly how one can use comparisons with normative data to make assumptions about the changes that occurred during development. Each of the examples that he provides, while not directly germane to the study of developmental dyslexia, has potential implications for future research on this topic. What is clear is that the field in general will surely benefit from a group effort to share MRI data from children with developmental dyslexia.

The ability of the brain to reorganize has long been considered one of the key features distinguishing the developing from the adult brain. For example, small strokes in the cerebral cortex of adults can result in profound disturbances in language and other cognitive skills, whereas an infant can lose his or her entire left hemisphere and still develop reasonably normal language. In recent years, however, researchers have been gaining an increased appreciation for the ability of the adult brain to reorganize in response to new stimuli. In this chapter, Hugo Théoret and Alvaro Pascual-Leone present exciting research detailing how the adult brain reorganizes following sensory deprivation. It appears that a brain that is deprived of sensory information can recruit underutilized primary sensory cortices when performing other sensory tasks. Thus, the visual cortex of blinded individuals is capable of processing tactile and auditory information. With regard to developmental dyslexia, there is a good deal of evidence that the most effective strategies are those that get language-related information into the brain via nonstandard pathways. We can hope that future therapies can take advantage of some of the knowledge now being gained about the plasticity of the adult brain to derive ways to "retrain the brain."

It is fitting we close this book with the chapter from Albert Galaburda. As mentioned in the preface, Galaburda organized the first "Extraordinary Brain" conference in 1987. In this chapter, he summarizes much of the research on the neurobiology of developmental dyslexia that has occurred in the ensuing years. This is more than a summary, however, as he continually points out the advantages of a cross-level approach to the study of this difficult issue. Citing research from his laboratory as well as those of other contributors to this book as an example, he points out the remarkable link between a purported dyslexia susceptibility gene, brain malformations, and behavior. It is clear that dyslexia is a complex disorder, and there are likely many different underlying etiologies. Galaburda's chapter strongly suggests a deep understanding of the biological substrates of developmental dyslexia will be expedited by a multidisciplinary approach. It is our hope that this book will inspire readers to discuss, collaborate, and investigate this important problem in that spirit.

Chapter • 15

MRI-based Morphometry in Human Developmental Disorders: Looking Back in Time

David N. Kennedy

SUMMARY

The human brain is a complex organ from both a structural and functional viewpoint. In order to arrive at its adult form, the brain undergoes a massively complex series of sequential developmental transformations, where each step is predicated on successful completion of the previous developmental stages. Using *in vivo* magnetic resonance imaging of the brain postnatally, we cannot see the preceding developments directly, but rather, we see the net accumulated consequences of the sequences of prior events. The integration of advanced imaging technology, with knowledge of developmental events, permits a rational reasoning system for looking into the past developmental history in order to better understand the anatomic consequences of normal and altered neuroanatomic development.

The author would like to acknowledge Verne Caviness, Nikos Makris, and Martha Herbert for years of collaborative work in the areas of neuroanatomy and neurodevelopment; Christian Haselgrove for his tireless work on the Internet Brain Volume Database; Sean McInerney for creating the volumetric visualization platform necessary for seeing volumetry clearly in three dimensions; Bruce Fischl and Anders Dale for collaboration in automation and the FreeSurfer environment; and Glenn Rosen and The Dyslexia Foundation for supporting scientific communication and collegiality in organizing and sponsoring the workshop where elements of this line of reasoning were presented.

INTRODUCTION

The morphology of the human brain is exceptionally complex, reflecting a myriad of inextricably intertwined systems of neuronal cell bodies, axons and other components. These systems have a structure, order, function, and composition that traverse and integrate many scales of size, cognitive and behavioral domains, genetic and epigenetic factors, and comprise the vary matrix of our essence and being. Morphometric analysis is the quantification of the morphologic properties such as size, shape, location, and composition of the brain and its component parts (Caviness, Lange, Makris, Herbert, & Kennedy, 1999). Magnetic resonance imaging (MRI) provides a highly efficacious means for observing the gross anatomic distribution of brain tissues that subserve its functional regions. MRI provides an unprecedented view of human neuroanatomy, permitting observation of cerebral and cerebellar cortex and white matter, as well as the deep gray matter structures and the ventricular system. Precise knowledge of the anatomic makeup of the brain is a fundamental cornerstone for such diverse applications as volumetric analysis, shape analysis, the analysis and quantification of intersubject variability, the localization of functional activation, and enhanced data visualization (Kennedy, Makris, Herbert, Takahashi, & Caviness, 2002).

Morphometric methods, in conjunction with neuropsychological, neurological, psychiatric observations, and functional neuroimaging, can be integrated to assess a number of broad classes of question including: (1) what neural operation is being performed at each location in the brain? (2) how do these localized processors interact spatially and temporally? and (3) how does the spatial deployment and operating characteristics of these processors change over time (with normal development and in the face of pathologic or developmental insults)?

Substantial effort has gone into building up the data and tools to create a concept of how big the human brain is (Caviness, Kennedy, Bates, & Makris, 1996; Durston et al., 2001). This is, of course, a dynamic question, and the answer depends on many factors, most notable, age. The application of morphometric methods typically focus on first defining the parameters of "normal" development, then subsequently identifying the deviation from normal in various pathological conditions. Characterization of normal development and aging represents a critical underpinning for the assessment of brain abnormalities. A large number of reports exist that summarize our current state of understanding regarding cerebral structures of the normal brain (see, for example, Caviness,

Kennedy, Richelme, Rademacher, & Filipek, 1996; Durston et al., 2001; Filipek, Richelme, Kennedy, & Caviness, 1994; Giedd et al., 1996; Jernigan, Trauner, Hesselink, & Tallal, 1991; Pfefferbaum et al., 1994). Despite methodological heterogeneity, the bulk of the literature, taken together, provides a reasonably comprehensive representation of the temporal developmental profile of the major brain structures from the age of four years on (see Figure 1).

Neuropathology, from the neuroimaging point of view, can be classified as "frank" lesion or abnormalities such as a tumor, multiple sclerosis, or stroke lesion (Caviness et al., 2002a, 2002b; Filipek, Kennedy, & Caviness, 1991; Kikinis et al., 1999), or as a "quiescent" lesion or abnormality, where there is no directly observable gross radiological finding. Quantitative volumetric analysis, while extremely useful for frank lesions, is essential in the assessment of individuals where the pathology provides no clinically appreciable evidence for localization. Examples of this class of observation in developmental disorders are reported (Courchesne, Townsend, & Saitoh, 1994) in the assessment of children with autism, attention deficit disorder (Filipek et al., 1997), dyslexia (Pennington et al., 1999), and schizophrenia (Seidman et al., 1999; Seidman et al., 2002; Shenton, Kikinis, Jolesz, et al., 1992), to name a few. In addition, numerous reports

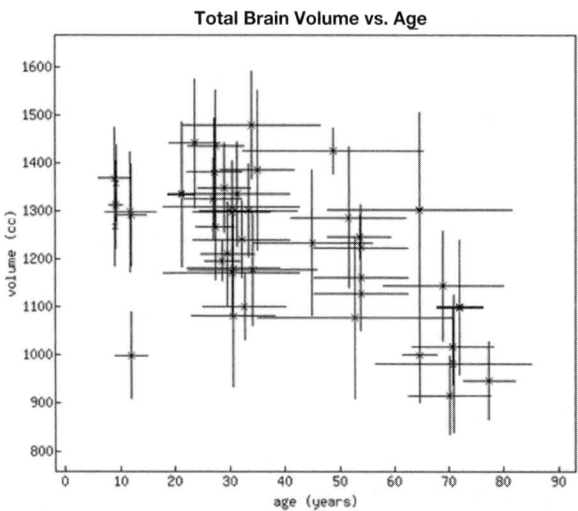

Figure 1. Total brain volume as a function of age as derived from the literature using the Internet Brain Volume Database (IBVD). See Methods for description.

in degenerative disorders such as Alzheimer's disease (Atiya, Hyman, Albert, & Killiany, 2003; Killiany et al., 2000; Killiany et al., 2002; Scheltens, Leys, Barkhof, et al., 1992; Seab et al., 1988), and Huntington's Disease (Rosas et al., 2001; Rosas et al., 2002), have shown where quantification of brain structure provides valuable information regarding the diagnosis, etiology, and time course of specific disease processes. Together, these application areas provide a valuable testbed for morphometric methods.

Starting from the current postnatal MRI-based point of view, however, is not completely satisfying, due to a number of factors. First, *in vivo* measures are age limited: numbers of subjects examined and precision of measurements falls off dramatically under the age of about three years, and are virtually nonexistent parentally for many technically challenging reasons. Most interesting developmental events occur well before this age of potential observation with current technology. Second, most developmental events occur on a much more anatomic and regionally specific fashion than the current regions of volumetric analysis.

The goal of this paper is to examine the points of inference that can be established in order to link these observable, postnatal structures, to the past, prenatal events that fundamentally set in motion the course of their development. We illustrate these points in the context of autism, gender-based dimorphism, and holoprosencephaly.

METHODS

Before analysis of brain morphology can be performed, the regions of interest of the brain must be robustly and efficiently identified. Historically, this task has been done by skilled technicians at great cost in time and money. One major thrust of recent research efforts has been the development of tools for accurate, robust, and efficient segmentation (Kennedy, Caviness, & Makris, 1996; Kennedy et al., 2002; Viergever et al., 2001; Wells, Grimson, Kikinis, & Jolesz, 1996).

Anatomic Framework

A framework for comprehensive anatomic analysis should include issues of anatomic specificity and precision, in conjunction with efficiency of operation, classes of observation, and clinical efficacy. Broadly speaking, there are voxel-based (or volumetric) (Ashburner & Friston, 2000; 2001; Bookstein, 2001; Filipek et al., 1994; Fischl et al., 2002) and surface-based classes of characteristics that can be commonly extracted from current MR images (Dale, Fischl, & Sereno, 1999; Fischl & Dale, 2000; Fischl, Sereno, & Dale, 1999; Fischl, Sereno, Tootell, & Dale, 1999; Thompson et al., 2000) (see Figure 2 in the four-color section on page 222-H).

We have developed and implemented a comprehensive and complete set of anatomic analysis routines that span virtually all levels of anatomic assessment available to the MR image of the living human brain from whole brain structures to fine-grained, topographically-defined, systems-related subdivisions of each major structure. We have developed these routines in a two-pronged fashion: (a) manual methods that maximize anatomic validity, and (b) automated methods that combine the *a priori* definitions imposed in the manual methods in a maximally efficient automated methodology for enhanced throughput. These methods, combined, provide maximum flexibility to the neuroscience user to select an appropriate level of anatomic analysis and cost benefit ratio. Figure 3 (see Figure 3 in the four-color section on page 222-H) provides an iconic guide to these developments: general segmentation (manual) (Filipek et al., 1994) and automated (Fischl et al., 2002; Worth, Makris, Meyer, Caviness, & Kennedy, 1998; Worth, Makris, Patti, et al., 1998), cortical parcellation (manual) (Caviness, Makris, Meyer, & Kennedy, 1996; Rademacher, Caviness, Steinmetz, & Galaburda, 1993; Rademacher, Galaburda, Kennedy, Filipek, & Caviness, 1992) and automated (Fischl et al., 2004), white matter parcellation (Makris, Meyer, Bates, Caviness, & Kennedy, 1999; Meyer, Makris, Bates, Caviness, & Kennedy, 1999), and cerebellum parcellation (surface-assisted, Makris et al., 2003). Many of these applications are developed in conjunction with the *FreeSurfer* surface-based analysis system (Dale et al., 1999; Fischl, Sereno, & Dale, 1999) in order to integrate "surface-assisted parcellation" schemes for enhancing ease of user operation and efficiency.

Volumetric Literature Search

The Internet Brain Volume Database (IBVD) is a Web-based database (publicly accessible at http://www.cma.mgh.harvard.edu/IBVD/) where the principle objective is to capture retrospective volumetric data and observations from the published literature. Volumetric observations are coded by publication, and the group and individual demographic, clinical, and volumetric descriptors reported. Data entry statistics for this site (as of 9/17/2004) include 160 publications, 469 subject groups, 2,300 group volume entries, 44 clinical diagnoses, 1,773 individuals, 8,619 individual structural volume entries, and 72 discrete brain structures. The site is continuously updated with respect to the published literature. The site supports searching based on diagnostic and anatomic criteria, and simple visualization for the query results. Also, complete linkage between the IBVD record and the PubMed literature citation, as well as any publicly available data about the subjects and groups, is supported. This utility is used in this report to demonstrate volumetric observations in the context of a large sample of the complete volumetric literature.

RESULTS

We now explore exemplar morphometric application areas that demonstrate the interaction of measurement and inference regarding unseen developmental events. These example areas include white matter specificity in autism, gender-based details of cortical volumetric dimorphism, and graded topological anomaly holoprosencephaly as a marker of abnormal development.

Application to Autism

Autism is associated with pervasive social and language behavioral consequences. However, qualitative brain imaging studies have shown no systematic abnormality. Over a decade of quantitative morphometric and volumetric studies have reported a number of specific alterations in the brains of children with autism (Courchesne et al., 2001; Courchesne, Townsend et al., 1994; Courchesne, Yeung-Courchesne, & Egaas, 1994; Courchesne, Yeung-Courchesne, Press, Hesselink, & Jernigan, 1988; Hardan, Minshew, Mallikarjuhn, & Keshavan, 2001; Piven, Saliba, Bailey, & Arndt, 1997). At the risk of oversimplifying the volumetric observations, one specific line of reasoning exemplifies the use of hierarchical partitioning of brain observation and the inferential power that can be applied to such data. In summary, there is volumetric evidence that children with autism have larger brains than controls (Hardan et al., 2001; Herbert et al., 2003). Also, this largeness is most pronounced in cerebral white matter. Figure 4 (see Figure 4 in the four-color section on page 222-I) uses the IBVD "paper view" methodology to highlight one specific paper that demonstrates the overall brain volume effect in autism (Herbert et al., 2003).

The cerebral white matter finding has been followed up with more specific regionalized white matter observation using the white matter parcellation scheme of Meyer (Makris et al., 1999; Meyer et al., 1999). In addition to providing a more fine-grained division of white matter anatomy, this level of anatomic observation permits reasoning with respect to developmental features of these anatomic regions. Specifically, each of the white matter regions measured can be related to observations in the literature regarding the initiation and duration of the myelination process during development. Thus, as alterations are identified with specific white matter subregions, the data can be interrogated for relationships between anatomic abnormality and commonality of parameters of development such as myelination features. In the study reported by Herbert et al. (2004), it was demonstrated that the white matter alteration was expressed almost exclusively in the peripheral (radiate) regions and later (and longer duration) myelinating regions showed greater volume increases compared to controls.

Application to Gender Dimorphism

A second example is drawn from the literature regarding the normative brain. Historically, *postmortem* results have indicated the presence of a subtle, 10% difference between the male and female brain (Filipek et al., 1994; Giedd et al., 1996; Reiss, Abrams, Singer, Ross, & Denckla, 1996). Again, changes of this magnitude are virtually imperceptible in qualitative or visual inspection of brain imaging data. Quantitative studies, however, have been quite successful at documenting this volumetric difference across many different studies with varying methodological design. Figure 5 (see Figure 5 in the four-color section on page 222-I) shows an IBVD plot for total brain volume for normal subjects, identified by gender where this dimorphic behavior is clearly evident across a wide age range.

This overall brain volume effect has been studied in detail by numerous groups, and found to be nonuniformly distributed across the various anatomic regions of the brain (Filipek et al., 1994; Kennedy, Lange, Makris, Bates, & Caviness, 1998). Within the cerebral cortex, for example, one theory of gender differentiation that may lead to regional volumetric differences relates to levels of sex steroid receptor in critical periods of brain development. Using the methods of fine-grained topographical cortical parcellation, a study by Goldstein et al. (2001) tested and confirmed the hypothesis that the predominant regions that are dimorphic are found in regions that have high developmental estrogen receptor density, consistent with this theory. Moreover, of the dimorphic regions in the cerebral hemisphere, the majority show female greater than male volumetric dimorphomism.

Application to Holoprosencephaly

As a final example, we consider holoprosencephaly (HPE), in which a dramatic developmental malformation is present in the central nervous system structures such that regions that are normally bilaterally represented in right and left halves of the forebrain are instead conjoined across the midline (Roessler & Muenke, 2001; Simon & Barkovich, 2001; Simon et al., 2001; Simon et al., 2000). Despite the extreme nature of the topological disorder, there are a number of general observations that can be made (Takahashi et al., 2003; Takahashi et al., 2004). First of all, the total brain volume of these subjects is dramatically reduced (only about 55% of normal volume in the "semilobar" variant of this disorder). Second, a spatially contiguous pattern to the midline anomaly can be observed and related to an "axis" of developmental specificity. The topological features of this anomaly include a midline gray matter "seam" (a rostro-caudally aligned midline gray matter confluence), fused midline structures, and alterations of the interhemispheric fissure. These observations are, however, related. The degree of brain volume decrease correlates with degree of topological anomaly. Thus, the more extensive the midline anomaly is, the smaller the overall volume of the brain. Figure 6 (see Figure 6 in the four-color section on page 222-I) includes volumetric renderings of some of these topological features of HPE.

DISCUSSION

Using quantitative, anatomically precise methods for analysis of anatomic features in the living brain, we have demonstrated the concept of using antenatal observations to infer consequences of prenatal events. This linkage of time frames requires linkage of knowledge (*a priori* information) across scales (much of our macroscopic inference comes from microscopic reasoning), species (much of our detailed knowledge about human development arises from other species), and modes of observation (little of our background knowledge comes from magnetic resonance volumetry). Specifically, we require the existence of MRI-based measurements based in an anatomic context that permits such knowledge linkage. The example volumetric observations reported here demonstrate this linkage using current state of the art MR imaging and morphometric analysis techniques. These are certainly only the "tip of the iceberg" of the classes of observation and application areas that have been reported to support this argument.

These example application areas also span morphologic severity. This includes volumetric alterations that are too subtle to see qualitatively (autism and gender dimorphism), to a topology that is so massively disrupted that, at first glance, it is difficult to even know what to measure to make sense of the anatomic representation (HPE). As above, observational order is imposed on these studies through the development of neurobiologically and neurodevelopmentally motivated metrics of quantitative assessment. In all of these studies, gross measurement of whole structure properties would miss the most informative aspects of these observations, and not provide suitable "next hypotheses" for follow-up studies.

While virtually all developmental disorders have received some morphometric treatment in the literature, there is wide variability regarding the detailed application of these measures as a function of disorder. Disorders such as schizophrenia, multiple sclerosis, and Alzheimer's disease have hundreds of publications each that utilize imaging and quantitative measurements. Conversely, dyslexia, along with Down, Turner's, William's, and Rett's syndromes, each have only tens of publications in quantitative morphometry at this time. In dyslexia specifically, asymmetry of language-related cortical features has been targeted in many studies. Example findings range from reduced brain volume and inferior frontal gyrus (pars triangularis) (Eckert et al., 2003), reduced temporal lobe gray matter volume (Eliez et al., 2000), rightward cerebral asymmetry with leftward asymmetry of the planum temporal and Sylvian fissure (Leonard et al., 2001; Leonard et al., 2002), and reduced insula volume with increased occipital cortex volume (Pennington et al., 1999). As yet, however, a comprehensive or compelling developmental story based on these observations is lacking. The technology for high-throughput, cost effective morphometry is becoming more accessible, and the internal consistency, power, specificity, and sensitivity that arise through widespread application is critical to developing a clear understanding of the subtle anatomic details and relationships of developmental anomalies that give rise to these disorders.

In this report, we concentrated on volumetric anatomic assessment of development as ascertained from T1-weighted MRI data. There is also a vast literature exploring other structural consequences (parameter mapping of T1, T2, proton density) (Jenkins et al., 1999), diffusion tensor and diffusion weighting (Makris et al., 1997; Neil et al., 1998, etc.), as well as functional (fMRI, PET, SPECT, etc.) ramifications and results of development in health and disease (Casey, Giedd, & Thomas, 2000; Casey & Munakata,

2002; Chiron, Raynaud, Maziere, et al., 1992; Chugani & Phelps, 1986; Chugani, Phelps, & Mazziotta, 1987; Sudikoff & Banasiak, 1998). Each of these classes of measurement make a unique comment regarding development, and represent a continued challenge to researchers regarding the appropriate and efficient integration across each of these classes of observation.

It is evident that morphometry and the myriad events of neurodevelopment can be linked. In this paper, we provided examples of this linkage in autism (linking early myelination pattern to white matter parcellation unit volume), gender dimorphism (linking early dimorphic receptor pattern to resultant pattern of regional cortical volume), and in HPE (linking disruption of the early pattern and timing of laterality encoding to resultant topographic anomalies). Each new study of *in vivo* morphometry has the opportunity to identify the ripple in the (neuroanatomic) space- (developmental) time continuum by matching precise observation with details of developmental knowledge. From a set of morphometric measures, what can be inferred about past history? As a final example of this, imagine the following "thought experiment" in the context of the HPE data presented above:

> There is a period of developmental time where right-left spatial differentiation is encoded into the "destiny" of the neural tissue. This lateral destiny gets "imprinted" sequentially along a rostral to caudal axis over the course of a specific critical time period. If this patterning mechanism fails for a short interval during this time period, the lateral destiny of the neural tissue that was supposed to be encoded during that time is disrupted. The longer the failure, the larger the resultant disruption; the location span of the eventual disruption is a "read out" of the time duration (size), and initiation and termination times of the failure relative to the critical period, and will determine the detailed location of the final disruption. Hence, we have a timing readout postnatally of a specific class of event (start time, stop time and duration) during early development.

As experiments are performed and interpreted in this class of developmental context, morphometric measurement will begin to play a more important role in the elucidation of the origins of the subtle (and not so subtle) anomalies associated with virtually all developmental disorders.

Address correspondence to: David N. Kennedy, MGH-CMA, 149 13th Street, Charlestown, MA 02129; E-mail: dave@cma.mgh.harvard.edu

REFERENCES

Ashburner, J., & Friston, K. J. (2000). Voxel-based morphometry—the methods. *Neuroimage, 11*(6 Pt 1), 805–821.
Ashburner, J., & Friston, K. J. (2001). Why voxel-based morphometry should be used. *Neuroimage, 14*(6), 1238–1243.
Atiya, M., Hyman, B. T., Albert, M. S., & Killiany, R. (2003). Structural magnetic resonance imaging in established and prodromal Alzheimer disease: A review. *Alzheimer Disease and Associated Disorders, 17*(3), 177–195.
Bookstein, F. L. (2001). "Voxel-based morphometry" should not be used with imperfectly registered images. *Neuroimage, 14*(6), 1454–1462.
Casey, B., Giedd, J., & Thomas, K. (2000). Structural and functional brain development and its relation to cognitive development. *Biological Psychology, 54*(1–3), 241–257.
Casey, B. J., & Munakata, Y. (2002). Converging methods in developmental science: An introduction. *Developmental Psychobiology, 40*(3), 197–199.
Caviness, V. S., Kennedy, D. N., Bates, J., & Makris, N. (1996). The developing human brain: A morphometric profile. In R. W. Thatcher, G. R. Lyon, J. Rumsey, & N. Krasnegor (Eds.), *Developmental neuroimaging: Mapping the development of brain and behavior* (pp. 3–14). New York: Academic Press.
Caviness, V. S., Kennedy, D. N., Richelme, C., Rademacher, R., & Filipek, P. (1996). The human brain age 7–11 years: A volumetric analysis based upon magnetic resonance images. *Cerebral Cortex, 6*(5), 726–736.
Caviness, V. S., Lange, N. T., Makris, N., Herbert, M. R., & Kennedy, D. N. (1999). MRI-Based brain volumetrics: Emergence of a developmental brain science. *Brain and Development, 21*(5), 289–295.
Caviness, V. S., Makris, N., Meyer, J., & Kennedy, D. (1996). MRI-based parcellation of human neocortex: An anatomically specified method with estimate of reliability. *Journal of Cognitive Neuroscience, 8*, 566–588.
Caviness, V. S., Makris, N., Montinaro, E., Sahin, N. T., Bates, J. F., Schwamm, L., et al. (2002a). Anatomy of stroke, Part I: An MRI-based topographic and volumetric system of analysis. *Stroke, 33*(11), 2549–2556.
Caviness, V. S., Makris, N., Montinaro, E., Sahin, N. T., Bates, J. F., Schwamm, L., et al. (2002b). Anatomy of stroke, Part II: Volumetric characteristics with implications for the local architecture of the cerebral perfusion system. *Stroke, 33*(11), 2557–2564.
Chiron, C., Raynaud, C., Maziere, B., et al. (1992). Changes in regional cerebral blood flow during brain maturation in children and adolescents. *Journal of Nuclear Medicine, 33*, 669–703.
Chugani, H. T., & Phelps, M. E. (1986). Maturational changes in cerebral function in infants determined by 18FDG positron emission tomography. *Science, 231*, 840–843.
Chugani, H. T., Phelps, M. E., & Mazziotta, J. C. (1987). Positron emission tomography study of human brain functional development. *Annals of Neurology, 22*, 487–497.
Courchesne, E., Karns, C., Davis, H., Ziccardi, R., Carper, R., Tigue, Z., et al. (2001). Unusual brain growth patterns in early life in patients with autistic disorder: An MRI study. *Neurology, 57*(2), 245–254.

Courchesne, E., Townsend, J., & Saitoh, O. (1994). The brain in infantile autism: Posterior fossa structures are abnormal. *Neurology, 44*(2), 214–223.

Courchesne, E., Yeung-Courchesne, R., & Egaas, B. (1994). Methodology in neuroanatomic measurement. *Neurology, 44*(2), 203–208.

Courchesne, E., Yeung-Courchesne, R., Press, G. A., Hesselink, J. R., & Jernigan, T. L. (1988). Hypoplasia of cerebellar vermal lobules VI and VII in autism. *The New England Journal of Medicine, 318*(21), 1349–1354.

Dale, A., Fischl, B., & Sereno, M. (1999). Cortical surface-based analysis. I. Segmentation and surface reconstruction. *NeuroImage, 9*, 179–194.

Durston, S., Hulshoff, P. H., Casey, B., Giedd, J., Buitelaar, J., & van Engeland, H. (2001). Anatomical MRI of the developing human brain: What have we learned? *Journal of the American Academy of Child and Adolescent Psychiatry, 40*(9), 1012–1020.

Eckert, M. A., Leonard, C. M., Richards, T. L., Aylward, E. H., Thomson, J., & Berninger, V. W. (2003). Anatomical correlates of dyslexia: Frontal and cerebellar findings. *Brain, 126*(Pt 2), 482–494.

Eliez, S., Rumsey, J. M., Giedd, J. N., Schmitt, J. E., Patwardhan, A. J., & Reiss, A. L. (2000). Morphological alteration of temporal lobe gray matter in dyslexia: An MRI study. *Journal of Child Psychology and Psychiatry, 41*(5), 637–644.

Filipek, P. A., Kennedy, D. N., & Caviness, V. S., Jr. (1991). Volumetric analyses of central nervous system neoplasm based on MRI. *Pediatric Neurology, 7*(5), 347–351.

Filipek, P. A., Richelme, C., Kennedy, D. N., & Caviness, V., Jr. (1994). The young adult human brain: An MRI-based morphometric analysis. *Cerebral Cortex, 4*(4), 344–360.

Filipek, P. A., Semrud-Clikeman, M., Steingard, R. J., Renshaw, P. F., Kennedy, D. N., & Biederman, J. (1997). Volumetric MRI analysis comparing subjects having attention-deficit hyperactivity disorder with normal controls. *Neurology, 48*(3), 589–601.

Fischl, B., & Dale, A. (2000). Measuring the thickness of the human cerebral cortex from magnetic resonance images. *Proceedings of the National Academy of Sciences, USA, 97*(20), 11050–11055.

Fischl, B., Salat, D. H., Busa, E., Albert, M., Dieterich, M., Haselgrove, C., et al. (2002). Whole brain segmentation: Automated labeling of neuroanatomical structures in the human brain. *Neuron, 33*(3), 341–355.

Fischl, B., Sereno, M., & Dale, A. (1999). Cortical surface-based analysis. II: Inflation, flattening, and a surface-based coordinate system. *NeuroImage, 9*, 195–207.

Fischl, B., Sereno, M., Tootell, R., & Dale, A. (1999). High-resolution intersubject averaging and a coordinate system for the cortical surface. *Human Brain Mapping, 8*, 272–284.

Fischl, B., van der Kouwe, A., Destrieux, C., Halgren, E., Segonne, F., Salat, D. H., et al. (2004). Automatically parcellating the human cerebral cortex. *Cerebral Cortex, 14*(1), 11–22.

Giedd, J. N., Snell, J. W., Lange, N., Rajapakse, J. C., Casey, B. J., Kozuch, P. L., et al. (1996). Quantitative magnetic resonance imaging of human brain development: Ages 4–18. *Cerebral Cortex, 6*, 551–560.

Goldstein, J. M., Seidman, L. J., Horton, N. J., Makris, N., Kennedy, D. N., Caviness, V. S., Jr., et al. (2001). Normal sexual dimorphism of the adult human brain assessed by in vivo magnetic resonance imaging. *Cerebral Cortex, 11*(6), 490–497.

Hardan, A., Minshew, N., Mallikarjuhn, M., & Keshavan, M. (2001). Brain volume in autism. *Journal of Child Neurology, 16*(6), 421–424.

Herbert, M. R., Ziegler, D. A., Deutsch, C. K., O'Brien, L. M., Lange, N., Bakardjiev, A., et al. (2003). Dissociations of cerebral cortex, subcortical and cerebral white matter volumes in autistic boys. *Brain, 126*(Pt 5), 1182–1192.

Herbert, M. R., Ziegler, D. A., Makris, N., Filipek, P. A., Kemper, T. L., Normandin, J. J., et al. (2004). Localization of white matter volume increase in autism and developmental language disorder. *Annals of Neurology, 55*(4), 530–540.

Jenkins, B. G., Chen, Y. I., Kyestermann, E., Makris, M., Nguyen, T. V., Kraft, E., et al. (1999). An integrated strategy for evaluation of metabolic and oxidative defects in neurodegenerative illness using magnetic resonance techniques. *Annals of the New York Academy of Science, 893*, 214–242.

Jernigan, T. L., Trauner, D. A., Hesselink, J. R., & Tallal, P. A. (1991). Maturation of human cerebrum observed in vivo during adolescence. *Brain, 114*, 2037–2049.

Kennedy, D. N., Caviness, V. S., & Makris, N. (1996). Structural morphometry in the developing brain. In R. W. Thatcher, G. R. Lyon, J. Rumsey, & N. Krasnegor (Eds.), *Developmental neuroimaging: Mapping the development of brain and behavior*. New York: Academic Press.

Kennedy, D. N., Lange, N., Makris, N., Bates, J., & Caviness, V. S. (1998). Gyri of the human neocortex: An MRI-based analysis of volumes and variance. *Cerebral Cortex, 8*(4), 372–384.

Kennedy, D. N., Makris, N., Herbert, M. R., Takahashi, T., & Caviness, V. S. (2002). Basic principles of MRI and morphometry studies of human brain development. *Developmental Science, 5*(3), 268–278.

Kikinis, R., Guttmann, C., Metcalf, D., Wells, W., Ettinger, H. L., Weiner, H., et al. (1999). Quantitative follow-up of patients with multiple sclerosis using MRI: Technical aspects. *Journal of Magnetic Resonance Imaging, 9*, 519–530.

Killiany, R. J., Gomez-Isla, T., Moss, M., Kikinis, R., Sandor, T., Jolesz, F., et al. (2000). Use of structural magnetic resonance imaging to predict who will get Alzheimer's disease. *Annals of Neurology, 47*(4), 430–439.

Killiany, R. J., Hyman, B. T., Gomez-Isla, T., Moss, M. B., Kikinis, R., Jolesz, F., et al. (2002). MRI measures of entorhinal cortex vs hippocampus in preclinical AD. *Neurology, 58*(8), 1188–1196.

Leonard, C. M., Eckert, M. A., Lombardino, L. J., Oakland, T., Kranzler, J., Mohr, C. M., et al. (2001). Anatomical risk factors for phonological dyslexia. *Cerebral Cortex, 11*(2), 148–157.

Leonard, C. M., Lombardino, L. J., Walsh, K., Eckert, M. A., Mockler, J. L., Rowe, L. A., et al. (2002). Anatomical risk factors that distinguish dyslexia from SLI predict reading skill in normal children. *Journal of Communication Disorders, 35*(6), 501–531.

Makris, N., Hodge, S. M., Haselgrove, C., Kennedy, D. N., Dale, A., Fischl, B., et al. (2003). Human cerebellum: Surface-assisted cortical parcellation and volumetry with magnetic resonance imaging. *Journal of Cognitive Neuroscience, 15*(4), 584–599.

Makris, N., Meyer, J., Bates, J., Caviness, V., & Kennedy, D. (1999). MRI-based topographic parcellation of human cerebral white matter and nuclei: II. Rationale and applications with systematics of cerebral connectivity. *NeuroImage, 9*(1), 18–45.

Makris, N., Worth, A. J., Sorensen, A. G., Papadimitriou, G. M., Wu, O., Reese, T. G., et al. (1997). Morphometry of in vivo human white matter association pathways with diffusion-weighted magnetic resonance imaging. *Annals of Neurology, 42*, 951–962.

Meyer, J. W., Makris, N., Bates, J. F., Caviness, V. S., & Kennedy, D. N. (1999). MRI-Based topographic parcellation of human cerebral white matter. *NeuroImage, 9*(1), 1–17.

Neil, J., Shiran, S., McKinstry, R., Schefft, G., Snyder, A., Almli, C., et al. (1998). Normal brain in human newborns: Apparent diffusion coefficient and diffusion anisotropy measured by using diffusion tensor MR imaging. *Radiology, 209*(1), 57–66.

Pennington, B. F., Filipek, P. A., Lefly, D., Churchwell, J., Kennedy, D. N., Simon, J. H., et al. (1999). Brain morphometry in reading-disabled twins. *Neurology, 53*(4), 723–729.

Pfefferbaum, A., Mathalon, D. H., Sullivan, E. V., Rawles, J. M., Zipursky, R. B., & Lim, K. O. (1994). A quantitative magnetic resonance imaging study of changes in brain morphology from infancy to late adulthood. *Archives of Neurology, 51*, 874–887.

Piven, J., Saliba, K., Bailey, J., & Arndt, S. (1997). An MRI study of autism: The cerebellum revisited. *Neurology, 49*(2), 546–551.

Rademacher, J., Caviness, V. S., Steinmetz, H., & Galaburda, A. M. (1993). Topographical variation of the human primary cortices: Implications for neuroimaging, brain mapping and neurobiology. *Cerebral Cortex, 3*, 313–329.

Rademacher, J., Galaburda, A. M., Kennedy, D. N., Filipek, P. A., & Caviness, V. S. (1992). Human cerebral cortex: Localization, parcellation, and morphometry with magnetic resonance imaging. *Journal of Cognitive Neuroscience, 4*, 352–374.

Reiss, A. L., Abrams, M. T., Singer, H. S., Ross, J. L., & Denckla, M. B. (1996). Brain development, gender and IQ in children. A volumetric imaging study. *Brain, 119*(Pt. 5), 1763–1774.

Roessler, E., & Muenke, M. (2001). Midline and laterality defects: Left and right meet in the middle. *Bioessays, 23*(10), 888–900.

Rosas, H. D., Goodman, J., Chen, Y. I., Jenkins, B. G., Kennedy, D. N., Makris, N., et al. (2001). Striatal volume loss in HD as measured by MRI and the influence of CAG repeat. *Neurology, 57*(6), 1025–1028.

Rosas, H. D., Liu, A. K., Hersch, S., Glessner, M., Ferrante, R. J., Salat, D. H., et al. (2002). Regional and progressive thinning of the cortical ribbon in Huntington's disease. *Neurology, 58*(5), 695–701.

Scheltens, P., Leys, D., Barkhof, F., et al. (1992). Atrophy of the medial temporal lobes on MRI in probable Alzheimer's disease and normal ageing: Diagnostic value and neuropsychological correlates. *Journal of Neurology, Neurosurgery, and Psychiatry, 55*, 967—972.

Seab, J. P., Jagust, W. J., Wong, S. T., Roos, M. S., Reed, B. R., & Budinger, T. G. (1988). Quantitative NMR measurement of hippocampal atrophy in Alzheimer's Disease. *Magnetic Resonance in Medicine, 8*, 200–208.

Seidman, L. J., Faraone, S. V., Goldstein, J. M., Goodman, J. M., Kremen, W. S., Toomey, R., et al. (1999). Thalamic and amygdala-hippocampal volume reductions in first-degree relatives of patients with schizophrenia: An MRI-based morphometric analysis. *Biological Psychiatry, 46*(7), 941–954.

Seidman, L. J., Faraone, S. V., Goldstein, J. M., Kremen, W. S., Horton, N. J., Makris, N., et al. (2002). Left hippocampal volume as a vulnerability indicator for schizophrenia: A magnetic resonance imaging morphometric study of nonpsychotic first-degree relatives. *Archives of General Psychiatry, 59*(9), 839–849.

Shenton, M., Kikinis, R., Jolesz, F., et al. (1992). Abnormalities of the left temporal lobe and thought disorder in schizophrenia: A quantitative MRI study. *The New England Journal of Medicine, 327*, 604—612.

Simon, E., & Barkovich, A. (2001). Holoprosencephaly: New concepts. *Magnetic Resonance in Imaging in Clinical North America, 9*(1), 149–164, viii–ix.

Simon, E., Hevner, R., Pinter, J., Clegg, N., Delgado, M., Kinsman, S., et al. (2001). The dorsal cyst in holoprosencephaly and the role of the thalamus in its formation. *Neuroradiology, 43*(9), 787–791.

Simon, E., Hevner, R., Pinter, J., Clegg, N., Miller, V., Kinsman, S., et al. (2000). Assessment of the deep gray nuclei in holoprosencephaly. *American Journal of Neuroradiology, 21*(10), 1955–1961.

Sudikoff, S., & Banasiak, K. (1998). Techniques for measuring cerebral blood flow in children. *Current Opinions in Pediatrics, 10*(3), 291–298.

Takahashi, T., Kinsman, S., Makris, N., Grant, E., Haselgrove, C., McInerney, S., et al. (2003). Semilobar holoprosencephaly with midline "seam": A topologic and morphogenetic model based upon MRI analysis. *Cerebral Cortex, 13*(12), 1299–1312.

Takahashi, T. S., Kinsman, S., Makris, N., Grant, E., Haselgrove, C., McInerney, S., et al. (2004). Holoprosencephaly—topologic variations in a liveborn series: A general model based upon MRI analysis. *Journal of Neurocytology, 33*(1), 23–35.

Thompson, P. M., Giedd, J. N., Woods, R. P., MacDonald, D., Evans, A. C., & Toga, A. W. (2000). Growth patterns in the developing brain detected by using continuum mechanical tensor maps. *Nature, 404*, 190–193.

Viergever, M., Maintz, J., Niessen, W., Noordmans, H., Pluim, J., Stokking, R., et al. (2001). Registration, segmentation, and visualization of multimodal brain images. *Computerized Medical Imaging and Graphics, 25*(2), 147–151.

Wells, W. M., Grimson, W. E. L., Kikinis, R., & Jolesz, F. A. (1996). Adaptive segmentation of MRI data. *IEEE Transactions on Medical Imaging, 15*(4), 429–442.

Worth, A. J., Makris, N., Meyer, J. W., Caviness, V. S., Jr., & Kennedy, D. N. (1998). Semiautomatic segmentation of brain exterior in magnetic resonance images driven by empirical procedures and anatomical knowledge. *Medical Image Analysis, 2*(4), 315–324.

Worth, A. J., Makris, N., Patti, M. R., Goodman, J. M., Hoge, E. A., Caviness, V. S., Jr., et al. (1998). Precise segmentation of the lateral ventricles and caudate nucleus in MR brain images using anatomically driven histograms. *IEEE Transactions on Medical Imaging, 17*(2), 303–310.

Chapter • 16

Cortical Plasticity: The Effects of Sensory Deprivation

Hugo Théoret and Alvaro Pascual-Leone

The study of blind individuals has revealed the exquisite ability of the human brain to reorganize following peripheral injury. Although it has long been believed that such plastic events were dependent on irreversible sensory deprivation occurring during a specific developmental period, recent evidence suggest that under certain experimental conditions, sensory interactions can be modified, thereby "creating" cross-modal plasticity. The idea that short-term behavioral interventions can modify brain organization could have far-reaching applications for conditions such as dyslexia. Here, we review the pertinent literature relating to plasticity in the brain of blind individuals and describe recent experiments conducted in our laboratory that show the surprising ability of the adult brain cortex to adapt to sensory deprivation.

BEHAVIORAL ADJUSTMENT TO BLINDNESS

Individuals who become blind during the course of their lifetime have to adjust to the striking demands of no longer being able to rely on vision to interact with their environment. Growing experimental evidence suggests that these adjustments not only implicate the remaining sensory modalities such as touch and hearing,

---

The authors gratefully acknowledge the support of the Canadian Institutes of Health Research (HT), the National Eye Institute, and National Institute of Mental Health (APL).

but also involve those parts of the brain once dedicated to vision itself. It appears that in the blind, brain areas commonly associated with the processing of visual information are not rendered "silent" by visual deprivation but rather are recruited in a compensatory cross-modal manner.

It is a common belief that the loss of vision is somehow compensated for by the remaining senses (Pons, 1996). Loss of visual input could lead to enhanced performance in the remaining sensory modalities through compensatory brain reorganization and attentional shifts. On the other hand, blindness may be detrimental to perception in the remaining senses because of the strong reliance on vision for the construction of spatial representations. Thus, the fundamental question in this regard is whether vision is required to calibrate other sensory modalities or if its loss confers a behavioral advantage that could be explained by compensatory plasticity.

Auditory Performance

The notion that blind individuals display superior auditory capabilities has garnered support from recent reports investigating sound localization abilities in early-blind subjects (Ashmead et al., 1998; Lessard, Pare, Lepore, & Lassonde, 1998; Muchnik, Efrati, Nemeth, Malin, & Hildesheimer, 1991; Röder et al., 1999). Lessard et al. (1998) showed that performance on a binaural sound localization task was similar in totally blind and sighted subjects, suggesting that vision is not necessary for the accurate development of three-dimensional spatial mapping of auditory space. The authors also showed that localizing sound sources monaurally was accompanied by a strong bias toward the unobstructed ear in sighted and half of their totally blind subjects. Indeed, sounds presented on the side of the obstructed ear were always localized on the opposite side. Most notably, half of the blind subjects were able to correctly localize sounds ipsilateral to the obstructed ear in almost 100% of the trials. Correct localization of sounds on the side of the obstructed ear was observed in none of the 36 sighted subjects tested. These data suggested the presence of functional compensation in response to absence of visual input. It was hypothesized that such compensations might occur in auditory structures such as the inferior colliculus or primary auditory cortex through increased use of spectral information. The unused visual cortex may also play a role as it could be recruited to perform auditory operations (Cohen et al., 1996; Sadato et al., 1996).

Further support for a behavioral advantage in blind individuals comes from an investigation of the spatial tuning curves within central and peripheral auditory space (Röder et al., 1999). Blind and sighted subjects were asked to identify infrequent deviant sounds emanating from the most peripheral or most central speaker out of an eight-speaker array placed on the horizontal azimuth. Subjects were to ignore sounds coming from all other speakers. The authors found that blind and sighted subjects performed equally well at detecting deviant stimuli coming from the central auditory space, again suggesting a noncritical role for vision in the development of this type of auditory behavior. However, when participants were asked to detect deviant sounds coming from the most peripheral speaker, blind subjects outperformed sighted subjects, hence demonstrating superior auditory capabilities in far-lateral space. In conjunction with the Lessard et al. (1998) study, these data underscore the striking ability of the brain to compensate for the loss of visual input. The findings also suggest that there might be specific differences in the likelihood of plastic reorganization affecting peripheral and central space. Possibly, differential connectivity between peripheral and central auditory space and visual cortex might underlay such findings. Recent data regarding anatomical connections between auditory and visual cortices in adult rhesus monkeys support such findings between peripheral and central space (Falchier, Clavagnier, Barone, & Kennedy, 2002).

The idea that visual feedback is not necessary for the development of adequate auditory processing has nonetheless recently been challenged. Zwiers, Van Opstal, and Cruysberg (2001a) hypothesized that monaural intensity judgments may explain the superior performance of blind individuals instead of increased use of spectral cues. The authors expanded the study of auditory ability to the vertical plane and added complex hearing conditions where background noise was added to the target while stimuli were presented in frontal space. Performance of blind subjects in a simple target localization task was similar to that of sighted subjects in both elevation and azimuth. When background noise was added, thereby increasing the difficulty of the task and simulating a more natural setting, blind subjects performed more poorly than sighted individuals at localizing auditory targets in the vertical plane. These data put into question previous reports of auditory hyperacuity in the blind (Lessard et al., 1998; Röder et al., 1999). Zwiers et al. (2001a) argued that visual feedback may be necessary in frontal space for accurate localization of sound since reliance on vision would be predominant in the central field. In peripheral space, where vision is much degraded, blind subjects may rely on motor, proprioceptive, or tactile feedback to calibrate the auditory system (Lewald, 2002; Zwiers, Van Opstal, & Cruysberg, 2001b). Furthermore, blind subjects may make better use of monaural intensity cues instead of spectral information, which could explain the results of Lessard et al. (1998) where stimuli were always presented at the same intensity. Lewald (2002) also proposed that the auditory performance of blind individuals may be explained by the use of audiomotor feedback rather than visual feedback. This implies that blind subjects do not have superior auditory capabilities *per se* but rather make better use of cues relating body position to auditory spatial information (Lewald, 2002).

Tactile Performance

Touch is of particular interest in the study of behavioral compensations occurring in the blind since many of these individuals learn to read Braille, a skill that requires great tactile accuracy. Braille reading requires the discrimination of subtle patterns of raised dots and the transformation of this spatial code into meaningful information. Furthermore, touch is used by the blind to navigate in near space and recognize objects. Early reports did not show differences in sensory thresholds between blind and sighted subjects (see Hollins, 1989). For example, Pascual-Leone and Torres (1993) reported no differences in sensory thresholds between 15 proficient blind Braille readers and 15 sighted volunteers with no Braille reading ability in response to electrical, touch (von Frey hairs), and two-point stimulation. No differences in sensory thresholds between the blind and sighted were also reported for grating ridge width using active scanning and grating discrimination using passive touch (Grant, Thiagarajah, & Sathian, 2000). In a Braille-like discrimination task, Blind subjects were shown to have lower thresholds than sighted volunteers (Grant et al., 2000). However, this behavioral advantage receded by the third or fourth session, indicating that blind people might not possess increased tactile sensitivity but rather use the available information in a more efficient way, in great part due to practice. In addition, it was shown that blind subjects who use several fingers to read Braille frequently misidentify which fingertip is being stimulated by a von Frey hair, suggesting maladaptive compensation in visually deprived individuals (Sterr et al., 1998).

Van Boven, Hamilton, Kauffman, Keenan, and Pascual-Leone (2000) recently compared the performance of early-blind subjects with that of sighted volunteers on a gratings orientation task (GOT). This task was chosen because comparing Braille discrimination performance can lead to confounds resulting from differential practice and familiarity effects as was reported by Grant et al. (2000). Furthermore, the GOT provides a quantitative measure of spatial acuity as subjects must discriminate between two orthogonal directions of varying groove widths. The authors found that the grating orientation threshold was significantly lower in blind individuals compared to sighted subjects, and that within the blind group, sensory thresholds were lower for the Braille-reading finger compared to the other fingers tested (see Figure 1 in the four-color section on page 222-J). The demonstration of heightened tactile acuity in the blind, coupled with other such reports (e.g., Hollins, 1989), suggests that increased practice in the blind results in plastic brain reorganizations (see below) that are functionally relevant. Furthermore, it would appear that the Braille reading skill can be generalized to some (e.g., grating orientation discrimination) but not all tactile activities as evidenced by the lack of tactile superiority in a wide variety of tasks (see Hollins, 1989). As in the auditory modality, it is evident that different tasks and populations (e.g., early-blind versus late-blind) can yield quite different accounts of behavioral compensations in response to blindness.

An interesting question relating to these issues is whether behavioral compensations in the blind are dependent on irreversible sensory deprivation occurring during a specific developmental period, or if under certain experimental conditions, these changes can be experimentally induced in normal adult subjects. As part of a larger study (Pascual-Leone & Hamilton, 2001), we wondered whether prolonged blindfolding would lead to increased tactile performance on a Braille reading task (Kauffman, Théoret, & Pascual-Leone, 2002). We compared the performance of sighted subjects on a Braille character discrimination task to that of normal participants blindfolded for a period of five days. Twenty-four subjects (mean age of approximately 25 years) were recruited and were randomized into four groups: blindfolded and stimulated, blindfolded and not stimulated, sighted and stimulated, sighted and not stimulated. The stimulated groups were enrolled in an intensive tactile stimulation program lasting for more than six hours a day including four hours of formal Braille instruction. To supplement their tactile stimulation, subjects also engaged in tactile games for at least two additional hours a day. For the Braille instruction, all subjects were taught to read using only their right index finger. Participants in the blindfolded/nonstimulated group were encouraged to use their sense of touch in their daily activities despite not receiving formal Braille training.

Braille recognition ability was tested in all subjects at day 1 (baseline), 3, and 5, and participants remained blindfolded throughout the testing sessions. Using a specially designed computer-driven Braille stimulator, testing of both the right and left index finger was carried out. Braille characters were presented to the pad of the index finger using six plastic rods (measuring 1 mm each in diameter and raising to a 1.5 mm height) arranged according to a typical Braille cell design and letter standard. When a Braille character was generated, the corresponding rods would push up and indent the skin of the resting finger pad. Pairs of Braille characters were presented, and a forced choice paradigm was used in which subjects were required to indicate whether a pair of characters were the same or different.

The main finding of this study was that through five days of complete visual deprivation, blindfolded subjects performed significantly better than sighted subjects in the Braille discrimination task (Figure 2). Indeed, of the blindfolded subjects, those that did not undergo intensive Braille training performed significantly better that the sighted and stimulated group. Thus, the superior performance of blindfolded individuals occurred despite equivalent practice between the two groups, suggesting that tactile differences between blind and sighted subjects do not entirely depend on prior experience and the learning of perceptual skills (Grant et al., 2000).

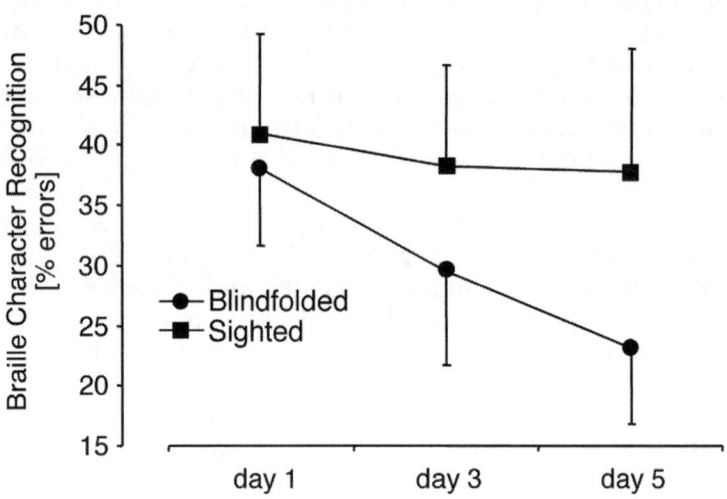

Figure 2. Compared to sighted subjects, blindfolded individuals learn Braille reading faster. After five days of blindfolding, subjects show marked decreases in Braille character recognition errors. (Adapted from Kauffman et al., 2002).

The demonstration of heightened perceptual abilities in the blind and blindfolded may reflect cortical plastic changes. Changes in behavior must be accompanied by a reorganization within the remaining modalities or through the deafferented visual cortex. Despite conflicting results relating to the behavioral capabilities of blind individuals, one must assume that the loss of visual input produces plastic changes in the brain. Indeed, the animal literature has taught us that sensory deprivation leads to major cortical and subcortical reorganization (Rauschecker, 1995). But what happens in the human brain in response to blindness?

NEUROPHYSIOLOGICAL ADJUSTMENT TO BLINDNESS

Somatosensory Cortex

Blind individuals need to extract crucial spatial information from available sensory modalities to function in their surroundings. The development of Braille as a written language is an excellent example of how the blind exploit their remaining sensory abilities to read and communicate effectively. In Braille reading, blind individuals learn to tactically explore patterns by sweeping their index finger over raised dots to extract meaningful language (proficient Braille readers often learn to scan with multiple fingers and both hands). Thus, it would be intuitive to think that sensory-motor systems would be a likely locus of neural reorganization in an individual learning to read Braille. Indeed, evidence from both animal and human studies have shown that tactile experience can modify the somatosensory representation of a body part such as the hand and its repeated use can lead to the enlargement of its cortical representation (Jenkins, Merzenich, Ochs, Allard, & Guic-Robles, 1990; Merzenich et al., 1984). Animal evidence also strongly suggests that changes in cortical representation may directly reflect perceptual ability (Recanzone, Allard, Jenkins, & Merzenich, 1990).

As was described earlier, sensory thresholds in blind Braille readers are similar in many respects to those of control subjects (Pascual-Leone & Torres, 1993). Despite the absence of widespread significant differences in peripheral sensory systems (but see Van Boven et al., 2000), several lines of evidence suggest that Braille reading in response to blindness is associated with plastic changes within the somatosensory cortex. Pascual-Leone and Torres (1993) recorded somatosensory evoked potentials from proficient Braille readers, and demonstrated that the cortical representation of the index finger was larger than that of sighted controls and blind non-Braille readers. In addition, the cortical representation of the Braille-reading finger was enlarged compared to the homologous finger of the opposite hand. Consistent with these findings, transcranial magnetic stimulation-induced suppression of tactile stimulus perception (Cohen et al., 1989) could be obtained through the stimulation of a larger number of sites over the sensorimotor cortex representation of the Braille reading finger of blind individuals compared to nonreading fingers or index fingers of control subjects (Pascual-Leone & Torres, 1993). At a behavioral level, these findings are consistent with the fact that blind individuals must quickly extract highly detailed spatial information for effective Braille reading. This expanded cortical representation may allow blind readers to carry out the complex task of Braille reading. The enlarged representation of the Braille reading finger in proficient Braille readers was further supported by a TMS mapping study in which motor evoked potentials in the first dorsal interosseus muscle of proficient blind Braille readers could be elicited through the stimulation of a larger area of motor cortex than that of the nonreading hand and both hands of control subjects (Pascual-Leone et al., 1993). These changes might be due to the fact that Braille reading creates new motor demands on the reading finger, resulting in cortical overrepresentations. It must be noted that longitudinal studies (over the course of one year) during the learning of Braille have shown cortical enlargements proceeding along two time scales: an initial, transient phase (lasting roughly six months) followed by a more stable period. The initial phase is characterized by a rapid and dramatic enlargement of cortical representation, likely due to the unmasking of existing connections and changes in synaptic efficacy, while the second phase is characterized by a more stable cortical representation of the reading finger reflecting enduring structural changes at multiple neuronal levels (Pascual-Leone, Hamilton, Tormos, Keenan, & Catala, 1999).

Proficient Braille readers often use more than one finger to read faster. As such, Sterr et al. (1998) investigated the effects of three-finger reading on somatotopic representations in Braille readers. The authors noticed that multiple finger readers made frequent mistakes in identifying which of their fingers was touched during a sensory threshold task. This behavior was not observed in single finger readers or in sighted controls. Could this change in perceptual behavior manifest itself at the cortical level? To investigate this issue, the authors used magnetic source imaging to demonstrate that the cortical representation of the reading fingers of blind individuals who are multiple finger readers is much more complex and appears disorganized compared to Braille readers who use one finger. The authors proposed that this pattern corresponds to the fusion of the cortical representation of the reading fingers caused by an increased level of simultaneous stimulation. This representational "smearing" of digital topography may explain the mislocalization of tactile stimuli. It is further argued that the fusing of digital input in multiple finger readers allows the incoming information to be processed more holistically, perhaps reflecting enhanced perceptual abilities and increased reading speed. A similar "smearing" of the homuncular representation of the digits has been described in dystonic patients, where altered processing of simultaneous sensory inputs was reported in a fMRI study (Sanger, Pascual-Leone, Tarsy, & Schlaug, 2002). The authors suggested that a nonlinear combination of each digit's activation patterns resulted in the dedifferentiation of tactile sensory fields, leading to impaired sensory perception. Interestingly, it was subsequently shown that Braille training for eight weeks increased tactile spatial acuity and decreased disability in dystonia patients (Zeuner et al., 2002). These data highlight the possibility that appropriately employed Braille reading may actually help "improve" or "restore" the homuncular representation, and may then lead to improved localization abilities for touch.

Taken together, these studies show that sensory and motor cortices undergo important adjustments in response to intensive tactile training. It is, however, difficult to estimate what role blindness plays in these plastic changes. It would be arduous to disentangle the respective contribution of sensory deprivation and practice in the development of enlarged reading finger cortical representations. Nevertheless, these results suggest that dramatic changes can occur in the brain of blind individuals.

Occipital Recruitment: Tactile

A pervasive question regarding the adjustment to blindness relates to what happens to the cortical areas normally associated with the processing of visual information. The occipital cortex is known to contain multiple representations of visual space (Felleman & Van Essen, 1991). In the striate cortex, visual information captured within the retina is transformed and decoded into meaningful spatial information and forwarded to extrastriate areas for further processing of feature-specific attributes of the visual scene such as form, color, and motion.

Wanet-Defalque et al. (1988) were among the first to report that occipital areas undergo functional changes in early blind subjects. Using cerebral metabolic rate for glucose (rCMRGlc) as a marker of neuronal function, the authors showed that long-standing visual deprivation (early-blind subjects) led to higher regional glucose utilization in striate and prestriate cortical areas compared to blindfolded sighted controls while carrying out object manipulation and auditory tasks. In a related study, Veraart et al. (1990) compared glucose metabolism in early- and late-blind (i.e., blinded after complete development of the visual system) individuals. They found that glucose utilization within the visual cortex of early-blind subjects was elevated and comparable to normal sighted controls (eyes open). In contrast, late-blind subjects showed glucose utilization just slightly lower than that observed in normal sighted controls (eyes closed). Uhl, Franzen, Lindinger, Lang, and Deecke (1991) presented further evidence of visual cortex reorganization in blind subjects by showing task-related (tactile) activations in the occipital cortex. Event-related EEG recordings showed sustained negative DC potential shifts over the occipital cortex in early-blind subjects while scanning Braille sentences. Furthermore, these shifts were more apparent when compared to passive scanning of random dot patterns and compared to sighted individuals carrying out the same task. Interestingly, the same group reported that tactile mental imagery in early-blind and sighted controls also led to occipital negative shifts as they imagined the feel of textures on the fingertips of their hand (Uhl et al., 1994). This finding is of particular interest when one considers that unlike sighted controls, the blind subjects had no prior visual perception. The authors suggested that despite visual deprivation, the occipital cortex of the blind is perhaps involved in a form of "tactile" imagery that employs similar neurophysiological mechanisms. In a follow-up study, Uhl, Franzen, Podreka, Steiner, and Deecke (1993) used SPECT and regional cerebral blood flow measurements to complement these findings, and found that occipital indices were higher in the blind than in sighted controls performing tasks of active (Braille reading) and passive (random dot patterns) touch. These findings strongly suggested that occipital cortical areas are not only active following sensory deprivation, but also may be recruited in a functional and meaningful way to carry out nonvisual tasks in the blind.

As the development and sensitivity of functional neuroimaging techniques improved, numerous groups readdressed the question of task-dependent functional participation of the occipital cortex in nonvisual function. Sadato et al. (1996) showed that the primary visual cortex is activated in early-blind subjects performing a Braille reading task (see Figure 3 in the four-color section on page 222-K). In the blind, bilateral activations were seen in the dorsal and ventral lobes of medial occipital cortex (area 17) with concomitant activity in extrastriate areas. Activation of the primary visual cortex was also evident in non-Braille tactile discrimination tasks (discrimination of angle, width, and Roman embossed characters encoded in Braille cells). There was also a pattern of activation in the blind subjects during the discrimination task involving suppression of the parietal operculum and activation of the ventral area of the occipital cortex. In the sighted controls carrying out the same tasks, the opposite pattern of activation occurred. As a control condition, passive sweeping of the finger over a homogeneous pattern of Braille dots (without responding) did not result in activation of the primary visual cortex in either the blind or sighted subjects. In explaining their findings, the authors suggested that visual imagery was unlikely to underlie the activation of visual cortex based on the fact that the blind subjects recruited in their study lost their vision early in life and had little visual mental recollections. Furthermore, Braille was often learned well after the complete loss of vision and, therefore, likely did not assist in their learning. In contrast, the authors suggested that occipital activations are likely related to other aspects of the task such as lexical processing.

The pattern of visual cortex activation in blind subjects was further investigated by Büchel, Price, Frackowiak, and Friston (1998) using PET. In contrast to the Sadato et al. (1996) study, activation of primary visual cortex was absent in congenitally blind subjects whereas extrastriate visual areas were activated during Braille reading. Conversely, primary visual cortex activations were observed in a group of late-blind individuals. The authors hypothesized that activation of area V1 in late-blind subjects was the result of visual imagery associated with early visual experience. Kossyln et al. (1999) have argued that visual perception and visual mental imagery share a similar neuroanatomical substrate. Indeed, the primary visual cortex is activated in normal sighted individuals during visual imagery and disruption of occipital cortex with TMS impairs the ability to carry out imagery tasks. It can be argued that the activation of occipital networks in the blind reflects the visual representations of stimuli generated by tactile stimulation. However, this argument does not seem hold true for congenitally blind individuals who, in many cases, do not have significant prior visual experience (Sadato et al., 1996).

These discrepant results sparked a series of studies that specifically address the issue of cross-modal plasticity as a function of age of blindness onset. Cohen et. al. (1999) showed that visual cortex activations during tactile discrimination tasks were weak or nonexistent in subjects who lost their vision after age 14, whereas primary and extrastriate visual areas were activated in both congenitally and early-blind individuals. This period of susceptibility to cross-modal plasticity was challenged by Burton et al. (2002) who showed clear activation of primary visual cortex during Braille reading in early- and late-blind subjects with fMRI. The low-level visual activations corresponded to retinotopically organized visual cortex, suggesting a functional role for this activity rather than reflecting pathological processes unrelated to Braille reading. It is important to note that high-level, well-defined visual areas were also activated in late- and early-blind subjects (V2, VP, $V4_V$, and LO). The only notable differences between late- and early-blind subjects occurred in MT/V5 and V8 where congenitally blind individuals showed more robust activations. It was hypothesized that Braille fluency differences might account for this different level of activity. Early-blind subjects were more fluent Braille readers and as such, might have used motion selective area MT/V5 (Tootell et al., 1995) more efficiently to process hand movements-related information across Braille cells. Sadato, Okada, Honda, and Yonekura (2002) reinvestigated the issue of critical periods and cross-modal plasticity associated with tactile processing. They showed increased primary visual cortex activity in subjects who lost their vision before 16 years of age whereas V1 activation decreased in late-blind individuals. As in previous reports, extrastriate visual areas were activated in both groups (Büchel et al. 1998; Burton et al., 2002; Cohen et al., 1999; Sadato et al., 1996).

The notion of a critical period of susceptibility to cross modal plasticity in the blind was again challenged by the presentation of striking pilot data. Pascual-Leone and Hamilton (2001) showed that a five-day period of complete blindfolding was enough to induce functionally relevant occipital recruitment in response to tactile processing in healthy adult subjects. These data imply that the activation of the occipital cortex during processing of nonvisual information may not necessarily be an exclusive feature of pathological conditions such as blindness. The recent demonstration of direct connections between A1 and V1 in monkeys (Falchier et al., 2002) supports this idea, and taken together, these data suggest that the issue of age of blindness onset should be readdressed in terms of functional connectivity changes. Finally, the fact that blindfolded subjects also show superior tactile abilities (Kauffman et al., 2002) supports the notion of occipital recruitment not only being functionally relevant but also conferring a behavioral advantage to the remaining sensory modalities.

Occipital Recruitment: Auditory

Studies in the blind have also demonstrated that functional reorganization occurs within the occipital cortex in response to auditory stimulation. Kujala, Alho, Paavilainen, Summala, and Naatanen (1992) compared the topography of event related potentials (ERP) in a sound localization task (pitch change discrimination) in blind and sighted subjects. They found that component signals were evident in posterior cortical areas of early-blind subjects. These results (later confirmed by MEG recordings by the same group) (see Kujala et al., 1995) suggested that in the blind, posterior brain regions (i.e., parietal and occipital cortices) may be involved in auditory, as well as tactile, processing. Following up on their initial findings, Kujala et al. (1997) investigated differences in scalp topography in early- and late-blind subjects with event-related potentials. In this study, both groups showed clear parietal-occipital activity, further suggesting that cross-modal recruitment of the occipital cortex may occur in the mature brain (contradictory to common belief that plastic changes occur only in early development). Furthermore, these changes appeared only during active but not passive detection of sound changes, consistent with their earlier findings (Kujala et al., 1992).

Similar to what has been reported in the tactile modality, the study of occipital activation in response to auditory stimulation has yielded robust results in blind individuals. For example, Leclerc, Saint-Amour, Lavoie, Lassonde, and Lepore (2000) studied four congenitally blind individuals who had previously demonstrated superior performance on an auditory discrimination task (Lessard et al., 1998). The authors measured scalp distributions of auditory event-related potentials during a sound localization task. The N1 and P3 component peaks of the evoked potentials were localized to the principle nodes of auditory processing in both blind and sighted subjects. Furthermore, these components were also clearly detected over the occipital pole in blind subjects (but not sighted). In another neuroimaging study, Weeks et al. (2000) used PET to demonstrate strong occipital activation in congenitally blind subjects performing an auditory localization task. Strong activation of the posterior parietal areas in both blind and sighted individuals was observed. However, right occipital cortical activation was only evident in the blind subjects despite the fact that behavioral data demonstrated that both groups performed similarly on the task. Using correlative analysis, extrastriate occipital areas corresponded to regions previously identified as visual spatial and motion-processing regions in experiments using sighted subjects. This similarity in foci of activation between visual processing in the sighted and auditory localization in the blind suggests that these areas may retain their functional and neuronal coding functions, despite processing different sensory modalities. Finally, the authors attributed the right-sided dominance of activation to the fact that spatial processing has often been attributed to the right hemisphere. Given the importance of audition to construct an internal representation of external space in the blind, it is possible that this stronger right-sided activity reflects consolidation of an occipital-parietal network implicated in effective auditory localization.

In summary, converging evidence suggests that cross-modal plasticity following sensory deprivation might be a general feature of the cerebral cortex. Indeed, the involvement of visual cortical areas in tactile and auditory processing has been clearly demonstrated, and activation of the *auditory* cortex was observed in a sample of profoundly *deaf* subjects in response to purely visual stimuli (Finney, Fine, & Dobkins, 2001). As such, it appears that following loss of sensory input to a unimodal primary sensory area, cortical activations evoked by information processing in other modalities are redistributed along the functional network to include the "unused" modality. Such a shift in connections and influences could be due to the establishment of new pathways or secondary to the unmasking of established ones. Fundamentally, the question is whether the activation detected in functional imaging studies is related to a top-down influence from multisensory areas, or whether there is direct input from other sensory modalities into primary visual cortical areas (Falchier et al., 2002). The speed at which occipital recruitment occurs in blindfolded subjects makes it unlikely that the establishment of new connections can entirely explain the phenomenon. Rather, it could be argued that latent pathways that participate in multisensory percepts in sighted subjects are unmasked and are potentiated in the event of complete loss of visual input. Further studies are needed to elucidate the mechanisms that underlie cross-modal plasticity in the blind.

FUNCTIONAL RELEVANCE OF NEUROPLASTIC CHANGES

Functional imaging studies have shown the plastic reorganization that occurs in response to blindness in unequivocal ways. Most notably, it appears the deafferented visual cortex is activated by tactile and auditory stimulation in blind subjects. Activity within occipital areas during nonvisual sensory processing does not necessarily mean that the visual cortex is directly involved in the completion of tactile and auditory behaviors. Indeed, the functional relevance of this "occipital recruitment" must be addressed to attach any behavioral significance to these activations and rule out the possibility that they are simply epiphenomena. The question of functional relevance has been addressed in two main ways: by use of transcranial magnetic stimulation (TMS) and with peripherally blind patients who suffered occipital damage.

Transcranial Magnetic Stimulation

The involvement of visual cortex in tactile behavior was first addressed by Cohen and collaborators (Cohen et al., 1996). They applied short trains of repetitive TMS (10 Hz, 3 seconds or 10Hz, 5 seconds) to different scalp positions while blind and sighted volunteers identified Braille and embossed Roman letters. It is believed that TMS can transiently disrupt performance when it is applied to a cortical region necessary for task completion through the introduction of "random noise" in the neural processes (Walsh & Cowey, 2000). As such, TMS can establish the causality between task performance and brain activation by interfering with cortical function. In blind subjects, magnetic stimulation of mid-occipital positions resulted in significant increases in Braille and Roman letter identification errors compared to sham stimulation (see Figure 4 in the four-color section on page 222-K). In the Braille condition, blind subjects reported "missing dots," "dots feeling faded," "phantom dots," "extra dots," and "dots not making sense" in response to visual cortex stimulation. In sighted volunteers, stimulation of mid-occipital cortex had no effect on identification of embossed Roman letters while somatosensory stimulation significantly increased the number of reporting errors. This was the first demonstration that blind individuals actively use their visual cortex to process somatosensory information. The functional relevance of occipital recruitment makes it possible that visual cortex activation can account in part for the behavioral improvements that have been reported in blind subjects (Lessard et al., 1998; Röder et al., 1999; Van Boven et al., 2000) or at least compensate for the loss of vision in the development of auditory and tactile abilities. Functionally relevant cross-modal plasticity in the blind was again demonstrated by Cohen et al. (1999) with a specific emphasis on determining a period of susceptibility during which occipital recruitment occurs and is related to behavior. As was detailed earlier, some data suggest that tactile to visual cross-modal plasticity is restricted to early-blind subjects. In addition to the absence of occipital activation during Braille reading in subjects who became blind after the age of 14 years, rTMS over the occipital pole did not induce reading errors in late-onset blind subjects. As such, the late-onset blind group behaved in much the same way as normal, sighted individuals.

The fact that blind subjects can detect tactile stimuli but have difficulties identifying them when the occipital pole is disrupted with TMS (Sadato et al., 1996) raises the intriguing possibility that the visual cortex is involved in the perception but not detection of tactile stimuli. Furthermore, great insight into the organization of the functional network subserving somatosensory processing in the blind would be gained by addressing the issue of timing the contribution of visual cortex to tactile processing. These questions were addressed by devising a task in which subjects must either detect or identify the presence of a Braille stimulus with the concomitant application of single-pulse TMS to somatosensory or visual cortex at different time intervals (Hamilton & Pascual-Leone, 1998). This particular design allows investigators to determine at what time a given cortical target makes a necessary contribution to task performance. For example, a single TMS pulse delivered over the occipital cortex can induce reporting errors of briefly flashed target letters in normal volunteers (Amassian et al., 1989). These errors are maximal when TMS is applied between 80 and 100 ms following visual stimulus presentation, implying that the occipital cortex makes a critical contribution to letter recognition only at these times since detection performance recovers quickly at later intervals. In a pilot study (Hamilton & Pascual-Leone, 1998), when single-pulse TMS was applied over the somatosensory cortex 20 to 40ms after Braille stimulus presentation to the index finger, blind subjects had difficulties detecting the peripheral stimulus and evidently could not identify it. In other words, subjects did not realize that a peripheral stimulus had been presented. This is in agreement with studies of TMS-induced tactile suppression in normal subjects (Cohen et al., 1989). Interestingly, when TMS was applied to the occipital cortex, detection was not affected but processing of the peripheral Braille stimulus (identification) was severely disrupted at interstimulus intervals of 50–80 ms. In other words, blind subjects knew a peripheral Braille stimulus had been presented but they could not discriminate whether it was real or nonsensical. In sum, these data show that (1) visual cortical areas in blind individuals are involved in the perception of tactile stimuli but are not involved in detection, and (2) the contribution of visual cortex to tactile processing occurs later than that of the somatosensory cortex.

Case Study

The reliance on visual cortex for the perception of tactile stimuli has recently been highlighted by the report of a blind woman who became alexic for Braille after a bilateral occipital stroke (Hamilton, Keenan, Catala, & Pascual-Leone, 2000). This subject was congenitally blind and started to read Braille at six years of age. She continued to use Braille extensively, approximately four to six hours a day, and showed remarkable reading speed. At 63, the patient suffered bilateral occipital ischemic strokes. Remarkably, upon recovery, she was unable to read Braille although she could still detect the presence of Braille stimuli on her fingertips, and reported no general impairment in touch or tactile sensitivity. MRI examination revealed no lesions in sensorimotor cortex or language areas, and sensory evoked potentials from the median nerve were normal. This case study strikingly resembles the effects of rTMS-induced "virtual lesions" of visual cortex in blind individuals where perception of tactile stimuli is compromised but detection is spared (Cohen et al., 1996; Hamilton & Pascual-Leone, 1998). This report further documents the plastic reorganizations that are thought to accompany blindness, most notably a shift of activity to posterior areas during tactile and auditory processing. It is reasonable to assume that parts of the tactile processing system in this patient were somehow reassigned to occipital areas and that the brain lesion disrupted this network component necessary for tactile perception. Tactile acuity tests were obviously not performed prior to stroke occurrence in this patient. As such, it is impossible to know if she displayed tactile hyperacuity comparable to that observed in a population of blind subjects (Van Boven et al., 2000). One might assume that if occipital recruitment is involved in behavioral enhancements, visual cortex lesions in blind subjects would have reverted this improved ability.

The study of causal relationships between visual cortex activity and tactile processing has provided important information relating to the organization of the functional network subserving sensory perception in blind individuals. Imaging data first suggested that the pathway for tactile and auditory discrimination changes with blindness. Then, disruptions in tactile processing following occipital TMS highlighted the functional relevance of occipital activations in blind humans. The notion that posterior areas are in effect "taken over" by the remaining sensory modalities puts into question the state of *visual* function within occipital cortex. This bears considerable importance when one considers the efforts made to develop visual cortex stimulation apparatus to restore rudimentary vision in the blind.

CONCLUSION

Studies in the blind have made it clear that areas once thought to be uniquely unimodal can process multimodal information under conditions of sensory deprivation. At the very least, visual cortical areas can process tactile and auditory signals, but further studies will show if the remaining sensory modalities (gustatory and olfactory) also recruit occipital cortex in blind individuals. One outstanding question is whether the multimodal properties of primary sensory areas are a unique feature of pathological conditions or if they can be expressed in normal subjects. Recent evidence suggests that cross-modal interactions do take place in primary sensory cortices of healthy subjects, and as such, it has been proposed that multisensory neurons within multimodal areas such as the parietal cortex can modulate the activity of visual neurons (Macaluso, Frith, & Driver, 2000). The demonstration of direct connections between area V1 and the parabelt areas of auditory cortex (Falchier et al., 2002), and studies in blindfolded subjects (Pascual-Leone & Hamilton, 2001) have added further support for multimodal processing in primary areas. Indeed, activation of primary auditory cortex was recently observed in normal subjects when viewing moving and static dots (Bavelier & Neville, 2002). This converging evidence highlights the need to reexamine the functional connectivity between primary and multimodal areas, and explore how unimodal areas interact to produce richly multimodal sensations.

Address correspondence to: Hugo Théoret, Département de psychologie, Université de Montréal, CP 6128, Succ Centre-Ville, Montréal, Qc, H3C 3J7 Canada; E-mail: hugo.theoret@umontreal.ca

REFERENCES

Amassian, V. E., Cracco, R. Q., Maccabee, P. J., Cracco, J. B., Rudell, A., & Eberle, L. (1989). Suppression of visual perception by magnetic coil stimulation of human occipital cortex. *Electroencephalography and Clinical Neurophysiology, 74*, 458–462.

Ashmead, D. H., Wall, R S., Ebinger, K. A., Eaton, S. B., Snook-Hill, M. M., & Yang, X. (1998). Spatial hearing in children with visual disabilities. *Perception, 27*, 105–122.

Bavelier, D., & Neville, H. J. (2002). Cross-modal plasticity: Where and how? *Nature Reviews Neuroscience, 3*, 443–452.

Büchel, C., Price, C., Frackowiak, R. S., & Friston, K. (1998). Different activation patterns in the visual cortex of late and congenitally blind subjects. *Brain, 121*, 409–419.

Burton, H., Snyder, A. Z., Conturo, T. E., Akbudak, E., Ollinger, J. M., & Raichle, M. E. (2002). Adaptive changes in early and late blind: A fMRI study of Braille reading. *Journal of Neurophysiology, 87*, 589–607.

Cohen, L. G., Bandinelli, S., Sato, S., Kufta, C., & Hallett, M. (1989). Attenuation in detection of somatosensory stimuli by transcranial magnetic stimulation. *Electroencephalography and Clinical Neurophysiology, 81*, 366–376.

Cohen, L. G., Celnik, P., Pascual-Leone, A., Corwell, B., Falz, L., Dambrosia, J., Honda, M., Sadato, N., Gerloff, C., Catala, M. D., & Hallett, M. (1996). Functional relevance of cross-modal plasticity in blind humans. *Nature, 389*, 180–183.

Cohen, L. G., Weeks, R. A., Sadato, N., Celnik, P., Ishii, K., & Hallett, M. (1999). Period of susceptibility for cross-modal plasticity in the blind. *Annals of Neurology, 45*, 451–460.

Falchier, A., Clavagnier, S., Barone, P., & Kennedy, H. (2002). Anatomical evidence of multimodal integration in primate striate cortex. *The Journal of Neuroscience, 22*, 5749–5759.

Felleman, D. J., & Van Essen, D. C. (1991). Distributed hierarchical processing in the primate cerebral cortex. *Cerebral Cortex, 1*, 1–47.

Finney, E. M., Fine, I., & Dobkins, K. (2001). Visual stimuli activate auditory cortex in the deaf. *Nature Neuroscience, 4*, 1171–1173.

Grant, A. C., Thiagarajah, M. C., & Sathian, K. (2000). Tactile perception in blind Braille readers: A psychophysical study of acuity and hyperacuity using gratings and dot patterns. *Perception and Psychophysics, 62*, 301–312.

Hamilton, R., & Pascual-Leone, A. (1998). Cortical plasticity associated with Braille learning. *Trends in Cognitive Sciences, 2*, 168–174.

Hamilton, R., Keenan, J. P., Catala, M. D., & Pascual-Leone, A. (2000). Alexia for Braille following bilateral occipital stroke in an early blind woman. *Neuroreport, 11*, 237–240.

Hollins, M. (1989). *Understanding blindness*. Hillsdale, NJ:Erlbaum.

Jenkins, W. M., Merzenich, M. M., Ochs, M. T., Allard, T., & Guic-Robles, E. (1990). Functional reorganization of primary somatosensory cortex in adult owl monkeys after behaviorally controlled tactile stimulation. *Journal of Neurophysiology, 63*, 82–104.

Kauffman, T., Théoret, H., & Pascual-Leone, A. (2002). Braille character discrimination in blindfolded human subjects. *Neuroreport, 13*, 571–574.

Kosslyn, S. M., Pascual-Leone, A., Felician, O., Camposano, S., Keenan, J. P., Thompson, W. L., Ganis, G., Sukel, K. E., & Alpert, N. M. (1999). The role of area 17 in visual imagery: Convergent evidence from PET and rTMS. *Science, 284*, 167–170.

Kujala, T., Alho, K., Paavilainen, P., Summala, H., & Naatanen, R. (1992). Neural plasticity in processing of sound location by the early blind: An event-related potential study. *Electroencephalography and Clinical Neurophysiology, 84*, 469–472.

Kujala, T., Huotilainen, M., Sinkkonen, J., Ahonen, A. I., Alho, K., Hamalainen, M. S., Ilmoniemi, R. J., Kajola, M., Knuutila, J. E., &

Lavikainen, J. (1995). Visual cortex activation in blind humans during sound discrimination. *Neuroscience Letters, 183,* 143–146.

Kujala, T., Alho, K., Huotilainen, M., Ilmoniemi, R. J., Lehtokoski, A., Leinonen, A., Rinne, T., Salonen, O., Sinkkonen, J., Standertskjold-Nordenstam, C. G., & Naatanen, R. (1997). Electrophysiological evidence for cross-modal plasticity in humans with early- and late-onset blindness. *Psychophysiology, 34,* 213–216.

Leclerc, C., Saint-Amour, D., Lavoie, M. E., Lassonde, M., & Lepore, F. (2000). Brain functional reorganization in early blind humans revealed by auditory event-related potentials. *Neuroreport, 11,* 545–550.

Lessard, N., Pare, M., Lepore, F., & Lassonde, M. (1998). Early-blind human subjects localize sound sources better than sighted subjects. *Nature, 395,* 278–280.

Lewald, J. (2002). Opposing effects of head position on sound localization in blind and sighted human subjects. *European Journal of Neuroscience, 15,* 1219–1224.

Macaluso, E., Frith, C. D., & Driver, J. (2000). Modulation of human visual cortex by cross modal spatial attention. *Science, 289,* 1206–1208.

Merzenich, M. M., Nelson, R. J., Stryker, M. P., Cynader, M. S., Schoppmann, A., & Zook, J. M. (1984). Somatosensory cortical map changes following digit amputation in adult monkeys. *The Journal of Comparative Neurology, 224,* 591–605.

Muchnik, C., Efrati, M., Nemeth, E., Malin, M., & Hildesheimer, M. (1991). Central auditory skills in blind and sighted subjects. *Scandinavica Audiologica, 20,* 19–23.

Pascual-Leone, A., & Hamilton, R. (2001). The metamodal organization of the brain. *Progress in Brain Research, 134,* 427–445.

Pascual-Leone, A., Cammarota, A., Wassermann, E. M., Brasil-Neto, J. P., Cohen, L. G., & Hallett, M. (1993). Modulation of motor cortical outputs to the reading hand of braille readers. *Annals of Neurology, 34,* 33–37.

Pascual-Leone, A., & Torres, F. (1993). Plasticity of the sensorimotor cortex representation of the reading finger in braille readers. *Brain, 116,* 39–52.

Pascual-Leone, A., Hamilton, R., Tormos, J. M., Keenan, J. P., & Catala, M. D. (1999). Neuroplasticity in the adjustement to blindness. In J. Grafman & Y. Christen (Eds), *Neuronal plasticity: Building a bridge from the laboratory to the clinic.* Berlin: Springer-Verlag.

Pons, T. (1996). Novel sensations in the congenitally blind. *Nature, 380,* 479–480.

Rauschecker, J. P. (1995). Compensatory plasticity & sensory substitution in the cerebral cortex. *Trends in Neuroscience, 18,* 36–43.

Recanzone, G. H., Allard, T. T., Jenkins, W. M., & Merzenich, M. M. (1990). Receptive-field changes induced by peripheral nerve stimulation in SI of adult cats. *Journal of Neurophysiology, 63,* 1213–1225.

Röder, B., Teder-Salejarvi, W., Sterr, A., Rosler, F., Hillyard, S. A., & Neville, H. J. (1999). Improved auditory spatial tuning in blind humans. *Nature, 400,* 162–166.

Sadato, N., Pascual-Leone, A., Grafman, J., Ibanez, V., Deiber, M. P., Dold, G., & Hallett, M. (1996). Activation of the primary visual cortex by Braille reading in blind subjects. *Nature, 380,* 562–568.

Sadato, N., Okada, T., Honda, M., & Yonekura, Y. (2002). Critical period for cross-modal plasticity in blind humans: A functional MRI study. *Neuroimage, 16*, 389–400.

Sanger, T. D., Pascual-Leone, A., Tarsy D., & Schlaug G. (2002). Nonlinear sensory cortex response to simultaneous tactile stimuli in writer's cramp. *Movement Disorders, 17*, 105–111.

Sterr, A., Muller, M. M., Elbert, T., Rockstroh, B., Pantev, C., & Taub, E. (1998). Perceptual correlates of changes in cortical representation of fingers in blind multifinger braille readers. *The Journal of Neuroscience, 18*, 4417–4423.

Tootell, R. B., Reppas, J. B., Kwong, K. K., Malach, R., Born, R. T., Brady, T. J., Rosen, B. R., & Belliveau, J. W. (1995). Functional analysis of human MT and related visual cortical areas using magnetic resonance imaging. *The Journal of Neuroscience, 15*, 3215–3230.

Uhl, F., Franzen, P., Lindinger, G., Lang, W., & Deecke, L. (1991). On the functionality of the visually deprived occipital cortex in early blind persons. *Neuroscience Letters, 124*, 256–259.

Uhl, F., Franzen, P., Podreka, I., Steiner, M., & Deecke, L. (1993). Increased regional cerebral blood flow in inferior occipital cortex and cerebellum of early blind humans. *Neuroscience Letters, 150*, 162–164.

Uhl, F., Kretschmer, T., Lindinger, G., Goldenberg, G., Lang, W., Oder, W., & Deecke, L. (1994). Tactile mental imagery in sighted persons and in patients suffering from peripheral blindness early in life. *Electroencephalography and Clinical Neurophysiology, 91*, 249–255.

Van Boven, R. W., Hamilton, R. H., Kauffman, T., Keenan, J. P., & Pascual-Leone, A. (2000). Tactile spatial resolution in blind Braille readers. *Neurology, 54*, 2230–2236.

Veraart, C., De Volder, A. G., Wanet-Defalque, M. C., Bol, A., Michel, C., & Goffinet, A. M. (1990). Glucose utilization in human visual cortex is abnormally elevated in blindness of early onset but decreased in blindness of late onset. *Brain Research, 510*, 115–121.

Walsh, V., & Cowey, A. (2000). Transcranial magnetic stimulation and cognitive neuroscience. *Nature Reviews Neuroscience, 1*, 73–79.

Wanet-Defalque, M. C., Veraart, C., De Volder, A., Metz, R., Michel, C., Dooms, G., & Goffinet, A. (1988). High metabolic activity in the visual cortex of early blind human subjects. *Brain Research, 446*, 369–373.

Weeks, R., Horwitz, B., Aziz-Sultan, A., Tian, B., Wessinger, C. M., Cohen, L. G., Hallett, M., & Rauschecker, J. P. (2000). A positron emission tomographic study of auditory localization in the congenitally blind. *The Journal of Neuroscience, 20*, 2664–2672.

Zeuner, K. E., Bara-Jimenez, W., Noguchi, P. S., Goldstein, S. R., Dambrosia, J. M., & Hallett, M. (2002). Sensory training for patients with focal hand dystonia. *Annals of Neurology, 51*, 593–598.

Zwiers, M. P., Van Opstal, A. J., & Cruysberg, J. R. (2001a). A spatial hearing deficit in early-blind humans. *Journal of Neuroscience, RC142*, 1–5.

Zwiers, M. P., Van Opstal, A. J., & Cruysberg, J. R. (2001b).Two-dimensional sound-localization behavior of early-blind humans. *Experimental Brain Research 140*, 206–222.

Chapter • 17

Dyslexia: Advances in Cross-level Research

Albert M. Galaburda

The history of dyslexia research comprises a series of successes as well as ongoing challenges. A remarkable expansion of our knowledge, spanning the fields of genetics, neurobiology, neurology, cognitive neuroscience, and education, has taken place since the first conference of the Extraordinary Brain series was inaugurated in Florence, Italy, almost 20 years ago. As the published volume from the Como Conference shows, we can say at this juncture that among those remarkable findings, there exists today for the condition known as developmental dyslexia at least one plausible known pathway between a genetic mutation and an abnormal behavior often associated with the diagnosis, including a rough description of the intervening neural structures involved. This is indeed a remarkable achievement that derives its strength mainly from cross-level approaches converging on the solution of the dyslexia problem. In the following pages, I will summarize relevant findings that lead to the above optimism, as well as bring up some still unanswered questions and remaining challenges.

FROM GENE TO BEHAVIOR: A CROSS-LEVEL AND MULTIDISCIPLINARY APPROACH

Everyone knows that complex behaviors can result from strong genetic predispositions without denying the fact that the environment helps to select among the possibilities presented by the genetic background. Thus, no complete program of research on a condition such as dyslexia could afford to ignore either the genetic background, described in the most detailed and mechanistic format permitted by current methodologies, or the cognitive and behavioral architectures that ultimately result from the interactions between genes and environment. The most laudable (but also the most challenging) goal of a dyslexia research program, which would also apply to most if not all disorders of perception, cognition, or behavior, would be to establish a clear and testable pathway between gene function and the perceptual, cognitive, and behavioral deficit. Such a research program requires a broad range of expertise amply found today, but generally in poorly bridged laboratories of genetics (molecular and above), neurobiology (systems, cell, and molecular), cognitive psychology, cognitive neuroscience, and education and rehabilitation. Praise should be given to the National Institutes of Health, especially the National Institute of Child Health and Human Development, for risking large amounts of taxpayer funds to promote cross-level research approaches, both in human populations and in animal models. Praise is also deserved by organizations like The Research Foundation, which has been pivotal in helping bring researchers together under pleasant surroundings to talk about their work and to foster growing numbers of cross-level collaborations. The Como Conference certainly is a case in point that will undoubtedly spawn quantities of interdisciplinary research as did the conferences that preceded it in Italy, Spain, South Africa, New Mexico, and Hawaii.

THE COMPLEXITY OF THE PROBLEM

The Dyslexic Mind

The problem of dyslexia is complex, where complex refers to deficits and dysfunctions describable at multiple levels: behavioral and educational (e.g., Lerner, 1989; Bashir & Scavuzzo, 1992; MacArthur, 1996; Snowling, 1996; Lyon & Moats, 1997; Tallal, Merzenich, Miller, & Jenkins, 1998; Rayner, Foorman, Perfetti, Pesetsky, & Seidenberg, 2001; Foorman, Breier, & Fletcher, 2003), cognitive (Stanovich, 1982; Frith, 1998; Lundberg, 1998; Coltheart, Rastle, Perry, Langdon, & Ziegler, 2001; Ramus, 2001; Rayner et al., 2001; McCandliss & Noble, 2003; Vellutino, Fletcher, Snowling, & Scanlon, 2004; and others), brain activation (e.g., Eden & Zeffiro, 1998; Connolly, D'Arcy, Lynn-Newman, & Kemps, 2000; Pugh et al., 2000; Demonet, 2002; Sarkari et al., 2002; Small & Burton, 2002), brain structure and brain development (c.f., Hynd & Semrud-Clikeman, 1989; Galaburda & Livingstone, 1993; Galaburda, 1993; Galaburda, Menard, & Rosen, 1994; Jenner, Rosen, & Galaburda, 1999; Eckert and Leonard 2000; Frenkel, Sherman, Bashan, Galaburda, & LoTurco, 2000; Pennington et al., 2000; Leonard et al., 2001; Nicolson, Fawcett, & Dean, 2001; Stein, 2001; Zeffiro & Eden, 2001; Foster, Hynd, Morgan, & Hugdahl, 2002; Rae et al., 2002; Eckert et al., 2003; Sheen & Walsh, 2003), and genes (Morris et al., 2000; Nopola-Hemmi et al., 2001; Fisher & DeFries, 2002; Francks, MacPhie, & Monaco, 2002; Grigorenko et al., 2003; Kaminen et al., 2003; Londin, Meng, & Gruen, 2003; Marino et al., 2003; Richardson, Leppänen, Leiwo, & Lyytinen, 2003; Marino et al., 2004; Peyrard-Janvid et al., 2004; and others). Furthermore, it is difficult at times to know when changes first occur (the initial states, see Mehler & Bever, 1967), what changes follow, and how changes first occurring at one level spread to other levels (Galaburda, 1994; Zilles et al., 1995; Luhmann, Raabe, Qu, & Zilles, 1998; Tallal et al., 1998; Frenkel et al., 2000; Lawn et al., 2000). Dyslexia most often is described in academic and behavioral terms, and the underlying cognitive representations and processes are less well known or even totally unknown. For example, dyslexics fail at reading tests and they have difficulty playing word games that require some intimacy with the way words can be broken down into its component sounds or phonemes (Bradley & Bryant, 1981; Snowling, 1981; Stanovich, 1982; Morais, Cluytens, & Alegria, 1984; Bertelson, 1986; Lundberg, 1998). It is assumed that these behavioral and educational problems arise from some corruption in underlying phonological representations and processes, but a clear idea of the nature of these subjacent cognitive structures does not exist. What is the fundamental nature of the phonology underlying the metaphonological and educational deficits disclosed by reading tests and word games? More research needs to be done to answer this basic question. Other behaviors are also implicated-visual perception and control of eye movements (Petri & Anderson, 1980; Pavlidis, 1985; Livingstone, Rosen, Drislane, & Galaburda, 1991; Fischer, Biscaldi, & Otto, 1993; Lovegrove, 1993; Kubova, Kuba, Peregrin, & Novakova, 1996; Slaghuis, Twell, & Kingston, 1996; Stein & Walsh, 1997; Rayner, 1998; Christenson, Griffin, & Taylor, 2001; Facoetti & Molteni, 2001; Facoetti, Turatto, Lorusso, & Mascetti, 2001; Laasonen, Service, & Virsu, 2001; Stein, 2001; Farrag, Khedr, & Abel-Naser, 2002; Williams, Stuart, Castles, & McAnally, 2003; Skoyles & Skottun, 2004), motor control (Wolff, Cohen, & Drake, 1984; Nicolson et al., 1999; Lyytinen et al., 2001; Eckert et al., 2003; Mati-Zissi & Zafiropoulou, 2003; Ramus, Pidgeon, & Frith,

2003), rapid naming tasks (Denckla & Rudel, 1976; Wolf, 1986; Wolff, Michel, & Ovrut, 1990; Waber, Wolff, Forbes, & Weiler, 2000), visual neglect (Witelson, 1977; Hari, Renvall, & Tanskanen, 2001), and again, the underlying cognitive architectures, presumable corrupted, are not known.

Some researchers (Galaburda & Eidelberg, 1982; Fitch, Tallal, Brown, Galaburda, & Rosen, 1994; Hari & Kiesila, 1996; Helenius, Uutela, & Hari, 1999; Clark, Rosen, Tallal, & Fitch, 2000; Benasich, 2002; Temple, 2002; but see also Conlon, Sanders, & Zapart, 2004; Tallal, this volume) believe that the presumed problem with phonology lying underneath the deficits in phonological awareness is a sensory-perceptual distortion that arises during development and affects the processing of certain types of sounds, which in turn, leads to abnormal phonological development, which in turn, explains metaphonological deficits at the behavioral and educational levels. There is an interesting debate regarding this proposed anomalous pathway, which is fueled by the observation that many dyslexics do not have the expected sensory-perceptual deficits, described by Tallal (Bailey & Snowling, 2002; Heiervang, Stevenson, & Hugdahl, 2002), and that some dyslexics often have sensory-perceptual deficits of a type not predicted by Tallal's hypothesis (Farrag, Khedr, & Abel-Naser, 2002; also see Ramus, this volume). One obvious problem here, which is amenable to experimental clarification, is that the intervening level of description—the cognitive, describing the state of affairs at phonological representations and processes—is not available with nearly enough detail in the mature or developing dyslexic to permit or exclude a possible link between sensory-perception and phonological awareness. The developmental perspective is important to stress here, whereby it is possible that initial states, effects of languages, effects of education and plasticity of and recovery from earlier deficits, all play important roles in modulating the final appearance of the dyslexic mind (for a case for developmental studies, see Thomas & Karmiloff-Smith, 2002).

The mind of a dyslexic contains other structures besides auditory and linguistic processes and representations, which include visual, motor, somesthetic, memory, attentional, motivations, and other executive functions, the roles of which are not known in dyslexia. Lip service is given to plausible roles of these functions in the behavioral expression of dyslexia, but lip service is also given to the implausibility of their roles. The fact is that reaching reading competence is a task complex enough to be likely to involve bottom-up and top-down processes that piggyback squarely on executive functions controlling motivation and planning, attention, motor control, mental imagery, and various forms of memory function affecting multiple modalities. It is difficult to believe that a single lesion at any focus of any of the many pathways involved could produce a devastating reading disorder, and the possibility that injury at multiple levels and in multiple pathways is to be found remains alive. That said, there is no other way but the empirical one to find out to what extent dysfunction in any combination of these mental functions contributes to the dyslexia behavioral phenotype. Moreover, the research has to be intrusive enough to take knowledge beyond mere associations and correlations into the realm of causality. Thus, for instance, if blind people cannot read regular print and adults with attention deficit disorders have poor reading comprehension (Loge, Staton, & Beatty, 1990; Johnson, 1995), it is not only possible but likely that disturbances in visual and attentional domains, and in the other above-mentioned domains, could be playing a role in the dyslexic reading deficits. Moreover, there is the pesky issue of comorbidity. For instance, conditions such as Attention Deficit Disorder are often difficult to diagnose, especially when mild, leading to the possibility that there may be significant numbers of undiagnosed comorbidities in our dyslexic populations that can explain the variability seen among dyslexic samples, which often leads to so much acrimonious debate about one cause or another (Semrud-Clikeman et al., 1992; Light & DeFries, 1995; Maughan, Pickles, Hagell, Rutter, & Yule, 1996; Purvis & Tannock, 1997; Richardson & Ross, 2000; King, Lombardino, Crandell, & Leonard, 2003; Toplak, Rucklidge, Hetherington, John, & Tannock, 2003).

The Dyslexic Brain

Any attempt to examine the brain in order to explain behavior is fraught with serious complications, from the philosophical (Fodor, 1981) to the methodological (Poeppel, 1996). Given the fact that we have no idea about how the brain produces or supports cognitive phenomena, and indirectly through them, behaviors, the problem is at present made easier and we can focus simply on the parts of the brain that seem to participate and the level of description that is most useful for building cross-level bridges. This phrenological approach has not changed in principle for 200 years where it concerns the types of cognitively based behaviors that interest us such as language, high-level vision, memory, attention, planning, motivation, and emotions. But even if we are better able to determine the parts of the brain involved, and even the useful level at which description should be carried out, we need to worry about time, because cognition and behavior have initial states and subsequent developmental courses. Plasticity changes after early injury could wreak havoc on the functional localization maps (for instance, Ojemann, 1979). Development, furthermore, may be accompanied by acquired injury at some point between childhood and senescence (because of stroke, head trauma, infection, trauma), and later still there can be added degenerative or involutional changes, which begin to take an insurmountable toll on structural and functional integrity. In other words, whatever brain structure is associated with a given behavior, and whatever anomaly in brain structure is associated with a given behavioral deficit, there is likely to come along comorbidities piggybacking along to make interpretation more difficult.

In the case of developmental disorders such as dyslexia, we assume that the initial state of brain structure is already altered, an assumption based on some supportive evidence (Galaburda, 1994; Galaburda & Cestnick, 2003). On top of that initial anomaly, there is also likely to occur additional developmental, acquired, involutional, and degenerative changes, likely to be similar to that occurring among good readers, but not necessarily so if plasticity differs between dyslexic and nondyslexic populations.

However, plasticity issues notwithstanding, the data thus far supports the presence of an abnormal initial state preceding reading acquisition, even language acquisition. The anomalies of cortical development seen in the dyslexic brain are traceable to fetal life (Galaburda & Kemper, 1979; Galaburda, Sherman, Rosen, Aboitiz, & Geschwind, 1985; Humphreys, Kaufmann, & Galaburda, 1990). Thus, we see nests of neurons and glia in the molecular layer of neocortex (called ectopias), representing errors of neuronal migration, which are located predominantly in perisylvian cortex and are found in greater numbers in the left hemisphere. Primary visual cortex is not affected by these malformations, although cortices known to be involved in high-level visual functions along the middle and inferior temporal lobes (e.g., area 37 of Brodmann) often show malformations. There are also frequent clusters in the superior temporal gyrus, on the planum temporale, in the inferior premotor and prefrontal cortex, and in the supramarginal and angular gyri (See Figure 1). These areas have been found to be implicated in dyslexics with the use of functional imaging techniques including the letter string, or word-form, area that overlaps with area 37 (Frith & Frith, 1996; Paulesu et al., 2001; Pugh et al., 2001; Shaywitz et al., 2002; Cohen & Dehaene, 2004). We have reason to suspect that the cortical lesions are related to the cognitive and metacognitive deficits demonstrable in many dyslexics in language and visual functions, but there is no way at present to prove this causality short of carrying out detailed transcranial magnetic stimulations experiments (see Théoret, this volume). Although one such study was performed by Branch Coslett in a patient with acquired alexia (Coslett & Monsul, 1994), I am not aware that the method has been applied to the study of developmental dyslexia. Experimental work in rodents would suggest that the anomalies can indeed cause disturbances in working memory and spatial maze functions (Schrott et al., 1993; Boehm, Sherman, Hoplight et al., 1996; Boehm, Sherman, Rosen, Galaburda, & Denenberg, 1996; Balogh et al., 1998; Hyde, Sherman, Stavnezer, & Denenberg, 2000; Hyde et al., 2001; Hyde, Stavnezer, Bimonte, Sherman, & Denenberg, 2002).

In addition to the cortical anomalies, there are abnormalities in the thalamus in the dyslexic brain, which consist of changes in the size of neurons in the medial and lateral geniculate nuclei. Such changes cannot be accurately dated since they may reflect functional events taking place later in life (Greenough, Larson, & Withers, 1985; Grossman et al., 2003). We have reason to believe that these changes cause auditory and visual temporal processing deficits, which are found in some dyslexics. This statement about causality represents an extrapolation from experiments carried out in animals (see below under "Help from animal studies").

Experimental work in rodents has helped establish a causal relationship between brain changes and behavior, which can be used to hypothesize about the situation in the human dyslexic. It is possible to induce cortical anomalies similar to those found in the dyslexic cortex (Rosen & Galaburda, 2000). Neuronal ectopias in the molecular layer and microgyria (both of which can be seen in the dyslexic brain) can be induced using a freezing probe near the end of neuronal migration to the cortex. Induction of these anomalies is associated with behavioral changes in the animal (Rosen, Waters, Galaburda, & Denenberg, 1995), but they also lead to secondary changes in the thalamus that mimic those found in the dyslexic brains (Herman, Galaburda, Fitch, Carter, & Rosen, 1997). This has lead us to postulate without direct evidence in the human that the cortical anomaly occurs first in the dyslexic brain, some time during mid gestation, which, in turn, causes secondary changes in the thalamus. The secondary changes in the thalamus, either directly or indirectly, cause the deficits in temporal processing in the animal. Thus, we have proposed that in the dyslexic brain, some factor, or perhaps several factors, can result in disordered neuronal migration. The latter then causes secondary changes in the thalamus, or alternatively the same factors that cause neuronal migration anomalies also cause changes in the thalamus (Galaburda & Duchaine, 2003). The changes in the cortex then lead to cognitive and metacognitive deficits, while the changes in the thalamus produce deficits in sensory-perceptual processing. But what causes the initial cortical anomaly in dyslexics? I will outline one plausible pathway from brain back to gene in the following section, but first I want to review some outstanding anatomical issues.

In the eight dyslexic brains examined, we found a comparable distribution of cortical anomalies, namely the left perisylvian cortex more so than the right, and more so than nonperisylvian cortex (Humphreys, Kaufmann, & Galaburda, 1990) (see Figure 1 in the four-color section on page 222-L). Why that distribution of lesions? One possibility that has been raised in discussion before is that the location of the lesions is such because we selected our cases for being dyslexic. Were we to have chosen cases with nonverbal learning disabilities, autism, mathematical learning disability, and the like, we would have found the same lesions somewhere else: a good phrenological hypothesis. However, although cortical ectopias are indeed described in other neurodevelopmental syndromes (Wisniewski, Dambska, Sher, & Qazi, 1983; Kotkoskie & Norton, 1988; Kuzniecky, 1994; Konovalov, Kovetsky, Bobryshev, & Ashwell, 1997; Barkovich, Kuzniecky, Jackson, Guerrini, & Dobyns, 2001; Komatsu, Sakata-Haga, Sawada, Hisano, & Fukui, 2001), they have not been found in specific learning disorders of the types listed above. It may indeed be the case that dyslexia is the only consequence of focally clustered ectopias in perisylvian cortex and that this is the only known distribution. We have no idea to date for this distribution, once we exclude a selection bias. There are other genetic disorders that produced uneven cortical pathology (Pilz et al., 1998), and several genes have been identified that act regionally in the brain to pattern cortical development (Bishop, Goudreau, & O'Leary, 2000; Grove & Fukuchi-Shimogori, 2003). The possibility exists that the fundamental causes of dyslexia interact in this way with other genes that are expressed regionally.

A second problem with our current knowledge about the anatomy of dyslexia relates to the planum temporale. This structure, which is an arbitrarily defined region on the superior temporal plane, contains bits and pieces of a variety of auditory regions, including those spilling out of Heschl's gyrus (BA 41 and 42), and caudal and lateral auditory associations cortices. This region is known to show a leftward bias in human populations and has been thought to be a marker for language lateralization to the left hemisphere (reviewed in Hugdahl, 2000). Deviations from this pattern have been described in dyslexia (Galaburda et al., 1985; Hugdahl et al., 1998; Eckert & Leonard, 2000) and other developmental disorders (Frangou et al., 1997; Sommer, Ramsey, Kahn, Aleman, & Bouma, 2001; Rojas, Bawn, Benkers, Reite, & Rogers, 2002), as well as in nonrighthanders (Foundas, Leonard, & Hanna-Pladdy, 2002). However, there is something more to the lack of asymmetry in the dyslexic planum temporale. We carried out experimental studies in rats that showed that there should be an inverse relationship between areal asymmetry and total size (Galaburda, Aboitiz, Rosen, & Sherman, 1986; Rosen, Sherman, Mehler, Emsbo, & Galaburda, 1989); that is, the sum of the two sides is greater the more symmetric an area is. Asymmetry, therefore, appears to be the curtailment of one side, rather than the enlargement of one side or a storage issue, whereby the left and right sides add up to a constant with population variation. However, in the presence of cortical malformations, this relationship breaks down and there is no longer a prediction about total size from degree of asymmetry (Rosen et al., 1989). There have been reports, for instance, that the plana are small in dyslexics even though they are more symmetric (Humphreys, Kaufmann, & Galaburda, 1990; Eckert & Leonard, 2000; Leonard et al., 2001). At present, we do not know the mechanism of interaction between asymmetry and brain malformation. We also do not know whether this abnormal symmetry in dyslexics (as opposed to a "normal" symmetry in left-handers and other normal individuals) plays a causative role in the behavioral profile of dyslexia.

HELP FROM ANIMAL STUDIES

From Brain to Behavior

Examination of autopsied brains in humans cannot address the issue of causality, and functional imaging studies in living dyslexics do not answer questions of etiology; that is, the reason for which the brain activates in the particular way that it does. Experimental work on rodents has been helpful in disclosing possible pathways between brain changes and behavior with the limitation that modeling human behaviors in rodents entails. Initially, the research in our laboratories focused on behaviors related to the cortical malformations. The first models, those of immune-defective mice with spontaneously occurring cortical ectopias (Sherman, Galaburda, & Geschwind, 1985; Sherman, Galaburda,

Behan, & Rosen, 1987), showed a range of behavioral anomalies, including many areas where affected animals were weaker than controls and some where they were more adept (Schrott et al., 1993; Boehm, Sherman, Hoplight et al., 1996; Boehm, Sherman, Rosen et al., 1996; Balogh, Sherman, Hyde, & Denenberg, 1998; Hyde et al., 2000; Hyde et al., 2002). Those findings were interesting in that they linked up nicely to the human data on dyslexics, which has from time to time mentioned cognitive deficits but also special skills (Rack, 1981; McNamara, Flannery, Obler, & Schacter, 1994; Wolff & Lundberg, 2002; von Karolyi, Winner, Gray, & Sherman, 2003).

Some of the deficits associated with the presence of cortical malformations could be assuaged if young animals were raised in enriched environments (cages with ramps, balls of yarn, and the like) (Schrott et al., 1992; Boehm, Sherman, Hoplight et al., 1996; Hoplight, Sherman, Hyde, & Denenberg, 2001). This, too, suggested a link to the situation in human dyslexics where it appeared that an enriched environment minimized the impact of risk (Foorman, Breier, & Fletcher, 2003). Such an effect had also begun to appear in the Alzheimer's literature, whereby individuals with more years of education were demonstrated to stave off the onset of Alzheimer symptoms for up to 10 years in some cases (Stern et al., 1994).

One problem with the cortical ectopias/behavioral correlations in the rodents was the absence of sex differences. Most studies on the prevalence of dyslexia indicated a sex bias, whereby boys were affected more often than girls (see recent study by Rutter et al., 2004). A selection bias was cited to explain this difference (Shaywitz, Shaywitz, Fletcher, & Escobar, 1990), but control for this factor still showed a male predominance, although perhaps not as high as previously thought (Rutter et al., 2004). Leaving aside a selection bias, how else to explain a sex difference such as this? One possibility is that the trait is Y-chromosome related, another is that it is X-linked and recessive, a third is the uneven effect of sex steroids in the causation of the disorder or its manifestations (Geschwind & Galaburda, 1985a, 1985b), acting directly or indirectly on the malformations. A fourth possibility is that the brains of males and females are fundamentally different at the initial state (Geschwind & Galaburda, 1985a, 1985b; Aboitiz et al., 1995; Wisniewski, 1998) so that any perturbation—congenital, acquired, degenerative—will have a different impact on the two sexes.

A Y-linked trait would never be expected to occur in females, so this possibility is easily excluded. An X-linked recessive trait would be expected to occur in females only rarely, which is not the case for dyslexia. The effects of hormones remain the most likely explanation for the observed sex difference. The possibility of lesions occurring with comparable frequency between the sexes but falling on a different brain substrate and thus leading to different effects is also an attractive one, but difficult to support by what we know about gender-based sex differences in the brain. In general, brain differences between the sexes have been demonstrated mainly in those parts of the brain that regulate reproductive behavior and not in regards to perceptual or cognitive behaviors, with rare exceptions (Wisniewski, 1998).

One more contrast to consider is whether lesions themselves occur at different rates between males and females (by any of the above-mentioned explanations), or whether differences in brain plasticity after the lesion account for the observed sex differences (Teskey, Hutchinson, & Kolb, 1999; Trentani et al., 2003). Soon after we started to introduce cortical malformations in newborn rat brains, Holly Fitch discovered that the males and females in the sample were not responding equally to the lesions when tested on one specific behavior: auditory temporal processing (Fitch, Brown, Tallal, & Rosen, 1997; Herman et al., 1997; Peiffer, Rosen, & Fitch, 2002b, 2004). Glenn Rosen, in our laboratory, went back and carefully analyzed the size and location of the lesions with the idea that perhaps the explanation lay in unplanned differences in the original lesions. However, no such differences were found. We had to conclude that the effect of the lesions on some auditory behaviors was different between the sexes. Following these early experiments, we have consistently found that the cortical lesions produce different effects in males and females in a range of auditory behaviors (also, see Fitch, this volume), and that this can be explained by changes that do not occur in the cerebral cortex but rather in the rat thalamus (Herman et al., 1997).

Two distinct anatomical findings were made in the dyslexic brains: cortical malformations and changes in cell distribution and size in the medial and lateral geniculate nuclei. After finding sex differences in auditory temporal processing in the rats with induced malformations, we went back and examined the geniculate nuclei of affected and control animals. The possibility existed that even though cortical malformations and cortical behaviors did not differentiate males and females, thalamic changes and auditory processing behaviors might, which turned out to be the case (Herman et al., 1997; Rosen, Burstein, & Galaburda, 2000; Peiffer, Rosen, & Fitch, 2002a). Numerous studies showed that the induction of cortical malformations in the rat lead to changes in the medial geniculate nucleus of male rats only, whereby there was a redistribution of neuronal sizes from larger to smaller, similar to the findings in the dyslexic brains. Female brains did not show these neuronal size changes, and female rats did not show temporal processing deficits, thus suggesting that the two were linked.

Are the sex differences seen in the dyslexia population related to thalamic cell changes and temporal processing deficits? The answer to this question is not as yet known and would be difficult to obtain. We can postulate that once a female is found to be dyslexic, she will be found to have the thalamic changes if the above suppositions are valid. The population of interest in this case would be the group of girls or women from dyslexic families who have cortical malformations, absence of thalamic changes, and absence of dyslexic symptoms, and another with both cortical malformations and thalamic changes, this group with dyslexia. We may expect to discover these individuals once structural MRI imaging technology is sufficiently developed to image cortical ectopias in living subjects. If the hypothesis is correct, we should expect to find girls or women from dyslexic families who have cortical malformations and no dyslexia, presumably due to a lack of thalamic change in response to the cortical malformations. To image in a living human subject the cell changes in the thalamus directly would require a technology not as yet available, even in its infancy.

To summarize, we find ourselves in a situation whereby the only sex difference we can demonstrate anatomically and behaviorally in animal models is one that links auditory temporal processing to changes in the thalamus, which in turn are secondary to induced cortical malformations. The cortical changes themselves, or the behaviors linked to them, do not show a sex bias. This can be taken to mean that fundamental to the sex differences seen in dyslexia is an underlying problem in auditory temporal processing defect, a statement that would be met with a great deal of resistance by some experts (see Ramus, this volume). However, another possibility is that we have not found the right level at which to analyze the cortical anatomy and cortically based behaviors and that sex differences are indeed to be found at those levels. Recently in our laboratory, Bettina Meples carried out two experiments (unpublished) that seem to indicate that subtle differences in the cortical lesions may exist between males and females. Relying on information from the field of cerebral palsy (Patkai et al., 2001; also see Gressens, this volume), she exposed pregnant females to the cytokine Interleukin-9. This substance was implicated in changing the size of the lesion in models of periventricular leukomalacia. Intraperitoneal injection of 60 μg/kg of IL-9 produced an enlargement of the area of microgyria induced by the usual method of cortical freezing, but this effect was found only in male rats. Experiments such as this demonstrate that there could be circulating factors such as IL-9 that can modify the severity of cortical a malformation in utero in dyslexic families so that females will end up with smaller lesions and possibly smaller behavioral effects.

Another finding made by Mesples in a second experiment (unpublished) designed to investigate the possibility that plasticity effects from induced cortical malformations that affected cell sizes in the thalamus involved sexually dimorphic differential cell death. Both decreased and increased survival has been reported in males versus female neurons (Nunez, Lauschke, & Juraska, 2001; Zhang et al., 2003). Mesples found that markers of cell death by Fluoro-Jade B staining after induction of a microgyrus in the barrel fields, characterized as small and large degenerating profiles in the ventrobasal complex, were qualitatively and quantitatively different in male and female rats, with males showing evidence of more cell death than females from presumably the same initial cortical freezing injury.

In summary, these findings do suggest that male-female differences may exist both in the cortex and in the thalamus in relation to cortical malformations and thalamic cell changes, which would help to explain sex differences in the prevalence of dyslexia between men and women. Despite the possibility that cortical sex differences play a role in this sex difference, most of the current evidence still points to differences in plasticity affecting the thalamus and resulting auditory processing deficits, which keeps the idea of this anatomical-behavioral complex alive as an important ingredient of the behavioral trait we call dyslexia.

From Genes to Brain

So far, I have reviewed with a broad brush the evidence linking brain changes, in the cortex and thalamus, to behaviors seen among individuals with developmental dyslexia. But how do the changes originate in the dyslexic brain? In the experimental animal model, we induce them with a freezing probe, but this is hardly the mechanism active in dyslexics. In a group of mutant mice, which includes spontaneous mutations as well as recombinant inbred strains and congenic animals, the cortical malformations arise without additional cortical manipulation at birth. There are potential chromosomal sites linked to the malformations, but not genes so far identified. On the other hand, progress has been made in the discovery of genes related to dyslexia in humans (see review by Cecilia Marino, this volume). Here I focus on a gene on Chromosome 15 recently proposed to be a dyslexia candidate gene, the so-called DYX1C1 gene (Taipale et al., 2003). As Joe LoTurco reports in this volume, Dyx1c1 is essential for neurons in the developing cerebral neocortex to migrate. Interference of Dyx1c1 in the fetal brain disrupts neuronal migration and creates malformations similar to those observed in the brains of dyslexics. The immediate malformation is neuronal migration arrest near the ventricular zone, followed later by evidence of cortical dysplasias. The region of Dyx1c1 previously associated with dyslexia susceptibility by mutation or deletion is necessary and sufficient to rescue disrupted migration. These results establish Dyx1c1 as a novel neuronal migration gene, and link a probable genetic cause of dyslexia with alterations in neuronal migration.

Even though Cecilia Marino and colleagues (this volume) did not find a link between DYX1C1 and dyslexia in her Italian cohorts, such a link was established in the Finish population published by Taippale and by others (Grigorenko et al., 1997; Schulte-Korne et al., 1998; Morris et al., 2000; Wigg et al., 2004), and one must entertain the possibility that different genes act in different ethnic groups. Several neuronal migration genes have been reported and it is likely that many others are still to be discovered. The finding that DYX1C1 is indeed a neuronal migration gene would serve to indicate that a plausible pathway exists between a specific gene mutation and the brain changes seen in dyslexia. There are likely to be others yet unspecified.

CONCLUSIONS

A plausible pathway now available to explain how a genetic mutation produces an abnormal behavior often, if not always, is associated with dyslexia. The pathway is the following: a gene mutation affecting a neuronal migration gene produces a cortical migration anomaly. This migration anomaly is associated with secondary changes in the thalamus and perhaps other subcortical structures. The data do not exclude the possibility that the genetic mutation also has a direct effect on the development of subcortical structures (although there are no present data for or against this possibility), and that the plasticity interactions between cortical and thalamic developments are additional to the underlying direct effects. As the abnormal genes and subsequent plasticity effects cause the brain changes, the latter are responsible for sensory-perceptual-motor low-level and cognitive and metacognitive deficits, attributable, respectively, to plasticity related thalamic and other subcortical changes as well as direct effects of the cortical malformation and secondary cortical changes. The direct pathway is, then, from gene to brain to behavior, although important details need to be worked out and other pathways, active in other subgroups of dyslexics, arising in different genes perhaps, need to be discovered.

The program of research on the fundamental causes of dyslexia has been successful so far to the extent that a pathway such as that outlined above has been possible to emerge from a broad collaboration of expertise on brain development, genetics, and behavioral science with healthy bridges among them. It is to my knowledge the first time a rough pathway has been presented for a complex abnormal trait in a complex species. But more work is needed to fully understand dyslexia and to make progress in other developmental disorders of behavior and cognition.

Address correspondence to: Albert M. Galaburda, M. D., Emily Fisher Landau Professor of Neurology and Neuroscience, Harvard Medical School, Chief, Division of Behavioral Neurology and Memory Disorders, Beth Israel Deaconess Medical Center, 330 Brookline Avenue, K-274, Boston, MA 02215; Tel: (617) 667-3235, Fax: (617) 667-7011

REFERENCES

Aboitiz, F., Ide, A., Navarrete, A., Pena, M., Rodriguez, E., Wolff, V., & Zaidel, E. (1995). The anatomical substrates for language and hemispheric specialization. *Biological Research, 28*(1), 45–50.

Bailey, P. J., & Snowling, M. J. (2002). Auditory processing and the development of language and literacy. *British Medical Bulletin, 63*, 135–146.

Balogh, S. A., Sherman, G. F., Hyde, L. A., & Denenberg, V. H. (1998). Effects of neocortical ectopias upon the acquisition and retention of a non-spatial reference memory task in BXSB mice. *Brain Research: Developmentak Brain Research, 111*(2), 291–293.

Barkovich, A. J., Kuzniecky, R. I., Jackson, G. D., Guerrini, R., & Dobyns, W. B. (2001). Classification system for malformations of cortical development: Update (2001). *Neurology, 57*(12), 2168–2178.

Bashir, A. S., & Scavuzzo, A. (1992). Children with language disorders: Natural history and academic success. *Journal of Learning Disabilities, 25*(1), 53–65; discussion 66–70.

Benasich, A. A. (2002). Impaired processing of brief, rapidly presented auditory cues in infants with a family history of autoimmune disorder. *Developmental Neuropsychology, 22*(1), 351–72.

Bertelson, P. (1986). The onset of literacy: Liminal remarks. *Cognition, 24* (1–2), 1–30.

Bishop, K. M., Goudreau, G., & O'Leary, D. D. (2000). Regulation of area identity in the mammalian neocortex by Emx2 and Pax6. *Science, 288*(5464), 344–349.

Boehm, G. W., Sherman, G. F., Hoplight, B. J., 2nd, Hyde, L. A., Waters, N. S., Bradway, D. M., Galaburda, A. M., & Denenberg, V. H. (1996). Learning and memory in the autoimmune BXSB mouse: Effects of neocortical ectopias and environmental enrichment. *Brain Research, 726*(1–2), 11–22.

Boehm, G. W., Sherman, G. F., Rosen, G. D., Galaburda, A. M., & Denenberg, V. H. (1996). Neocortical ectopias in BXSB mice: Effects upon reference and working memory systems. *Cerebral Cortex, 6*(5), 696–700.

Bradley, L., & Bryant, P. (1981). Visual memory and phonological skills in reading and spelling backwardness. *Psychological Research, 43*(2), 193–199.

Brunswick, N., McCrory, E., Price, C. J., Frith, C. D., & Frith, U. (1999). Explicit and implicit processing of words and pseudowords by adult developmental dyslexics: A search for Wernicke's Wortschatz? *Brain, 122*(Pt. 10), 1901–1917.

Christenson, G. N., Griffin, J. R., & Taylor, M. (2001). Failure of blue-tinted lenses to change reading scores of dyslexic individuals. *Optometry, 72*(10), 627–633.

Clark, M. G., Rosen, G. D., Tallal, P., & Fitch, R. H. (2000). Impaired processing of complex auditory stimuli in rats with induced cerebrocortical microgyria: An animal model of developmental language disabilities. *Journal of Cognitive Neuroscience, 12*(5), 828–839.

Cohen, L., & Dehaene, S. (2004). Specialization within the ventral stream: The case for the visual word form area. *Neuroimage, 22*(1), 466–476.

Coltheart, M., Rastle, K., Perry, C., Langdon, R., & Ziegler, J. (2001). DRC: A dual route cascaded model of visual word recognition and reading aloud. *Psychological Review, 108*(1), 204–256.

Conlon, E., Sanders, M., & Zapart, S. (2004). Temporal processing in poor adult readers. *Neuropsychologia, 42*(2), 142–157.

Connolly, J. F., D'Arcy, R. C., Lynn Newman, R., & Kemps, R. (2000). The application of cognitive event-related brain potentials (ERPs) in language-impaired individuals: Review and case studies. *International Journal of Psychophysiology, 38*(1), 55–70.

Coslett, H. B., & Monsul, N. (1994). Reading with the right hemisphere: Evidence from transcranial magnetic stimulation. *Brain and Language, 46*(2), 198–211.

Demonet, J. F. (2002). Developmental dyslexias: Use of functional neuroimaging. *Archives of Pediatrics, 9*(Suppl. 2), 268s–270s.

Denckla, M. B., & Rudel, R. G. (1976). Rapid "automatized" naming (R.A.N): Dyslexia differentiated from other learning disabilities. *Neuropsychologia, 14*(4), 471–479.

Eckert, M. A., & Leonard, C. M. (2000). Structural imaging in dyslexia: The planum temporale. *Mental Retardation and Developmental Disabilities Research Reviews, 6*(3), 198–206.

Eckert, M. A., Leonard, C. M., Richards, T. L., Aylward, E. H., Thomson, J., & Berninger, V. W. (2003). Anatomical correlates of dyslexia: Frontal and cerebellar findings. *Brain, 126*(Pt. 2), 482–494.

Eden, G. F., & Zeffiro, T. A. (1998). Neural systems affected in developmental dyslexia revealed by functional neuroimaging. *Neuron, 21*(2), 279–282.

Facoetti, A., & Molteni, M. (2001). The gradient of visual attention in developmental dyslexia. *Neuropsychologia, 39*(4), 352–357.

Facoetti, A., Turatto, M., Lorusso, M. L., & Mascetti, G. G. (2001). Orienting of visual attention in dyslexia: Evidence for asymmetric hemispheric control of attention. *Experimental Brain Research, 138*(1), 46–53.

Farrag, A. F., Khedr, E. M., & Abel-Naser, W. (2002). Impaired parvocellular pathway in dyslexic children. *European Journal of Neurology, 9*(4), 359–363.

Fischer, B., Biscaldi, M., & Otto, P. (1993). Saccadic eye movements of dyslexic adult subjects. *Neuropsychologia, 31*(9), 887–906.

Fisher, S. E., & DeFries, J. C. (2002). Developmental dyslexia: Genetic dissection of a complex cognitive trait. *Nature Reviews Neuroscience, 3*(10), 767–780.

Fitch, R. H., Brown, C. P., Tallal, P., & Rosen, G. D. (1997). Effects of sex and MK-801 on auditory-processing deficits associated with developmental microgyric lesions in rats. *Behavioral Neuroscience, 111*(2), 404–412.

Fitch, R. H., Tallal, P., Brown, C. P., Galaburda, A. M., & Rosen, G. D. (1994). Induced microgyria and auditory temporal processing in rats: A model for language impairment? *Cerebral Cortex, 4*(3), 260–270.

Fodor, J. A. (1981). The mind-body problem. *Scientific American, 244*(1), 114–120, 122–123.

Foorman, B. R., Breier, J. I., & Fletcher, J. M. (2003). Interventions aimed at improving reading success: An evidence-based approach. *Developmental Neuropsychology, 24*(2–3), 613–639.

Foster, L. M., Hynd, G. W., Morgan, A. E., & Hugdahl, K. (2002). Planum temporale asymmetry and ear advantage in dichotic listening in developmental dyslexia and attention-deficit/hyperactivity disorder (ADHD). *Journal of the International Neuropsychological Society, 8*(1), 22–36.

Foundas, A. L., Leonard, C. M., & Hanna-Pladdy, B. (2002). Variability in the anatomy of the planum temporale and posterior ascending ramus: Do right- and left-handers differ? *Brain and Language, 83*(3), 403–424.

Francks, C., MacPhie, I. L., & Monaco, A. P. (2002). The genetic basis of dyslexia. *Lancet Neurology, 1*(8), 483–490.

Frangou, S., Aylward, E., Warren, A., Sharma, T., Barta, P., & Pearlson, G. (1997). Small planum temporale volume in Down's syndrome: A volumetric MRI study. *American Journal of Psychiatry, 154*(10), 1424–1429.

Frenkel, M., Sherman, G. F., Bashan, K. A., Galaburda, A. M., & LoTurco, J. J. (2000). Neocortical ectopias are associated with attenuated neurophysiological responses to rapidly changing auditory stimuli. *Neuroreport 11*(3), 575–579.

Frith, C., & Frith, U. (1996). A biological marker for dyslexia. *Nature 382*(6586), 19–20.

Frith, U. (1998). Cognitive deficits in developmental disorders. *Scandinavian Journal of Psychology, 39*(3), 191–195.

Galaburda, A., & Livingstone, M. (1993). Evidence for a magnocellular defect in developmental dyslexia. *Annals of the New York Academy of Sciences, 682*, 70–82.

Galaburda, A. M. (1993). Neuroanatomic basis of developmental dyslexia. *Neurologic Clinics, 11*(1), 161–173.

Galaburda, A. M. (1994). Developmental dyslexia and animal studies: At the interface between cognition and neurology. *Cognition, 50*(1–3), 133–149.

Galaburda, A. M., Aboitiz, F., Rosen, G. D., & Sherman, G. F. (1986). Histological asymmetry in the primary visual cortex of the rat: Implications for mechanisms of cerebral asymmetry. *Cortex, 22*(1), 151–160.

Galaburda, A. M., & Cestnick, L. (2003). Developmental dyslexia. *Revista de Neurología, 36*(Suppl. 1), S3–S9.

Galaburda, A. M., & Duchaine, B. C. (2003). Developmental disorders of vision. *Neurologic Clinics, 21*(3), 687–707.

Galaburda, A. M., & Eidelberg, D. (1982). Symmetry and asymmetry in the human posterior thalamus. II. Thalamic lesions in a case of developmental dyslexia. *Archives of Neurology, 39*(6), 333–336.

Galaburda, A. M., & Kemper, T. L. (1979). Cytoarchitectonic abnormalities in developmental dyslexia: A case study. *Annals of Neurology, 6*(2), 94–100.

Galaburda, A. M., Menard, M. T., & Rosen, G. D. (1994). Evidence for aberrant auditory anatomy in developmental dyslexia. *Proceedings of the National Academy of Sciences USA, 91*(17), 8010–8013.

Galaburda, A. M., Sherman, G. F., Rosen, G. D., Aboitiz, F., & Geschwind, N. (1985). Developmental dyslexia: Four consecutive patients with cortical anomalies. *Annals of Neurology, 18*(2), 222–233.

Georgiewa, P., Rzanny, R., Gaser, C., Gerhard, U. J., Vieweg, U., Freesmeyer, D., Mentzel, H. J., Kaiser, W. A., & Blanz, B. (2002). Phonological processing in dyslexic children: A study combining functional imaging and event related potentials. *Neuroscience Letters, 318*(1), 5–8.

Geschwind, N., & Galaburda, A. M. (1985a). Cerebral lateralization. Biological mechanisms, associations, and pathology: I. A hypothesis and a program for research. *Archives of Neurology, 42*(5), 428–459.

Geschwind, N., & Galaburda, A. M. (1985)b. Cerebral lateralization. Biological mechanisms, associations, and pathology: II. A hypothesis and a program for research. *Archives of Neurology, 42*(6), 521–552.

Greenough, W. T., Larson, J. R., & Withers, G. S. (1985). Effects of unilateral and bilateral training in a reaching task on dendritic branching of neurons in the rat motor-sensory forelimb cortex. *Behavioral and Neural Biology, 44*(2), 301–314.

Grigorenko, E. L., Wood, F. B., Golovyan, L., Meyer, M., Romano, C., & Pauls, D. (2003). Continuing the search for dyslexia genes on 6p. *American Journal of Medical Genetics, 118B*(1), 89–98.

Grigorenko, E. L., Wood, F. B., Meyer, M. S., Hart, L. A., Speed, W. C., Shuster, A., & Pauls, D. L. (1997). Susceptibility loci for distinct components of developmental dyslexia on chromosomes 6 and 15. *American Journal of Human Genetics, 60*(1), 27–39.

Grossman, A. W., Churchill, J. D., McKinney, B. C., Kodish, I. M., Otte, S. L., & Greenough, W. T. (2003). Experience effects on brain development: Possible contributions to psychopathology. *Journal of Child Psychology and Psychiatry and Allied Disciplines, 44*(1), 33–63.

Grove, E. A., & Fukuchi-Shimogori, T. (2003). Generating the cerebral cortical area map. *Annual Review of Neuroscience, 26*, 355–380.

Hari, R., & Kiesila, P. (1996). Deficit of temporal auditory processing in dyslexic adults. *Neuroscience Letters, 205*(2), 138–140.

Hari, R., Renvall, H., & Tanskanen, T. (2001). Left minineglect in dyslexic adults. *Brain, 124*(Pt. 7), 1373–1380.

Heiervang, E., Stevenson, J., & Hugdahl, K. (2002). Auditory processing in children with dyslexia. *Journal of Child Psychology and Psychiatry and Allied Disciplines, 43*(7), 931–938.

Helenius, P., Uutela, K., & Hari, R. (1999). Auditory stream segregation in dyslexic adults. *Brain, 122*(Pt. 5), 907–913.

Herman, A. E., Galaburda, A. M., Fitch, R. H., Carter, A. R., & Rosen, G. D. (1997). Cerebral microgyria, thalamic cell size and auditory temporal processing in male and female rats. *Cerebral Cortex, 7*(5), 453–464.

Hoplight, B. J., Sherman, G. F., Hyde, L. A., & Denenberg, V. H. (2001). Effects of neocortical ectopias and environmental enrichment on Hebb-Williams maze learning in BXSB mice. *Neurobiology of Learning and Memory, 76*(1), 33–45.

Hugdahl, K. (2000). Lateralization of cognitive processes in the brain. *Acta Psychologica (Amsterdam) 105*(2–3), 211–235.

Hugdahl, K., Heiervang, E., Nordby, H., Smievoll, A. I., Steinmetz, H., Stevenson, J., & Lund, A. (1998). Central auditory processing, MRI morphometry and brain laterality: Applications to dyslexia. *Scandinavian Audiology (*Suppl.)*49*, 26–34.

Humphreys, P., Kaufmann, W. E., & Galaburda, A. M. (1990). Developmental dyslexia in women: Neuropathological findings in three patients. *Annals of Neurology, 28*(6), 727–738.

Hyde, L. A., Hoplight, B. J., Harding, S., Sherman, G. F., Mobraaten, L. E., & Denenberg, V. H. (2001). Effects of ectopias and their cortical location on several measures of learning in BXSB mice. *Developmental Psychobiology, 39*(4), 286–300.

Hyde, L. A., Sherman, G. F., Stavnezer, A. J., & Denenberg, V. H. (2000). The effects of neocortical ectopias on Lashley III water maze learning in New Zealand black mice. *Brain Research, 887*(2), 482–483.

Hyde, L. A., Stavnezer, A. J., Bimonte, H. A., Sherman, G. F., & Denenberg, V. H. (2002). Spatial and nonspatial Morris maze learning: Impaired behavioral flexibility in mice with ectopias located in the prefrontal cortex. *Behavioral Brain Research, 133*(2), 247–259.

Hynd, G. W., & Semrud-Clikeman, M. (1989). Dyslexia and brain morphology. *Psychological Bulletin, 106*(3), 447–482.

Jenner, A. R., Rosen, G. D., & Galaburda, A. M. (1999). Neuronal asymmetries in primary visual cortex of dyslexic and nondyslexic brains. *Annals of Neurology, 46*(2), 189–196.

Johnson, D. J. (1995). An overview of learning disabilities: Psychoeducational perspectives. *Journal of Child Neurology, 10*(Suppl. 1), S2–S5.

Kaminen, N., Hannula-Jouppi, K., Kestila, M., Lahermo, P., Muller, K., Kaaranen, M., Myllyluoma, B., Voutilainen, A., Lyytinen, H., Nopola-Hemmi, J., & Kere, J. (2003). A genome scan for developmental dyslexia confirms linkage to chromosome 2p11 and suggests a new locus on 7q32. *Journal of Medical Genetics, 40*(5), 340–345.

King, W. M., Lombardino, L. J., Crandell, C. C., & Leonard, C. M. (2003). Comorbid auditory processing disorder in developmental dyslexia. *Ear and Hearing, 24*(5), 448–456.

Komatsu, S., Sakata-Haga, H., Sawada, K., Hisano, S., & Fukui, Y. (2001). Prenatal exposure to ethanol induces leptomeningeal heterotopia in the cerebral cortex of the rat fetus. *Acta Neuropathologica (Berlin), 101*(1), 22–26.

Konovalov, H. V., Kovetsky, N. S., Bobryshev, Y. V., & Ashwell, K. W. (1997). Disorders of brain development in the progeny of mothers who used alcohol during pregnancy. *Early Human Development, 48*(1–2), 153–166.

Kotkoskie, L. A., & Norton, S. (1988). Prenatal brain malformations following acute ethanol exposure in the rat. *Alcoholism: Clinical and Experimental Research, 12*(6), 831–836.

Kubova, Z., Kuba, M., Peregrin, J., & Novakova, V. (1996). Visual evoked potential evidence for magnocellular system deficit in dyslexia. *Physiological Research, 45*(1), 87–89.

Kuzniecky, R. I. (1994). Magnetic resonance imaging in developmental disorders of the cerebral cortex. *Epilepsia, 35*(Suppl. 6), S44–S56.

Laasonen, M., Service, E., & Virsu, V. (2001). Temporal order and processing acuity of visual, auditory, and tactile perception in developmentally dyslexic young adults. *Cognitive, Affective, and Behavioral Neuroscience, 1*(4), 394–410.

Lawn, N., Londono, A., Sawrie, S., Morawetz, R., Martin, R., Gilliam, F., Faught, E., & Kuzniecky, R. (2000). Occipitoparietal epilepsy, hippocampal atrophy, and congenital developmental abnormalities. *Epilepsia, 41*(12), 1546–1553.

Leonard, C. M., Eckert, M. A., Lombardino, L. J., Oakland, T., Kranzler, J., Mohr, C. M., King, W. M., & Freeman, A. (2001). Anatomical risk factors for phonological dyslexia. *Cerebral Cortex, 11*(2), 148–157.

Lerner, J. W. (1989). Educational interventions in learning disabilities. *Journal of the American Academy of Child and Adolescent Psychiatry, 28*(3), 326–331.

Light, J. G., & DeFries, J. C. (1995). Comorbidity of reading and mathematics disabilities: Genetic and environmental etiologies. *Journal of Learning Disabilities, 28*(2), 96–106.

Livingstone, M. S., Rosen, G. D., Drislane, F. W., & Galaburda, A. M. (1991). Physiological and anatomical evidence for a magnocellular defect in developmental dyslexia. *Proceedings of the National Academy of Sciences USA, 88*(18), 7943–7947.

Loge, D. V., Staton, R. D., & Beatty, W. W. (1990). Performance of children with ADHD on tests sensitive to frontal lobe dysfunction. *Journal of the American Academy of Child and Adolescent Psychiatry, 29*(4), 540–545.

Londin, E. R., Meng, H., & Gruen, J. R. (2003). A transcription map of the 6p22.3 reading disability locus identifying candidate genes. *BMC Genomics, 4*(1), 25.

Lovegrove, W. (1993). Weakness in the transient visual system: A causal factor in dyslexia? *Annals of the New York Academy of Sciences, 682*, 57–69.

Luhmann, H. J., Raabe, K., Qu, M., & Zilles, K. (1998). Characterization of neuronal migration disorders in neocortical structures: Extracellular in vitro recordings. *European Journal of Neuroscience, 10*(10), 3085–3094.

Lundberg, I. (1998). Why is learning to read a hard task for some children? *Scandinavian Journal of Psychology, 39*(3), 155–157.

Lyon, G. R., & Moats, L. C. (1997). Critical conceptual and methodological considerations in reading intervention research. *Journal of Learning Disabilities, 30*(6), 578–588.

Lyytinen, H., Ahonen, T., Eklund, K., Guttorm, T. K., Laakso, M. L., Leinonen, S., Leppänen, P. H., Lyytinen, P., Poikkeus, A. M., Puolakanaho,

A., Richardson, U., & Viholainen, H. (2001). Developmental pathways of children with and without familial risk for dyslexia during the first years of life. *Developmental Neuropsychology, 20*(2), 535–554.

MacArthur, C. A. (1996). Using technology to enhance the writing processes of students with learning disabilities. *Journal of Learning Disabilities, 29*(4), 344–354.

Marino, C., Giorda, R., Vanzin, L., Molteni, M., Lorusso, M. L., Nobile, M., Baschirotto, C., Alda, M., & Battaglia, M. (2003). No evidence for association and linkage disequilibrium between dyslexia and markers of four dopamine-related genes. *European Child and Adolescent Psychiatry, 12*(4), 198–202.

Marino, C., Giorda, R., Vanzin, L., Nobile, M., Lorusso, M. L., Baschirotto, C., Riva, L., Molteni, M., & Battaglia, M. (2004). A locus on 15q15-15qter influences dyslexia: Further support from a transmission/disequilibrium study in an Italian speaking population. *Journal of Medical Genetics, 41*(1), 42–46.

Mati-Zissi, H., & Zafiropoulou, M. (2003). Visuomotor coordination and visuospatial working memory of children with specific reading disabilities: A study using the Rey-Osterrieth Complex Figure. *Perceptual and Motor Skills, 97*(2), 543–546.

Maughan, B., Pickles, A., Hagell, A., Rutter, M., & Yule, W. (1996). Reading problems and antisocial behaviour: Developmental trends in comorbidity. *Journal of Child Psychology and Psychiatry and Allied Disciplines, 37*(4), 405–418.

McCandliss, B. D., & Noble, K. G. (2003). The development of reading impairment: A cognitive neuroscience model. *Mental Retardation and Developmental Disabilities Research Reviews, 9*(3), 196–204.

McNamara, P., Flannery, K. A., Obler, L. K., & Schachter, S. (1994). Special talents in Geschwind's and Galaburda's theory of cerebral lateralization: An examination in a female population. *International Journal of Neuroscience, 78*(3–4), 167–176.

Mehler, J., & Bever, T. G. (1967). Cognitive capacity of very young children. *Science, 158*(797), 141–142.

Morais, J., Cluytens, M., & Alegria, J. (1984). Segmentation abilities of dyslexics and normal readers. *Perceptual and Motor Skills, 58*(1), 221–222.

Morris, D. W., Robinson, L., Turic, D., Duke, M., Webb, V., Milham, C., Hopkin, E., Pound, K., Fernando, S., Easton, M., Hamshere, M., Williams, N., McGuffin, P., Stevenson, J., Krawczak, M., Owen, M. J., O'Donovan, M. C., & Williams, J. (2000). Family-based association mapping provides evidence for a gene for reading disability on chromosome 15q. *Human Molecular Genetics, 9*(5), 843–848.

Nicolson, R. I., Fawcett, A. J., Berry, E. L., Jenkins, I. H., Dean, P., & Brooks, D. J. (1999). Association of abnormal cerebellar activation with motor learning difficulties in dyslexic adults. *Lancet, 353*(9165), 1662–1667.

Nicolson, R. I., Fawcett, A. J., & Dean, P. (2001). Developmental dyslexia: The cerebellar deficit hypothesis. *Trends in Neuroscience, 24*(9), 508–511.

Nopola-Hemmi, J., Myllyluoma, B., Haltia, T., Taipale, M., Ollikainen, V., Ahonen, T., Voutilainen, A., Kere, J., & Widen, E. (2001). A dominant gene for developmental dyslexia on chromosome 3. *Journal of Medical Genetics, 38*(10), 658–664.

Nunez, J. L., Lauschke, D. M., & Juraska, J. M. (2001). Cell death in the development of the posterior cortex in male and female rats. *The Journal of Comparative Neurology, 436*(1), 32–41.

Ojemann, G. A. (1979). Individual variability in cortical localization of language. *Journal of Neurosurgery, 50*(2), 164–169.

Patkai, J., Mesples, B., Dommergues, M. A., Fromont, G., Thornton, E. M., Renauld, J. C., Evrard, P., & Gressens, P. (2001). Deleterious effects of IL-9-activated mast cells and neuroprotection by antihistamine drugs in the developing mouse brain. *Pediatric Research, 50*(2), 222–230.

Paulesu, E., Demonet, J. F., Fazio, F., McCrory, E., Chanoine, V., Brunswick, N., Cappa, S. F., Cossu, G., Habib, M., Frith, C. D., & Frith, U. (2001). Dyslexia: Cultural diversity and biological unity. *Science, 291*(5511), 2165–2167.

Pavlidis, G. T. (1985). Eye movement differences between dyslexics, normal, and retarded readers while sequentially fixating digits. *American Journal of Optometry and Physiologic Optics, 62*(12), 820–832.

Peiffer, A. M., Rosen, G. D., & Fitch, R. H. (2002a). Rapid auditory processing and MGN morphology in microgyric rats reared in varied acoustic environments. *Brain Research: Developmental Brain Research, 138*(2), 187–193.

Peiffer, A. M., Rosen, G. D., & Fitch, R. H. (2002b). Sex differences in rapid auditory processing deficits in ectopic BXSB/MpJ mice. *Neuroreport, 13*(17), 2277–2280.

Peiffer, A. M., Rosen, G. D., & Fitch, R. H. (2004). Sex differences in rapid auditory processing deficits in microgyric rats. *Brain Research: Developmental Brain Research, 148*(1), 53–57.

Pennington, B. F., Filipek, P. A., Lefly, D., Chhabildas, N., Kennedy, D. N., Simon, J. H., Filley, C. M., Galaburda, A., & DeFries, J. C. (2000). A twin MRI study of size variations in human brain. *Journal of Cognitive Neuroscience, 12*(1), 223–232.

Petri, J. L., & Anderson, M. E. (1980). Eye and head movements in reading-disabled and normal children. *American Journal of Occupational Therapy, 34*(12), 801–808.

Peyrard-Janvid, M., Anthoni, H., Onkamo, P., Lahermo, P., Zucchelli, M., Kaminen, N., Hannula-Jouppi, K., Nopola-Hemmi, J., Voutilainen, A., Lyytinen, H., & Kere, J. (2004). Fine mapping of the 2p11 dyslexia locus and exclusion of TACR1 as a candidate gene. *Human Genetics, 114*(5), 510–516.

Pilz, D. T., Matsumoto, N., Minnerath, S., Mills, P., Gleeson, J. G., Allen, K. M., Walsh, C. A., Barkovich, A. J., Dobyns, W. B., Ledbetter, D. H., & Ross, M. E. (1998). LIS1 and XLIS (DCX) mutations cause most classical lissencephaly, but different patterns of malformation. *Human Molecular Genetics, 7*(13), 2029–2037.

Poeppel, D. (1996). A critical review of PET studies of phonological processing. *Brain and Language, 55*(3), 317–351, discussion 352–385.

Pugh, K. R., Mencl, W. E., Jenner, A. R., Katz, L., Frost, S. J., Lee, J. R., Shaywitz, S. E., & Shaywitz, B. A. (2000). Functional neuroimaging studies of reading and reading disability (developmental dyslexia). *Mental Retardation and Developmental Disabilities Research Reviews 6*(3), 207–213.

Pugh, K. R., Mencl, W. E., Jenner, A. R., Katz, L., Frost, S. J., Lee, J. R., Shaywitz, S. E., & Shaywitz, B. A. (2001). Neurobiological studies of reading and reading disability. *Journal of Communication Disorders, 34*(6), 479–492.

Purvis, K. L., & Tannock, R. (1997). Language abilities in children with attention deficit hyperactivity disorder, reading disabilities, and normal controls. *Journal of Abnormal Child Psychology, 25*(2), 133–144.

Rack, L. (1981). Developmental dyslexia and literary creativity: Creativity in the area of deficit. *Journal of Learning Disabilities, 14*(5), 262–263.

Rae, C., Harasty, J. A., Dzendrowskyj, T. E., Talcott, J. B., Simpson, J. M., Blamire, A. M., Dixon, R. M., Lee, M. A., Thompson, C. H., Styles, P., Richardson, A. J., & Stein, J. F. (2002). Cerebellar morphology in developmental dyslexia. *Neuropsychologia, 40*(8), 1285–1292.

Ramus, F. (2001). Outstanding questions about phonological processing in dyslexia. *Dyslexia 7*(4), 197–216.

Ramus, F., Pidgeon, E., & Frith, U. (2003). The relationship between motor control and phonology in dyslexic children. *Journal of Psychology and Psychiatry and Allied Disciplines, 44*(5), 712–722.

Rayner, K. (1998). Eye movements in reading and information processing: 20 years of research. *Psychological Bulletin, 124*(3), 372–422.

Rayner, K., Foorman, B. R., Perfetti, C. A., Pesetsky, D., & Seidenberg, M. S. (2001). How psychological science informs the teaching of reading. *Psychological Science, 2*(Suppl. 2), 31–74.

Richardson, A. J., & Ross, M. A. (2000). Fatty acid metabolism in neurodevelopmental disorder: A new perspective on associations between attention-deficit/hyperactivity disorder, dyslexia, dyspraxia and the autistic spectrum. *Prostaglandins, Leukotrienes & Essential Fatty Acids, 63*(1–2), 1–9.

Richardson, U., Leppänen, P. H., Leiwo, M., & Lyytinen, H. (2003). Speech perception of infants with high familial risk for dyslexia differ at the age of 6 months. *Developmental Neuropsychology, 23*(3), 385–397.

Rojas, D. C., Bawn, S. D., Benkers, T. L., Reite, M. L., & Rogers, S. J. (2002). Smaller left hemisphere planum temporale in adults with autistic disorder. *Neuroscience Letters, 328*(3), 237–240.

Rosen, G. D., Burstein, D., & Galaburda, A. M. (2000). Changes in efferent and afferent connectivity in rats with induced cerebrocortical microgyria. *The Journal of Comparative Neurology, 418*(4), 423–440.

Rosen, G. D., & Galaburda, A. M. (2000). Single cause, polymorphic neuronal migration disorders: An animal model. *Developmental Medicine and Child Neurology, 42*(10), 652–662.

Rosen, G. D., Sherman, G. F., Mehler, C., Emsbo, K., & Galaburda, A. M. (1989). The effect of developmental neuropathology on neocortical asymmetry in New Zealand black mice. *International Journal of Neuroscience, 45*(3–4), 247–254.

Rosen, G. D., Waters, N. S., Galaburda, A. M., & Denenberg, V. H. (1995). Behavioral consequences of neonatal injury of the neocortex. *Brain Research, 681*(1–2), 177–189.

Rutter, M., Caspi, A., Fergusson, D., Horwood, L. J., Goodman, R., Maughan, B., Moffitt, T. E., Meltzer, H., & Carroll, J. (2004). Sex differences in developmental reading disability: New findings from 4 epidemiological studies. *Journal of the American Medical Association, 291*(16), 2007–2012.

Sarkari, S., Simos, P. G., Fletcher, J. M., Castillo, E. M., Breier, J. I., & Papanicolaou, A. C. (2002). Contributions of magnetic source imaging to the understanding of dyslexia. *Seminars in Pediatric Neurology, 9*(3), 229–238.

Schrott, L. M., Denenberg, V. H., Sherman, G. F., Waters, N. S., Rosen, G. D., & Galaburda, A. M. (1992). Environmental enrichment, neocortical ectopias, and behavior in the autoimmune NZB mouse. *Brain Research: Developmental Brain Research, 67*(1), 85–93.

Schrott, L. M., Waters, N. S., Boehm, G. W., Sherman, G. F., Morrison, L., Rosen, G. D., Behan, P. O., Galaburda, A. M., & Denenberg, V. H. (1993). Behavior, cortical ectopias, and autoimmunity in BXSB-Yaa and BXSB-Yaa+ mice. *Brain, Behavior, and Immunity, 7*(3), 205–223.

Schulte-Korne, G., Grimm, T., Nothen, M. M., Muller-Myhsok, B., Cichon, S., Vogt, I. R., Propping, P., & Remschmidt, H. (1998). Evidence for linkage of spelling disability to chromosome 15. *American Journal of Human Genetics, 63*(1), 279–282.

Semrud-Clikeman, M., Biederman, J., Sprich-Buckminster, S., Lehman, B. K., Faraone, S. V., & Norman, D. (1992). Comorbidity between ADDH and learning disability: A review and report in a clinically referred sample. *Journal of the American Academy of Child and Adolescent Psychiatry, 31*(3), 439–448.

Shaywitz, B. A., Shaywitz, S. E., Pugh, K. R., Mencl, W. E., Fulbright, R. K., Skudlarski, P., Constable, R. T., Marchione, K. E., Fletcher, J. M., Lyon, G. R., & Gore, J. C. (2002). Disruption of posterior brain systems for reading in children with developmental dyslexia. *Biological Psychiatry, 52*(2), 101–110.

Shaywitz, S. E., Shaywitz, B. A., Fletcher, J. M., & Escobar, M. D. (1990). Prevalence of reading disability in boys and girls. Results of the Connecticut longitudinal study. *Journal of the American Medical Association, 264*(8), 998–1002.

Sheen, V. L., & Walsh, C. A. (2003). Developmental genetic malformations of the cerebral cortex. *Current Neurology and Neuroscience Reports, 3*(5), 433–441.

Sherman, G. F., Galaburda, A. M., Behan, P. O., & Rosen, G. D. (1987). Neuroanatomical anomalies in autoimmune mice. *Acta Neuropathologia (Berlin) 74*(3), 239–242.

Sherman, G. F., Galaburda, A. M., & Geschwind, N. (1985). Cortical anomalies in brains of New Zealand mice: A neuropathologic model of dyslexia? *Proceedings of the National Academy of Sciences USA, 82*(23), 8072–8074.

Skoyles, J., & Skottun, B. C. (2004). On the prevalence of magnocellular deficits in the visual system of non-dyslexic individuals. *Brain and Language, 88*(1), 79–82.

Slaghuis, W. L., Twell, A. J., & Kingston, K. R. (1996). Visual and language processing disorders are concurrent in dyslexia and continue into adulthood. *Cortex, 32*(3), 413–438.

Small, S. L., & Burton, M. W. (2002). Functional magnetic resonance imaging studies of language. *Current Neurology and Neuroscience Reports, 2*(6), 505–510.

Snowling, M. J. (1981). Phonemic deficits in developmental dyslexia. *Psychological Research, 43*(2), 219–234.

Snowling, M. J. (1996). Annotation: Contemporary approaches to the teaching of reading. *Journal of Child Psychology and Psychiatry and Allied Disciplines, 37*(2), 139–148.

Sommer, I., Ramsey, N., Kahn, R., Aleman, A., & Bouma, A. (2001). Handedness, language lateralisation and anatomical asymmetry in schizophrenia: Meta-analysis. *British Journal of Psychiatry, 178*, 344–351.

Stanovich, K. E. (1982). Individual differences in the cognitive processes of reading: II. Text-level processes. *Journal of Learning Disabilities, 15*(9), 549–554.

Stein, J. (2001). The magnocellular theory of developmental dyslexia. *Dyslexia, 7*(1), 12–36.

Stein, J., & Walsh, V. (1997). To see but not to read. The magnocellular theory of dyslexia. *Trends in Neuroscience, 20*(4), 147–152.

Stern, Y., Gurland, B., Tatemichi, T. K., Tang, M. X., Wilder, D., & Mayeux, R. (1994). Influence of education and occupation on the incidence of Alzheimer's disease. *Journal of the American Medical Association, 271*(13), 1004–1010.

Taipale, M., Kaminen, N., Nopola-Hemmi, J., Haltia, T., Myllyluoma, B., Lyytinen, H., Muller, K., Kaaranen, M., Lindsberg, P. J., Hannula-Jouppi, K., & Kere, J. (2003). A candidate gene for developmental dyslexia encodes a nuclear tetratricopeptide repeat domain protein dynamically regulated in brain. *Proceedings of the National Academy of Sciences USA, 100*(20), 11553–11558.

Tallal, P., Merzenich, M. M., Miller, S., & Jenkins, W. (1998). Language learning impairments: Integrating basic science, technology, and remediation. *Experimental Brain Research 123*(1–2), 210–219.

Temple, E. (2002). Brain mechanisms in normal and dyslexic readers. *Current Opinions in Neurobiology, 12*(2), 178–183.

Teskey, G. C., Hutchinson, J. E., & Kolb, B. (1999). Sex differences in cortical plasticity and behavior following anterior cortical kindling in rats. *Cerebral Cortex, 9*(7), 675–682.

Thomas, M., & Karmiloff-Smith, A. (2002). Are developmental disorders like cases of adult brain damage? Implications from connectionist modelling. *Behavioral and Brain Sciences, 25*(6), 727–750, discussion 750–787.

Toplak, M. E., Rucklidge, J. J., Hetherington, R., John, S. C., & Tannock, R. (2003). Time perception deficits in attention-deficit/ hyperactivity disorder and comorbid reading difficulties in child and adolescent samples. *Journal of Child Psychology and Psychiatry and Allied Disciplines, 44*(6), 888–903.

Trentani, A., Kuipers, S. D., te Meerman, G. J., Beekman, J., ter Horst, G. J., & den Boer, J. A. (2003). Immunohistochemical changes induced by repeated footshock stress: Revelations of gender-based differences. *Neurobiology of Disease, 14*(3), 602–618.

Vellutino, F. R., Fletcher, J. M., Snowling, M. J., & Scanlon, D. M. (2004). Specific reading disability (dyslexia): What have we learned in the past four decades? *Journal of Child Psychology and Psychiatry and Allied Disciplines, 45*(1), 2–40.

von Karolyi, C., Winner, E., Gray, W., & Sherman, G. F. (2003). Dyslexia linked to talent: Global visual-spatial ability. *Brain and Language, 85*(3), 427–431.

Waber, D. P., Wolff, P. H., Forbes, P. W., & Weiler, M. D. (2000). Rapid automatized naming in children referred for evaluation of heterogeneous learning problems: How specific are naming speed deficits to reading disability? *Neuropsychology, Development and Cognition, Section C, Child Neuropsychology, 6*(4), 251–261.

Wigg, K. G., Couto, J. M., Feng, Y., Anderson, B., Cate-Carter, T. D., Macciardi, F., Tannock, R., Lovett, M. W., Humphries, T. W., & Barr, C.

L. (2004). Support for EKN1 as the susceptibility locus for dyslexia on 15q21. *Molecular Psychiatry*, 1–11.

Williams, M. J., Stuart, G. W., Castles, A., & McAnally, K. I. (2003). Contrast sensitivity in subgroups of developmental dyslexia. *Vision Research, 43*(4), 467–477.

Wisniewski, A. B. (1998). Sexually-dimorphic patterns of cortical asymmetry, and the role for sex steroid hormones in determining cortical patterns of lateralization. *Psychoneuroendocrinology 23*(5), 519–547.

Wisniewski, K., Dambska, M., Sher, J. H., & Qazi, Q. (1983). A clinical neuropathological study of the fetal alcohol syndrome. *Neuropediatrics, 14*(4), 197–201.

Witelson, S. F. (1977). Developmental dyslexia: Two right hemispheres and none left. *Science, 195*(4275), 309–311.

Wolf, M. (1986). Rapid alternating stimulus naming in the developmental dyslexias. *Brain and Language, 27*(2), 360–379.

Wolff, P. H., Cohen, C., & Drake, C. (1984). Impaired motor timing control in specific reading retardation. *Neuropsychologia, 22*(5), 587–600.

Wolff, P. H., Michel, G. F., & Ovrut, M. (1990). Rate variables and automatized naming in developmental dyslexia. *Brain and Language, 39*(4), 556–575.

Wolff, U., & Lundberg, I. (2002). The prevalence of dyslexia among art students. *Dyslexia, 8*(1), 34–42.

Zeffiro, T., & Eden, G. (2001). The cerebellum and dyslexia: perpetrator or innocent bystander? *Trends in Neuroscience, 24*(9), 512–3.

Zhang, L., Li, P. P., Feng, X., Barker, J. L., Smith, S. V., & Rubinow, D. R. (2003). Sex-related differences in neuronal cell survival and signaling in rats. *Neuroscience Letters, 337*(2), 65–68.

Zilles, K., Qu, M., Schleicher, A., Schroeter, M., Kraemer, M., & Witte, O. W. (1995). Plasticity and neurotransmitter receptor changes in Alzheimer's disease and experimental cortical infarcts. *Arzneimittelforschung, 45*(3A), 361–366.

Author Index

A

Abbott, R. D., 12, 13, *17*
Adams, K., 13, *19*
Adams, M. J., 13, *17*
Andreason, P. A., 28, 29, 30, 34, *45*
Anzivino, M. J., 245, 246, 247, 249, 250, *253*, *257*
Atkins, P., 32, 39, *42*

B

Badian, N., 10, *17*
Bailey, A., 87, *93*
Ball, E. W., 25, *41*
Balogh, S. A., 79, *93*, 335, *343*
Balota, D. A., 35, *42*
Barnes, G., 26, 27, *44*
Beck, I. L., 14, *17*
Becker, J., 35, *43*
Behrmann, M., 27, *41*
Beig, S., *41*
Bell, L., 23, 25, *44*
Belliveau, J. W., 39, *42*
Berninger, V. W., 12, 13, *17*
Bertram, E., 245, 246, 247, 249, 250, *253*, *257*
Bhadha, B., 10, *18*
Blachman, B. A., 25, *41*
Black, S. E., 27, *41*

Billingsley, F., 12, 13, *17*
Bookstein, F. L., *43*
Booth, J. R., 26, 28, 33, 34, *41*, *44*
Bowers, P. G., 10, *17*, *19*
Bradley, L., 24, 25, 40, *41*
Brady, S., *41*, *44*
Breier, J. I., 23, 25, 30, *41*, *45*
Bronen, R. A., 27, *44*
Bruck, M., 23, 24, 25, *41*
Brunswick, N., 28, 30, *41*, *44*
Bryant, P., 24, 25, 40, *41*
Buckner, R. L., 39, *42*
Burgaya, F., 156, *160*
Burman, D. D., 26, 28, 33, *41*

C

Cappa, S. F., 28, 41, *44*
Carnine, D. W., 14, *18*
Carpenter, P. A., *43*
Carter, B., 23, 24, 25, *42*, *43*
Castellanos, F. X., 87, *94*
Castillo, E. M., 25, 30, *45*
Chanoine, V., 28, 41, *44*
Chen, Z.-F., 245, 246, 247, 249, 250, *253*, *257*
Chochon, F., 26, *42*
Cohen, L., 26, *42*
Cohen, Y., 12, *17*

Coltheart, M., 32, 39, *42*
Constable, R. C., 27, 29, 33, 34, 35, *43*, *44*, *45*
Cornelissen, P. L., 24, 26, 27, *42*, *44*, *46*
Cossu, G., 28, 41, *44*
Crino, P. B., 163, 195, 196, 197, 198, 199, 202, 203, *205*
Curtis, B., 32, 39, *42*

D

Dale, A. M., 39, *42*
Deacon, T., 6, *18*
Defries, J. C., 40, *44*
Dehaene, S., 6, 26, *18*, *42*
Demonet, J.-F., 28, *41*, *44*
Denckla, M. B., 9, *18*
Desmond, J. E., 27, *44*
Dixon, R. C., 14, *18*
Dobrich, W., 24, *45*, 54, *72*
Doi, L. M., 10, *18*
Donnelly, K., 13, *19*
Donohue, B. C., 28, 29, 30, 34, 39, *43*, *45*
Drummond, J., 245, 246, 247, 249, 250, *253*, *257*

E

Eden, G. F., 10, 25, *18*, *42*
Eliez, S., 77, *94*

F

Fazio, F., 28, *41*, *44*
Felton, R. H., 11, *18*
Ferrer, I., 195, 202, *206*, 223, *239*
Fiebach, C. J., 27, 28, 34, 35, *42*
Fiez, J. A., 27, 35, *42*
Filipek, P. A., 25, *42*
Fiscal, B. R., 39, *42*
Fischer, W., 23, 24, 25, *42*, *43*
Fisher, S. E., 90, *95*, 167, 172, *190*

Fitch, R. H., 262, 264, 266, 267, 269, *281*
Fletcher, J., 23, 24, 25, 29, *42*, *44*
Fletcher, J. K., 25, *42*
Fletcher, J. M., 25, 27, 29, 33, 34, *43*, *45*
Foorman, B. R., 13, 25, *19*, *42*
Fowler, A. E., 23, 24, 25, *42*
Frachowiak, R. S. J., 27, *44*
Francis, D., 25, *42*
Francis, D. J., 23, 24, 25, *42*
Freund, H.-J., *45*
Friederici, A. D., 27, 28, 34, 35, *42*
Frijters, J. C., 10, 13, *18*
Friston, K., 28, *42*
Frith, C. D., 28, 30, *41*, *44*
Frith, U., 28, 30, *41*, *44*
Frost, R., 39, *42*, *43*
Frost, S. J., 10, *19*, 22, 23, 25, 28, 29, 32, 33, 34, 35, 37, 39, *42*, *43*, *45*
Fukuyama, H., 41, *44*
Fulbright, R., 27, 29, 33, 34, 35, *43*, *44*, *45*

G

Gabrieli, J. D., 27, 40, *43*, *44*
Galaburda, A. M., vii, *viii*, 25, *42*, 76, 78, 79, 80, 81, 82, 83, 84, 85, 86, 87, 88, 89, 90, *94*, *95*, 331, 334, 335, 336, 337, 338, 339, *345*
Gatenby, J. C., *43*
German, D. J., 14, *18*
Geschwind, N., 9, *18*
Gilger, J. W., 40, *44*
Giraud, A. L., 38, *44*
Gitelman, D. R., 26, 28, 33, *41*
Gleeson, J., 122, 123, 124, 125, *128*, 133, *140*
Glover, G. H., 27, *44*

Good, R. H., 10, 11, *18*
Goodman, G., 13, *19*
Gore, J. C., 27, 29, 33, 34, *43*, *44*
Goswami, U., 13, *18*
Grady, C. L., *43*
Gressens, P., 209, 210, 216, 217, 218, *220*, *221*
Grigorenko, E. L., 22, 24, 40, *42*, *43*, 110, 112, *117*, 172, *188*, 331, *342*

H
Habib, M., 25, 28, *43*, *44*
Halgren, E., 39, *42*
Haller, M., 32, 39, *42*
Hampson, M., *43*
Hanakawa, T., 41, *44*
Hansen, P. C., 24, 26, 27, *42*, *44*
Harasaki, Y., 26, 28, 33, *41*
Harm, M. W., 38, *43*
Harn, B. A., 10, 11, *18*
Hart, L. A., 40, *42*
Haxby, J. V., *43*
Hedehus, M., 40, *43*
Herbster, A., 35, *43*
Hirano, S., 41, *44*
Ho Chan, D., 10, *18*
Holliday, I., 26, 27, *44*
Honda, M., 41, *44*
Horwitz, B., 29, 30, 39, *43*, *45*
Humphreys, G. W., 38, *44*

I
Inoue, H., 41, *44*
Ito, J., 41, *44*

J
Jacobs, K. M., *222f*, 265
Jeffrey, J., 13, *19*
Jenner, A. R., 22, 23, 25, 28, 29, 32, 33, 34, 37, 39, *43*, *44*

Joffe, T., 13, *19*
Just, M. A., *43*

K
Kame'enui, E. J., 10, 11, 14, *18*
Kapur, J., 245, 246, 247, 249, 250, *253*, *257*
Katz, L., 22, 23, 24, 25, 27, 28, 29, 32, 33, 34, 35, 37, 39, *42*, *43*, *44*, *45*
Katzir-Cohen, T., 8, 12, *19*
Keller, T. A., *43*
Kennedy, D. N., 292, 295, *301*, *302*, *303*
Kiesila, P., 26, 28 30, 34, *45*
Kinard, C. L., 245, 246, 247, 249, 250, *253*, *257*
Klingberg, T., 40, *43*
Kringelbach, M. L., 26, 27, *44*
Krisch, S. D., 26, 27, *44*

L
Lacadie, C., 27, 29, *44*
Lee, J. R., 22, 23, 25, 28, 29, 32, 33, 34, 37, 39, *43*, *44*
Lee, K. S., 245, 246, 247, 249, 250, *253*, *257*
Lee, S.-H., 10, 35, *18*, *43*
Lehericy, S., 26, *42*
Lemer, C., 26, *42*
Lewine, J. D., 39, *42*
Liberman, A. M., 22, *43*
Liberman, I. Y., 23, 24, 25, *42*, *43*
Liu, A. K., 39, *42*
LoTurco, J. J., 120, 121, *126*, *127*, 132, *138*, *159*, *256*, 272, 273, *283*, 331, *345*
Lovett, M., 13, *19*
Lovett, M. W., 10, 13, *18*
Lukatela, G., 25, *43*
Lyon, G. R., 15, *18*

M

Machizawa, M., 245, 246, 247, 249, 250, *253*, *257*
Maisog, J. M., 28, 29, 30, 34, *45*
Manis, F. R., 10, *18*
Marchione, K. E., 29, 33, 34, *43*, *44*
Marino, C., 112, 115, *117*
Mason, S. A., 29, 33, 34, 35, *43*, *45*
Matsuda, T., 41, *44*
McClelland, J., 13, *19*
McIntosh, A. R., *42*, *43*
McKeown, M. G., 14, *17*
McCrory, E., 28, 30, *41*, *44*
Mehta, P., 25, *42*
Mencl, W. E., 10, *19*, 22, 23, 25, 28, 29, 32, 33, 34, 35, *37*, *39*, *43*, *44*, *45*
Mesulam, M. M., *41*
Meyer, M. S., 11, *18*, 40, *42*
Miller, L., 13, *19*
Mintun, M., 35, *43*
Misra, M., 10, *18*
Moats, L., 10, 13, 15, *18*
Mody, M., 41, *44*
Molteni, M., 112, 115, *117*
Moore, C. J., 38, *44*
Moore, D., 10, *19*
Moore, D. L., 35, *45*
More, C. J., 38, *44*
Morris, R., 13, *19*
Moseley, M. E., 40, *43*
Mueller, K., 27, 28, 34, 35, *42*

N

Nace, K. L., 28, 29, 30, 34, *45*
Nagy, W., 12, 13, *17*
Nakamura, K., 41, *44*
Nebes, R., 35, *43*
Nopola-Hemmi, J., 117, *118*, *128*, 172, *188*, *189*
Noppeney, U., 38, *44*

O

O'Brien, B., 13, *19*
Oga, T., 41, *44*

P

Pammer, K., 26, 27, *44*
Papanicolaou, A. C., 22, 23, 25, 30, *41*, *45*
Paramasivam, M., 82, 89, *101*
Parrish, T. B., *41*
Pascual-Leone, A., 314, 322, *325*, *326*, 335
Paulesu, E., 28, *41*, *44*
Pauls, D. L., 40, *42*, *44*
Peiffer, A. M., 79, 85, *98*, 121, *127*, 268, 270, *281*, *285*
Pennington, B. F., 40, *44*
Perfetti, C. A., 14, *17*, 23, 25, 30, *44*
Petersen, S. E., 27, 35, *42*
Peterson, B. S., *43*
Pinker, S., 8, *18*
Plaisant, F., 215, 216, *222*
Plaut, D. C., 34, *44*
Poldrack, R. A., 27, 40, *43*, *44*
Price, C., 28, 30, *41*
Price, C. J., 22, 23, 25, 26, 27, 28, 29, 32, 37, 38, 39, *44*
Prull, M. W., 27, *44*
Pugh, K. R., 10, *19*, 22, 27, 29, 33, 34, 35, *43*, *44*, *45*

R

Raichle, M. E., 35, *42*
Ramus, F., 51, 57, 61, *71*, *72*, 75, 77, 84, 85, *98*, *99*, 330, 331, 332, *351*
Rivaud, S., 26, *42*
Rosen, G. D., 19, 49, 51, 61, 72, 76, 77, 78, 79, 80, 81, 84, 89, 92, *94*, *99*, 120, 121, *127*, 129, 130, *139*, 152, 167, 224, *244*, 263, 264, 265, 266, 267, 268,

269, 270, 271, 272, 276, 277, *281, 282, 285, 286*
Rudel, R. G., 9, *18*
Rumsey, J. M., 28, 29, 30, 34, 39, *43, 45*
Rueckl, J. G., 29, 33, 34, 35, 36, *43, 45*

S

Salonen, O., 26, 28, 30, 34, *45*
Salmelin, R., 26, 28, 30, 34, *45*
Saltz, T., 40, *43*
Sandak, R., 10, *19*, 29, 33, 34, 35, *43*
Sarkari, S., 25, 30, *45*
Sawamoto, N., 41, *44*
Scarborough, H., 24, *45*, 54, 72
Schatschneider, C., 25, *42*
Schmandt-Besserat, D., 6, *19*
Schmitz, F., *45*
Schottler, F., 245, 246, 247, 249, 250, *253, 257*
Schnitzler, A., *45*
Segal, D., 14, *19*
Seidenberg, M., 13, *19*
Seidenberg, M. S., 38, *43*
Service, E., 26, 28, 30, 34, *45*
Shankweiler, D. P., 23, 24, 25, 29, *42, 43, 44*
Shaywitz, B. A., 22, 23, 24, 25, 27, 28, 32, 33, 34, 37, 39, *42, 44*
Shaywitz, S. E., 22, 23, 24, 25, 27, 28, 32, 33, 34, 37, 39, *42, 44*
Shibasaki, H., 41, *44*
Shuster, A., 40, *42*
Simmons, D. C., 10, 11, *18*
Simos, P. G., 22, 23, *25, 30*, 41, *44, 45*
Skudlarski, P., 27, 29, 33, 34, *43, 44*
Smith, S. A., 40, *44*

Smith, S. D., 40, *44*
Speed, W. C., 40, *42*
Stanovich, K. E., 23, 24, 25, *46*, 330, 331, *353*
Steinbach, K. A., 10, 13, *18*
Strain, E., 35, *46*
Studdert-Kennedy, M., 41, *44*
Stuebing, K. K., 23, 24, 25, *42*

T

Tagamets, M. A., 27, 33, *46*
Tallal, P., 41, *46*, 61, *72*, 76, *100*, 193, 259, 260, 261, 262, 263, 264, 265, 267, 268, 274, 276, *280, 281, 282, 285, 287*
Tan, L. H., 41, *46*
Tarkiainen, A., 27, *46*
Temple, E., 40, *43*
Théoret, H., 335
Torgesen, J. K., 25, *47*
Trotter, S., 245, 246, 247, 249, 250, *253, 257*
Tsang, S.-M., 10, *18*
Tsuchitani, S., 245, 246, 247, 249, 250, *253, 257*
Turkeltaub, P. E., 28, 33, *47*
Turvey, M. T., 25, *43*

U

Uutela, K., 26, 28, 30, 34, *45*

V

Van Santen, F. W., 26, 28, 33, *41*
von Cramon, D. Y., 27, 28, 34, 35, *42*

W

Wagner, A. D., 27, *44*
Wang, Y., 82, 89, *101, 139*, 145
Williams, C., 245, 246, 247, 249, 250, *253, 257*

Williams, R., 181, *187*, *188*, *189*, *190*
Winterburn, D., 38, *44*
Wise, R. J. S., 27, 28, 29, 34, 38, *44*, *45*
Wolf, M., 8, 10, 12, 13, 14, *17*, *19*
Wood, F. B., 40, *42*

Z

Zeffiro, T. A., 10, 25, *47*, 330, 331, *344*, *354*
Zhang, F., 245, 246, 247, 249, 250, *253*, *257*
Zouridakis, G., 23, *41*
Zsombok, A., *222f*, 265

Subject Index

A
Alphabetic principle, 7
Altered circuits in reading disability, 28–30
Analysis of the DYX1 candidate region
  Affymetrix arrays, 176–177
  analysis of array data, 178–180
  comparing across scales, 183
  detecting cooperating pair of QTLs, 185–186
  genetic covariance, 180–181
  interval mapping of DYX candidate genes, 184–185
  mRNA processing and measurement, 177–178
  QTL analysis of DYX candidates, 184
  significance of genetic correlations, 181–183
  Chr 15q21.2, 174–175
  criteria for the DYX1 candidates, 173–174
  gene network, 175–176
Animal models
  auditory processing deficits, 270–272
  cognitive and memory effects, 272–274
  cortical development, 191–193
  cortical effects on auditory processing, 277–278
  focal cortical anomalies, 278–279
  linking behavioral and anatomical features of language disability, 265
  microgyria, auditory processing, and thalamic morphology, 265–270
  sex differences, 274–276
Attention deficits hyperactivity (ADHD), 57, 85, 87
Auditory processing deficits and language disability, 259–262
  auditory modality, 261

AUDITORY PROCESSING DEFICITS (*continued*)
cross modal investigation, 261
phonological processing deficit, 262
temporal processing variables, 260–262
visual modality, 261

B

Basic reading processes model, 9
Behavioral studies of reading disability, 23–25
Blindness
adjustment to, 308–309, 313–315
auditory occipital recruitment, 319–320
auditory performance, 308–310
neuroplastic changes, 320–321
somatosensory cortex, 313–315
tactile occipital recruitment, 315–318
tactile performance, 310–313
Transcranial Magnetic Stimulation (TMS), 321–324
Boustrphon directional style, 6
Brain anomalies in other developmental disorders, 87–88
Brain plasticity
application to autism, 296–297
application to gender dimorphism, 297
application to holoprosencephaly, 298
a priori information, 298–300
morphometric analysis, 292
morphometric methods of research, 292–294
surface-based classes of characteristics, 294–295
volumetric literature search, 295–296
voxel based classes of characteristics, 294–295

C

Clinical implications
cognitive impairments, 90–91
comprehensive diagnostic approach, 91
diagnostic categories, 90–91
hypothesis of a specific cognitive deficit, 92–93
sensory explanation of dyslexia, 92–93
Complex behavior of dyslexia
animal studies, 337
from brain to behavior, 337–341
from genes to brain, 341–342
cross-level and multidisciplinary approach, 329–330
dyslexic brain, the, 333–337
dyslexic mind, the, 330–333
Cortical malformations
behavioral deficits in the tish rat, 251

Eight-arm radial maze,
  252–253
Morris Water Maze
  (MWM), 251
development of the tish
  neocortex, 246–248
heterozygous phenotype,
  253–255
overview of the tish rat,
  245–246
seizure prone tish rats,
  249–250
Cortical reading systems,
  25–28

D
Development view of developmental reading disabilities, 58–60
Double-Deficit Hypothesis, 1, 10–11, 15, 51

E
Egyptian hieroglyphic writing, 6
Epileptogenic microgyria
  cellular mechanisms,
    235–236
  dyslexia and epilepsy,
    236–238
  methods, 225–227
  results, 227–233
    postsynaptic currents
      on microgyral rats,
      229–233
Etiology of development
  dyslexia,
  extension of the model to
    other developmental
    disorders, 85–86
Excitotoxic lesions
  effects of IL-9, 216–217
  effects of inflammatory
    cytokines, 214–216
  effects of trophic factors
    and neuroprotective
    molecules, 217–220
  role of brain
    macrophages, 213
  role of preoligodendrocytes, 213–214
  successive steps of brain
    development, 210–213

F
Fast ForWord, 63–64, 66–67
Focal anomalies and the
  phonological deficit,
  80–82
Functional genomics and
  complexity of dyslexia
  animal models, 170
  genetic complexity,
    168–169
  Huntington disease,
    170
  locus versus gene, 168
  summary of the DYX loci,
    169–170, 172f
Functional Magnetic
  Resonance Imaging
  (fMRI), 1, 9, 22, 31,
  34–36, 39, 66–67, 137,
  276, 299, 315, 318, see
  also Neuroimaging
  technologies

G
Genetics of dyslexia
  basis of, 89–90
  chromosome 15,
    110–117
  cortical development,
    103
  developmental dyslexia,
    107–110
  DYX1C1, 111–117
Graphemes, 7

H
Heterogeneity and comorbidity, 86–87
Huntington disease, 170
Hypothesized role of component circuits, 37f

I
Imagistic logographic symbols, 6
Insights from anatomical studies and animal models, 77–80
Interstimulus interval, 58, 275

J
Joubert syndrome, 136–138

L
Language Learning Impairment (LLI), 2, 50–51, 59, 61–63, 259–262, 264
Language to literacy, 66–67
Lateral geniculate nucleus (LGN),
Left-hemisphere (LH) systems
 adaptive learning, 35–36
 extending research, 40–41
 further partitioning, 33–34
 implications of findings, 36–38
 phonological priming, 34
 reading-related tasks, 25–28, 33–38
 tradeoffs between Phonology and Semantics, 34–35

M
Magnetoencephology (MEG), 22, see also Neuroimaging technologies
Malformations of cortical development, 195–196
Markers of fetal hormonal conditions, 89
Medial geniculate nucleus, 78, 83–84, 264
Molecular neurobiology of focal MCD, 197–204

N
Neurobiological effects of successful reading remediation, 31–32
Neuroimaging technologies
 development of, 39–40
 functional Magnetic Resonance Imaging (fMRI), 1, 9, 22, 31, 34–36, 39, 66–67, 137, 276, 299, 315, 318
 magnetoencephology (MEG), 22
 positron Emission Tomography (PET), 22, 29, 39, 299, 317, 319, 222-K
Neuronal migration and brain wiring
 brain wiring defect in Joubert syndrome, 136–138
 defects associated with mutations in microtubule-associate proteins, 131–136
Neuronal migration and neocortical development
 cellular dynamics of DYX1C1 protein, 126
 DYX1C1 and neuronal migration, 123–125
 genetic disruption of neuronal migration in neocortex, 122–123

ectopias and neocortical function, 120–121
neocortical malformation, 120
overview, 121–122
No Child Left Behind, 50
Nonimpaired (NI) readers, 24, 25, 28, 29, 30, 32, 35, 60, *see also* Reading disabled (RD) individuals

P

Phonemes, 2, 7, 13, 52, 54–56, 64, 66, 331
Plasticity and remediation, 63–66
Positron Emission Tomography (PET), 22, 29, 39, 299, 317, 319, *222-K*
Postmortem analysis of dyslexic brains, 263–265
Potentially compensatory processing, 30–31
Preliminary model of neurobiology of word recognition, 32–33

R

Rapid auditory processing, 24, 58–59, 61, 64, 67, 193, 261–262, 276, 279–280
RAVE-O program, 1, 11, 13–14, 16–17
Rebus principle, 6
Reading-disabled (RD) individuals, 23–26, 28–32, 34, 37–38, *see also* Nonimpaired (NI) readers
Reading network, the, 37*f*

S

Sex differences in the occurrence of language disability, 262–263

Sex hormones and the sensorimotor syndrome, 82–85
Sex-ratio, 88
Signaling at the cortical plate
 Alex3, 153–155
 cDNA subtraction, 145–146
 clone 3F3, 151
 future prospects of cloning, 157–158
 generation of cDNA libraries, 146–147
 library screening, 147–148
 Podocalyxin, 151–153
 subtracted clones studied, 148–151
 Tspan5, 155–157
Sources of reading breakdown, 10–11
Speech processing, 57, 60–62
Speech sounds represented in the brain
 central auditory process disorders, 54
 temporal order judgment, 57
 tone onset time (TOT), 56–57
 voice onset time, 56–57
Specific language impairments (SLI), 50–54, 61–62, 76–77, 83, 85–86, 90–91
Symbolic representation, 6–7
Sumerian cuneiform system, 6

T

Targeted therapy for epilepsy in MCD, 204